Theoretical Models in Biology

Preface

Whenever I pick up a scientific book in a bookshop, the first thing I want to know is, 'Will I be able to understand it?'. To put prospective readers' minds at rest (or possibly confirm their worst fears), I will state at the outset what background is expected.

This book uses information and techniques from more fields than is typical of most books on science. The main purpose of the book is to expose the reader to a sampling of quantitative, theoretical models drawn from three main areas in biology: the origin of life, the immune system, and the brain. However, although the main subject of the book is biology, the reader is not expected to know much of anything about it, beyond the sort of general impressions that might be gleaned from watching a nature documentary on television. Although a book of this size cannot give its readers a comprehensive background in biology, enough information is presented for the biologically naïve reader to understand what it is that the theories considered in this book are trying to explain.

The main background assumed of the reader is in applied mathematics. The general level expected is that of second year mathematics in a North American or British university. Familiarity with calculus up to the level of partial differentiation and multiple integrals, an acquaintance with vectors and matrices up to some basic facts on eigenvalues and eigenvectors, and some exposure to differential equations are all expected. All of these topics are normally required of students taking degrees in mathematics or the physical and engineering sciences.

Two other topics would be useful for readers of this book: statistics and computer science. It has been my experience that many students who have the required background in mathematics have omitted these two topics from their education. As it would be unreasonable to expect too much of my readers, I have included appendices in which the basics of these topics are summarized. Because of the nature of many of the models, it has not been possible to describe them without considerable reliance on statistical and probabilistic arguments, so the reader ignorant of probability and statistics should strive to learn something of the subject before approaching these chapters.

Many of the models described in this book rely heavily on computer simulations. To fully understand how such models work, readers would be well advised to write some of their own computer simulations. I have, however, written the book in such a way that readers without any knowledge of computers can follow all the main chapters, provided they are willing to accept the results of a computer model on faith. For those with knowledge of a structured computer language such as Pascal, C, or Fortran 90, an appendix is included in which some guidelines are given for writing a large computer simulation. Also included is a complete program (in C) for simulating one of the models in the main part of the book.

Although mathematics is used in several of the models presented here, this book is *not* a book *about* mathematics. Any mathematics that appears in a model in this book is there because it is required to develop a model which is explicitly devised to explain a *biological* system. This emphasis may puzzle some readers, so a bit of explanation may be helpful.

The idea of applying mathematical and computational methods to construct theoretical models of biological systems is a fairly recent one. The relative youth of the subject means that most of the researchers in the field known as *theoretical biology* had their training in another discipline.[1] These researchers naturally bring into theoretical biology the skills they had acquired and developed during their training and work in their original field, resulting in a great variety of approaches to the problems of constructing models of living systems. The motives of these researchers for studying biology are as varied as their methods. Some are genuinely interested in explaining how biological systems work. Others have found analogues in biology of systems familiar to them in their original fields, and therefore analyse biology with a view to furthering knowledge in another area. Models of the latter sort, although often resulting in fundamental insights into areas of science such as mathematics, computer architecture, or physics, frequently do not tell us much of direct relevance to biology.

For example, several differential and difference equations occurring in population biology (the study of how populations of organisms interact with each other) give rise to intricate, chaotic (in the mathematical sense of the word) solutions for certain values of their parameters, although these parameters may be totally unrealistic biologically. The solution of these equations in these parameter ranges is, therefore, of little interest to a theoretical biologist, although it may be of great significance to a mathematician.

In the field of brain theory, the structure of the human brain has been the inspiration for a new generation of computers (the parallel processors) and computer languages (artificial intelligence). Although the motivation for these developments in computer science came from studies of the organization of natural nervous tissue, research in these areas has diverged into

---

[1] The author of this book is no exception—my training is in physics.

two streams: those interested in explaining how the human brain (sometimes known as 'wetware') works, and those interested in constucting new computers and designing new computer languages. Work in the latter stream has a rapidly decreasing relevance to the study of biological intelligence, although, of course, it is providing a highly sophisticated computer technology.

This book is concerned only with models that seek to explain specifically biological phenomena. The models that we examine are, for the most part, complex enough that they require computer simulation. Although there are many models in biology that do not use computer simulation[2] (except possibly for numerical solution of differential or difference equations), it is the author's belief that these will form an ever-shrinking minority of those models that are capable of genuine application to biology. This is for two reasons. First, fast, powerful and cheap computational power is now available to almost anyone who needs it. Second, biological systems are inherently more complex than the inanimate systems of physics and chemistry, so that models that do not take account of this complexity cannot be considered realistic.

There is still a lot of resistance to this view. Researchers trained in the classical, analytical approach to mathematics or the physical sciences often feel that computer simulations cannot provide rigorous results, or that the 'brute force' approach excludes a more elegant, compact solution to the problem. Although it is true that, in the 300 years since Newton, most of theoretical science has been done using the rigorous, analytical approach, the reason for that is simply that that is the only kind of science that *could* be done, since for most of that time, electronic computers did not exist. The lack of computational power meant that researchers could only answer questions that had clean, elegant solutions. Because these analytical methods had such great success in formulating models of the world, it was natural to believe that all the unsolved problems had neat, clean solutions as well. It is only now that we have the ability to do complex calculations and simulations that we are discovering that a great many systems seem to have an inherent complexity that cannot be simplified. But we have only been able to do these sorts of calculations for about one-tenth the time that has been spent on the more classical approach. After another 300 years, we will no doubt feel as comfortable using computer simulations to analyse nature as scientists today feel using Newton's laws of motion to describe the trajectory of a falling stone.

Having delivered my soliloquy, it is time to address the issue of the aims and objectives of this book. My goal is to give the reader a sample of the sorts of models that have been constructed to gain a theoretical un-

---

[2] A comprehensive survey of such models is given in the book by Murray (1989).

derstanding of several diverse biological systems. Although the three areas of biology chosen for study may appear to be quite disconnected from each other, several common themes will be seen to recur. Methods or ideas developed in one area have been applied fruitfully in other areas, leading to some hope that a unified biological theory may not be as far-fetched as we might have thought. Darwin's principle of evolution by natural selection (the idea that species produce offspring of variable fitness, the best of which are selected by the environment to carry on) has an obvious application to the origin of life, but we find that it is a useful idea when applied to the immune system, and we even encounter a model of brain function in which evolution figures prominently. The concept of distributed memory, originally designed to model the brain, finds an application in the immune system. Ideas borrowed from the physics of magnetic substances find applications in all three areas of biology.

Many readers will have come upon this book after several years studying the physical sciences. Fields such as physics, chemistry, and mathematics have several centuries of rigorous achievements on which textbooks have been written. One may read these works with a confidence that what they say about the world is, for the most part, correct. Even if a scientific revolution should overturn, say, quantum theory, the description of the world provided by quantum theory cannot be entirely wrong, if for no other reason than its very success at predicting with astounding accuracy the behaviour of the subatomic world.

Theoretical biology has no such pedigree. Although many of the principles of biology have qualitative theories which are no longer seriously questioned, such as the theory of evolution, the security provided by a quantitative theory is lacking. This is not the place to embark on a philosophical discussion as to why this is the case, but the reader should keep in mind that the theories and models presented in this book must not be accepted as the last word on how life works. Indeed, in many cases, they are only the first words in the subject.

The main aim of this book, then, is to provide the reader with a snapshot of some of the ideas and techniques that are currently being used by biological modellers in attempts to build a quantitative theoretical biology. I have tried to do this by presenting a cross-section of several areas in biology spanning systems from the most primitive (the origin of life) through a cellular system (the immune system) up to the most complex organization of matter known to man (the brain). In doing so, I have had to omit many areas of theoretical biology in which substantial progress has been made. Even within each field that has been included, I have chosen only five or six models for study.

In the case of the origin of life, the selection of models for inclusion in the book was fairly simple, because there are relatively few such models in existence. Models of the origin of life attempt to explain an event which presumably took place on the Earth several billion years ago, in an environment very different from that around us today. Because the origin of life took place so long ago, and took so long to come about, it is very difficult to compare a model with experimental data. However, besides being interesting for its own sake, models of the origin of life introduce several techniques and concepts useful in other areas of theoretical biology.

When we move to the immune system, we find a much larger body of both experimental data and theoretical models. The immune system is, in one sense, much easier to model than the origin of life because we have an abundance of working systems to study. However, the study of these 'real-life models' shows that it is a very complex system indeed. Within this complexity, we will discover an evolving ecosystem in miniature, so that the ideas used in some origin of life models prove useful here as well.

The brain presents the ultimate challenge to both the laboratory and computer researcher. Again, we find an abundance of data from the experimentalists, but from the theoretician's point of view, this data has some aggravating gaps in it. These gaps have not stopped the modellers from practising their craft, however, and we find a veritable cornucopia of models from which to choose. The variety is so great that we must ration ourselves to models from one specialized area of brain research—that of memory. Even here, there are many more models than we can comfortably handle in a book this size. I have tried to choose models of memory that have some relation to the models we have encountered in the other two sections of the book, so that the reader can see some sort of continuity.

The chapters in the book may be read in almost any order, although the first chapter in each of the three parts of the book (the first two chapters in the case of the third part) provides some biological background which motivates the models that follow. The models within each part of the book are presented in a way which will lead the reader from simpler to more complex models, although most of the models can be understood on their own.

I had originally intended to provide some problems at the end of each chapter, but the more I considered this idea, the more I realized that it was not practical. Most of the models rely heavily on computer simulation, so the best way for readers to bring the subject matter to life would be to write some of the simulations for themselves. Specially contrived problems which may be solved with pencil and paper detract from, rather than add to, the reader's understanding of the purpose of these models.

In writing this book, I have had advice and assistance from many people. I will try to acknowledge their contributions personally here.

Thanks go to Michael Pullen for writing the program used to generate the results shown in Chapter 4. For taking the time to read parts of the manuscript and offering comments, I would like to thank Scott Findlay, Petra Leimich, Neil McIntyre, Stephen Scrimgeour, and Jenny Pocock, as well as several anonymous referees. For endless patience and invaluable assistance on all aspects of computing, from the unravelling of the intricacies of LATEX to providing a map through the minefields of numerical analysis packages, I would like to thank the past and present members of the computing staff in the Department of Mathematics and Computer Science at the University of Dundee: Eric Fraga, Colin Macleod, Alastair Davie, and Nick Dawes. Finally, my thanks to the staff at Oxford University Press, who guided this book from its inception to the final form you hold in your hands.

Dundee   *G.W.A.R.*
May 1993

Contents

II   THE IMMUNE SYSTEM

III   THE BRAIN

Part I

The Origin of Life

1

The molecular basis of life

1.1   Introduction

It seems appropriate to begin a book on theoretical models in biology with
a look at some of the theories that have been proposed to explain the origin
of life. In one sense, such theories are the simplest of biological models, because in dealing with primitive organisms we need not consider most of the
complex properties of higher plants and animals such as intelligence, immunity to infection, the structure and function of organs and muscles, and
so on. We can concentrate on 'life-forms' that are simply single molecules
possessing only the ability to reproduce.

However, building an accurate model of the origin of life is difficult
because we are dealing with something that happened in the distant past
(probably more than 3 billion years ago) on an Earth with very different
properties than it has today. There are very little data about the Earth at
that time that are universally accepted, so we cannot be sure what sort of
environment an early organism would face. The theories and models are
even harder to test experimentally, for the chemical and physical processes
that led to life beginning probably took millions of years.

The best we can hope to do, then, is to build models which show that
systems possessing certain properties can, under a wide range of environ-
ments, give rise to systems that have some of the general properties of life.
It would be unrealistic at this stage to expect a theory that will predict,
starting from the molecular level some three to four billion years ago, the
existence of cedar trees or duck-billed platypuses.

Before we can present any quantitative theories of the origin of life,
we must make a survey of some of the more general properties of life as
it exists today. It is reasonable that any properties that are common to
all organisms are in some way fundamental and essential to life in general.
As such, they were likely to have been present in those molecular systems
with which it all began thousands of millenia ago. If we can identify these
properties, we will have some idea of the sorts of things our models must
include.

Despite the remarkable diversity of living things on the Earth today, there are a few common themes that run through all forms of them. All organisms extract energy in some form from their environment in order to maintain themselves from one moment to the next. The uses to which this energy is put are many and varied, from a single-celled paramecium beating its flagella to move, to humans producing works of art and literature. Organisms have become highly efficient in channelling energy in ways that prolong their lives. However, sooner or later something will happen to any organism which none of its clever defences can withstand, and it will die.

If all living things could do was process energy in ways that helped them survive from one day to the next, eventually all life would die out. To perpetuate the species beyond an individual's death requires that the organism has some way of producing a copy of itself. A method of reproduction is another essential property of life.

The interplay of these two aspects of survival—short term through processing energy (*metabolism*), and long term through *reproduction*—is at the heart of the theory of natural selection, or 'survival of the fittest'. Those organisms that are best equipped to deal with the vagaries of the environment will be those that leave the most offspring, and thus such well-adapted creatures must ultimately dominate the life in their area.

If we envision the earliest life as little more than bare molecules, their short term survival depended on nothing more than the chemical stability in their molecular structure. A molecule which is more stable to collisions with other molecules and various forms of radiation will tend to last longer. However, no matter how stable a molecule is, it is useless as a precursor to life if it cannot replicate itself. On the molecular level, then, this is where the crux of the problem lies: finding a molecular structure which allows reproduction.

The discovery of the details of the method of reproduction used by all life was one of the great triumphs of twentieth century biology. The remarkable fact that, on the molecular level, all organisms use essentially the same method of copying themselves is one of the strongest pieces of evidence for the theory that all life has evolved from a common ancestor in the distant past. The universality of this method strongly suggests that we must incorporate this molecular mechanism in any theory of the origin of life. We will therefore devote some space to explaining how the information for reproduction is stored and transmitted in living organisms.

1.2   How life reproduces

During the following description of molecular reproductive methods, the reader should keep in mind that the 'modern' organism is the result of hundreds of millions of years of fine tuning through the processes of evolution. We cannot expect that primitive systems had many of the advantages of the elegant and seemingly custom-made biochemical processes that guide the reproductive process in highly evolved life. For this reason we shall take a bare-bones approach to reproductive biochemistry, describing only those processes that seem central to reproduction rather than those that merely serve to streamline it or improve its accuracy and reliability. Besides, a comprehensive survey of even this one aspect of molecular biology would fill several books the size of this one.

It has been known for some time that the information necessary to create a copy of an organism is passed down from parent to offspring in terms of genes. The composition of genes and how the information is stored and transmitted were mysteries until the last half of the twentieth century. In a series of ingenious experiments many of these problems were solved, but our understanding of the reproductive process is still incomplete. (A very readable account of this work can be found in Stent and Calendar (1978).)

1.2.1   DNA, RNA, and proteins

In every organism that has been studied so far, the genetic information is stored in the chemical structure of the molecule deoxyribonucleic acid (DNA) or, in some simpler creatures such as certain viruses, the related molecule ribonucleic acid (RNA). The elucidation of the structure and some of the resulting functions of DNA were worked out in the 1950s by Francis Crick and James Watson. An entertaining account of this discovery was written by Watson (1981) in his book *The Double Helix*. A comprehensive account of the biochemistry of DNA can be found in any modern textbook on molecular biology (for example, Darnell *et al.* (1986) or Stryer (1988)).

Despite the fact that the *information* needed to build an organism is stored in the DNA, DNA is a relatively inert molecule. As a result, it is not much use when it comes to performing those services that keep an organism alive from one moment to the next. The real workhorse molecules are the proteins. Proteins come in an enormous variety of forms: some can form links with each other so that they can be used to build strong, resilient body parts (such as skin and hair), while others (the enzymes) serve as catalysts that can speed up reaction rates by many orders of magnitude.

Among all the myriad tasks for which proteins are responsible is that of mediating the replication of the DNA molecule itself. The DNA molecule contains the information required for the construction of all proteins, including those that replicate the DNA. Thus the quality of information stored in a DNA molecule determines not only the fate of the organism in which it resides but the fate of future generations of the DNA itself. It has been said by Richard Dawkins (1976) that the organism is merely the gene's

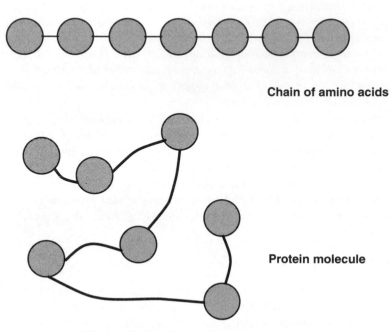

Chain of amino acids

Protein molecule

Figure 1.1   The structure of a protein molecule.

way of producing another gene. In other words, all of the functions in a
creature's life are mere embellishments to improve the efficiency of reproduction. On its simplest level, then, life may be viewed as a two-component
cycle: the DNA produces the proteins which are needed to replicate the
DNA which produces more proteins, and so on.

To understand how a DNA molecule stores the information required to
produce a protein, we must first know a little about the structure of proteins. Although a protein molecule can have almost any three-dimensional
shape (it is largely the shape of a protein that determines its function), it is
essentially nothing more than a linear molecule (like a piece of string) that
has been folded up onto itself in a particular way. The bends and folds are
held in place by chemical bonds between different parts of the molecule,
so that the three-dimensional structure of the protein is not a haphazard
affair. If one looks a bit more closely (Fig. 1.1) at the 'string' from which
the protein is made, it will be seen that this string actually looks more like
a pearl necklace, where each pearl can be one of 20 different kinds of *amino
acid*. The detailed chemical structure of an amino acid is not important
for our purposes—it may be thought of as nothing more than a pearl of a

Amino acids	
Ala	Alanine
Arg	Arginine
Asn	Asparagine
Asp	Aspartic Acid
Cys	Cysteine
Glu	Glutamic Acid
Gln	Glutamine
Gly	Glycine
His	Histidine
Ile	Isoleucine
Leu	Leucine
Lys	Lysine
Met	Methionine
Phe	Phenylalanine
Pro	Proline
Ser	Serine
Thr	Threonine
Trp	Tryptophan
Tyr	Tyrosine
Val	Valine

Table 1.1   Amino acids used in modern proteins.

certain size and shape. The 20 amino acids used in modern proteins are listed in Table 1.1.

Once the order of amino acids in a protein molecule is specified (once it is stated in what order the various pearls are to be strung onto the necklace), the protein will automatically fold up into a precise three-dimensional structure. Since the three-dimensional structure determines the function of the protein, and the sequence of amino acids determines the three-dimensional structure, the amino acid sequence of a protein determines its function. Thus to store the information needed to perform a certain function in a living organism, all that needs to be done is to store the sequence of amino acids that is used to build the protein that has that function. Protein sizes vary, but a typical protein contains on the order of 100 amino acids.

The DNA molecule, like a protein, is also a linear molecule. Unlike a protein, however, DNA consists not of a single strand, but of two parallel strands that spiral around each other to form a double helix. The two strands of the helix are weakly bonded to each other by a series of molecular bridges, so that the overall structure closely resembles a spiral staircase:

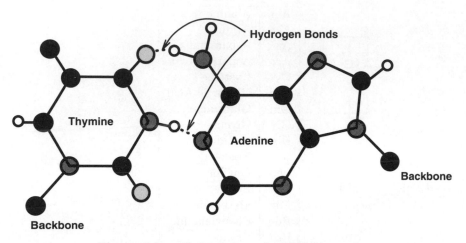

Figure 1.2   The structure of a DNA base pair.

the two strongly bound 'backbones' of the molecule are analogous to the
spiral supports which hold the individual steps in place, while the molecular
bridges correspond to the steps themselves. At warm temperatures (around
50°C), the two strands of the double helix will separate from each other,
with each of the bridges or steps splitting roughly in the middle. The effect
is rather like the molecule 'unzipping' down the middle.

The information storing capacity of DNA is contained not in the two
helical backbones, but in the bridges between them. Each bridge is composed of two smaller molecules. Each of these small molecules is firmly
anchored at one end to one of the helical backbones, while the other end
sticks out, meeting its partner, the other small molecule, sticking out from
the other backbone. The shapes of these two smaller molecules are such
that where they meet in the middle of the double helix, they fit together
like two pieces of a jigsaw puzzle. A weak chemical bond forms at this
meeting place.

Each of these smaller molecules (which are called 'bases' because of their
chemical nature) can be one of four types: adenine, guanine, cytosine, or
thymine, abbreviated as A, G, C, or T respectively. Again, the detailed
structures of these molecules are not important, save in one respect. The
precise meshing together of two of these molecules in the middle of the
bridge between the two helical strands will occur only if the two molecules
are paired off in a certain way. If one of the molecules is an adenine,
its partner must be a thymine (Fig. 1.2), while if one is a guanine, the
other must be a cytosine. Thus A always pairs with T, and C with G.

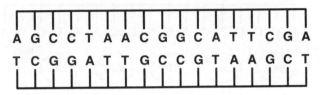

Figure 1.3   The complementary nature of the two strands of a DNA molecule.

The order in which the molecules are placed along one of the backbone strands is arbitrary, but once the order on one strand has been decided upon, the order on the other strand is automatically determined by the pairing requirements.

For example, if the order of 10 bases along one strand is ATGCG-TAATT, then the order on the other (often called the *complementary* strand) must be TACGCATTAA (Fig. 1.3).

This structure elegantly solves both the information storage and reproduction problems at a single stroke. Since the order of the bases on one strand is arbitrary, any amount of information can be stored in the base sequence of a DNA molecule, although it may take a very long molecule to store any significant amount of information (the total amount of DNA in each human cell is of the order of 10^9 bases). Also, since proteins are made from 20 different kinds of amino acids and DNA is made from 4 different kinds of bases, there cannot be a one-to-one correspondence between base and amino acid. In fact, each triplet of bases on a DNA strand corresponds to a single amino acid. There are 64 possible triplets, or 'codons' as they have become known, and it is now known that 61 of them code for one of the 20 amino acids (so that some amino acids have more than one codon coding for them), while the remaining 3 codons are 'stop signs', in that they mark the end of the region that codes for a particular protein in much the same way as a full stop indicates the end of a sentence.

Reproduction of a DNA molecule takes advantage of the complementarity of the two strands. Special proteins (called DNA polymerases) exist that can separate the DNA strands in a small region and manufacture a complementary copy for each of the two strands. These proteins work their way down a DNA molecule so that when they reach the end, the original double helix has been split in half and a new complementary strand has been built on each original strand. The molecule has given rise to two identical offspring. The polymerases are so sophisticated that they even have a proof-reading ability—they test each addition they make to the new

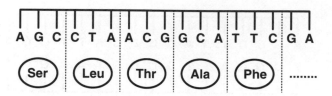

Figure 1.4   Each codon in DNA codes for one amino acid in a protein.

strands to be sure it correctly matches its partner on the original strand.

1.2.2   How proteins are made

As mentioned in the last section, the information needed to build a protein
molecule is stored in the sequence of bases in a length of DNA, or, in some
cases, RNA. Each triplet of bases, or codon, in the DNA molecule codes
for one of the 20 amino acids used to construct a protein (Fig. 1.4). The
'dictionary' giving the translations between codons and amino acids is the
genetic code, shown in Table 1.2.

For a given codon, locate the first base in the codon in the left-most
column in the table. This narrows down the choice of amino acid to one
block of four rows. The second base in the codon decides the column and
the third base decides which of the four rows to choose. For example, given
the codon ATG, the table tells us that it codes for Met.

The three-letter abbreviations in Table 1.2 stand for the full names of
each amino acid as shown in Table 1.1.

In Table 1.1, three codons (TAA, TAG, and TGA) are listed as corresponding to a 'stop' signal. These codons act as termination symbols,
telling the enzymes reading the DNA when the code for a particular protein stops. The codon ATG, which codes for the amino acid methionine,
also acts as a 'start' signal in certain circumstances. The precise mechanism by which the beginning of a protein coding section is recognized
is quite complicated, and varies considerably with the particular protein.
This complexity serves a purpose, however, since there must be some way
of regulating when a protein is produced and how much of it is made when
it is being produced. If all that needs to be done to produce a protein is
to have a DNA-reading enzyme find the start signal and begin grinding
out proteins, the cell would quickly be swamped with unwanted proteins,
or else run out of amino acids with which to produce them. Although we
shall not concern ourselves here with the various ways in which regulation
of protein production is accomplished, the subject is a fascinating one and

First pos'n	Second position				Third pos'n
	T	C	A	G	
T	Phe	Ser	Tyr	Cys	T
	Phe	Ser	Tyr	Cys	C
	Leu	Ser	Stop	Stop	A
	Leu	Ser	Stop	Trp	G
C	Leu	Pro	His	Arg	T
	Leu	Pro	His	Arg	C
	Leu	Pro	Gln	Arg	A
	Leu	Pro	Gln	Arg	G
A	Ile	Thr	Asn	Ser	T
	Ile	Thr	Asn	Ser	C
	Ile	Thr	Lys	Arg	A
	Met	Thr	Lys	Arg	G
G	Val	Ala	Asp	Gly	T
	Val	Ala	Asp	Gly	C
	Val	Ala	Glu	Gly	A
	Val	Ala	Glu	Gly	G

Table 1.2   The Genetic code.

the reader is urged to explore it further. A good introduction can be found in Darnell *et al.* (1986).

1.2.3 Protein synthesis

Protein synthesis begins with the reading of the section of the DNA molecule that codes for the required protein. As usual with any biochemical process, every step of the way is mediated by an array of enzymes that make everything go quickly and smoothly, but the central enzyme is *RNA polymerase*, which is responsible for building an RNA copy of the DNA code.

RNA is structurally similar to DNA, in that a single strand of RNA consists of a strongly bonded backbone to which are attached a series of bases in an arbitrary order. Unlike DNA, however, RNA does not tend to form double helices. It is possible for mutually complementary parts of a single strand of RNA to pair with each other, so that the single strand doubles back on itself. This is an important aspect of such molecules as transfer RNA, which will be discussed below. One other difference between RNA and DNA is that RNA uses the base uracil, abbreviated U, in place of thymine. Since uracil is similar in structure to thymine, it is also capable of pairing with adenine inside a double helix structure.

When conditions are right for a copy of a protein to be made, RNA polymerase will locate the ATG start signal codon and attach itself to the DNA at that point. The double helix structure of the DNA is locally loosened up so that the enzyme can gain access to the bases inside. Starting with the ATG codon, a copy of the DNA is made by constructing an RNA molecule with the same sequence as the DNA, except that all thymines in DNA are replaced with uracils in the RNA. (For this reason, genetic code tables are often given with U instead of T.) The transcription process continues until a stop signal is reached, at which point a complete RNA copy of the DNA gene has been created. This RNA molecule is called *messenger RNA* (or just *mRNA*) since it carries the message of how to construct a protein from the library (the DNA) to the place where the protein is actually built (the ribosome, which we will get to in a minute).

Once the complete mRNA is formed, it must form a complex with several other molecules so that translation of the genetic message from RNA to protein can begin. Two other structures that we have not met so far are important in the translation process: transfer RNA and ribosomes.

A transfer RNA molecule, or tRNA for short, is a single-stranded molecule approximately 70 bases in length. Transfer RNAs come in many different forms, but the structure of all of them is roughly the same (Fig. 1.5).

The base sequence of a tRNA is such that the molecule can, by folding back on itself, form complementary bonds between parts of itself for short distances (around 4 or 5 bases in each case). This folding results in the tRNA being shaped rather like a distorted cross. The two free ends of the molecule join together, with the middle section folding so as to create three complementary loop structures.

The tRNA is the key to the translation process, since one of the loops (the one opposite the joined free ends) is capable of recognizing one particular codon in an mRNA molecule, while the part of the molecule where the two free ends are joined together can bind the amino acid that corresponds to that codon. The mRNA codon is recognized by the specific sequences of bases in the middle loop of the tRNA, a loop known as the *anti-codon*, since the base sequence of the middle three bases in the loop is complementary to the codon which it recognizes. Actually, the correspondence between tRNA and codon is not one-to-one, since one tRNA can often match with more than one codon for a given amino acid, provided that the codons differ only in the third base, as is often the case (refer to the genetic code table above). The reason for this is that tRNAs often contain non-standard bases, different from the normal A, U, C, and G used in ordinary RNA. These modified bases allow more flexibility in the base-pairing rules. Thus, although there are 61 different codons that code for amino acids, fewer than this number of tRNAs are needed to recognize all the codons.

In order for the tRNA molecules to perform the translation process, they must be provided with an environment in which all the parts required

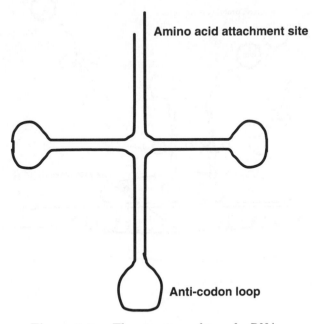

Figure 1.5   The structure of transfer RNA.

(mRNA, amino acids, tRNAs, and assorted proteins) can be positioned correctly. This is provided by the structure known as the ribosome. A ribosome is a complex structure composed of yet another version of RNA, called ribosomal RNA or rRNA, and up to 50 different types of proteins. A ribosome acts much like a tape reader, where the input tape is the mRNA molecule and the output is a newly built protein molecule.

To begin the translation, the first codon on the mRNA (an AUG, corresponding to a transcribed ATG from the DNA) attaches to a ribosome (Fig. 1.6).

A tRNA of the correct type, that is, one that can recognize an AUG codon, attaches to the ribosome in such a way that its anti-codon loop lies next to the codon on the mRNA. In order for the tRNA to bind, it must first be *activated*, that is, it must have an amino acid of the correct type bound to its free end. Since the AUG codon codes for methionine, the corresponding tRNA must be able to match the AUG sequence with its anti-codon, and have a methionine bound to its free end. With the first codon and corresponding tRNA in place, the second codon in the mRNA is positioned so that the corresponding activated tRNA can drift in and bind

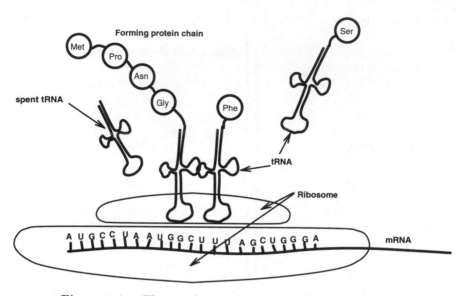

Figure 1.6   The translation of messenger RNA into protein.

its anti-codon to the codon. Suppose this second codon is CUG, which
corresponds to the amino acid leucine. The second tRNA to attach must
then have an anti-codon which can match the sequence CUG, and it must
have a leucine molecule bound to its free end. Now the methionine from
the first tRNA is bound to the leucine on the second tRNA, creating an
amino acid chain of two units in length—the beginning of the new protein
molecule. The methionine now detaches from the first tRNA molecule,
which in turn is now freed to drift away from the ribosome. The mRNA
is shunted over one space so that the second tRNA molecule now occupies
the place vacated by the first, with the third codon in the place formerly
occupied by the second. At this stage the leucine tRNA has a two amino-
acid chain attached to its free end. A new activated tRNA molecule is
now brought in to match the third codon, the amino acid chain from the
leucine tRNA is bound to the new amino acid and the whole chain, now
consisting of 3 amino acids, is shifted over to the newest tRNA. The process
is continued until the end of the mRNA is reached, at which point the new
protein molecule, now complete, detaches from the last tRNA and folds up
into its active form, ready for service.

Since many mRNA molecules are quite long, it is possible for several
ribosomes to translate the same mRNA simultaneously. Once one ribosome has progressed sufficiently far down the mRNA, a second ribosome

can attach itself at the initiation end (the AUG codon) and proceed independently of the first. The production of protein can be speeded up this way.

The reader may have noticed that the production of proteins involves not just the participation of various forms of nucleic acids, but also requires the services of proteins at many stages. The polymerases that make the mRNA copy of the DNA, the various initiation factors necessary to allow the mRNA to bind to a ribosome, and the proteins necessary to give the ribosome its structure are all integral parts of the transcription and translation processes. Yet all of these proteins must themselves be produced by the same processes. Even those proteins not directly involved in transcription or translation can influence the process through various kinds of feedback. Often a protein is capable of binding to that stretch of DNA that codes for it, thus inhibiting any further transcription, so that once a certain amount of the protein has been produced, the supply is cut off. When the stock of protein falls as the molecules degrade, the gene coding for the protein is freed up and production can resume.

The DNA–RNA-protein chain is thus not a sequence of events with a definite beginning and end—rather it is a cycle, where each link in the chain has an effect on all future repetitions of the cycle.

1.3 Modelling the origin of life

A comprehensive model of the origin of life should explain how the molecular machinery of DNA replication and protein production can arise spontaneously from simple precursors. However, no such comprehensive theory yet exists, simply because the processes involved are so complex and the number of variables so immense.

To approach the problem of life's origins we will examine in the following chapters a few models which attempt to show how general molecular species having some of the properties of nucleic acids and proteins can self-organize to form systems with some of the properties of life. In modern organisms, the replication of DNA depends on numerous proteins and the proteins depend on the codes in the DNA. In attempting to model the origin of such a system, we are faced with a chicken-and-egg problem: which came first, the DNA or the protein? Or did they arise simultaneously?

There are proponents of all three possibilities. Some researchers think that proteins formed small globules called 'proto-cells' which gradually assimilated the other biomolecules, including nucleic acids, to form the first truly living cells. Others think that a primitive form of nucleic acid was able to reproduce itself without the aid of proteins, but eventually the link between the base sequence of a DNA molecule and the amino acid sequence of a protein was established, and the proteins became part of the catalytic cycle because they speeded up the replication of DNA. Still others think that primitive nucleic acids and proteins existed together on the early Earth and managed to form a partnership at the very beginning. There is even a plausible theory (Cairns-Smith (1982,1985)) that the first life-forms were composed of clay minerals, since such minerals have a crystalline structure with the ability to replicate themselves, and clays are common minerals on the Earth.

Is it reasonable to assume that nucleic acids and amino acids could form spontaneously? The answer to this seems to be a guarded 'yes'. A classic series of experiments by Stanley Miller and Harold Urey in the 1950s (see Miller (1953); also review articles by Miller and Urey (1959) and Miller (1986)), based on ideas put forward by Oparin (1938), showed that for a system of water and an atmosphere consisting of the gases that were thought to be common on the pre-biological Earth, electrical discharges (similar to lightning) or ultraviolet radiation resulted in the formation of some amino acids and nucleotides, although not in the same proportions as they exist at present. Other experiments by Sidney Fox and coworkers (Harada and Fox (1964)) have shown that heat can also create amino acids from non-biological compounds. Virtually all 20 amino acids used in modern proteins were created this way. Thus the theories assuming the existence of the building blocks of DNA and proteins seem to have something going for them.

One problem that faces any model is that of finding an environment in which the concentrations of the various reactants, whatever they are assumed to be, can reach high enough levels for interactions to occur fairly often. For example, one calculation done by Hull (1960) showed that if the processes in a Miller-type experiment did occur on the primitive Earth, it is unlikely that the concentrations of even the most abundant amino acids would exceed 10^{-12} moles per litre. In addition, Hull argues that the very processes used to create these biomolecules (electric discharges and ultraviolet radiation) are even more efficient at destroying them.

Hull's arguments are based on the assumption that these biomolecules are more or less evenly distributed over the Earth, and that no mechanism exists for isolating and concentrating them before they become so widely dispersed, or destroyed. In a rebuttal to Hull's article published in the same journal, Bernal (1960) shows that many such mechanisms exist for concentrating rare substances on the Earth (consider the existence of gold mines) and that, given such mechanisms, the scenario of amino acids developing and combining into more complex molecules is not so far-fetched.

One possibility is that of life beginning in some shallow pool, possibly in the intertidal region of a seashore. Charles Darwin envisioned life beginning in a 'warm little pond' in which precursors of biomolecules could accumulate until a murky primordial or prebiotic 'soup' is formed. Such a process could occur, for example, in pools that alternately fill and then dry out, leaving behind the reactants which grow in concentration each time round. Another possibility that has been suggested is that the molecules accumulated on water droplets in the atmosphere, for example in clouds.

A criticism often levelled at the DNA-first camp by the protein-first team is that, even if enough nucleic acid could be produced and concentrated for some primitive self-replicating system to form, DNA or RNA do not possess a way of maintaining and increasing the concentration levels so that some serious evolving can get started. It is claimed that proteins have the ability to form primitive cell-like structures, inside which is a protected environment in which biomolecules can accumulate and evolve unmolested by the outside world. The difficulty with such a model is that it is not clear how the information needed to build the 'right' proteins is maintained without a molecule such as DNA or RNA.

Most quantitative theoretical models of early biochemistry tend to assume that the DNA-first scenario is correct. This has the advantage that such systems are easier to model, because DNA-like molecules have the self-replication property, so it is easy to construct a system that evolves over time. A model involving proteins, which cannot self-replicate, must invoke some external agent (such as DNA) to allow indirect replication of the proteins. This complicates the model considerably. (Having said this, it must be noted that Kauffman (1986) proposed that an autocatalytic set of proteins could form, which is self-sufficient.)

Although models of a DNA-first system are not difficult to construct (we will encounter one in the next chapter), they all assume that short strands of DNA or RNA are already present, and that these snippets will readily polymerize into longer strings. However, it is not obvious that DNA will spontaneously form without some catalytic help. Many experiments have been done over the last 30 years, by Leslie Orgel (see Orgel, 1973) and others, in attempts to determine what conditions are necessary for individual nucleotides to polymerize into a single strand of a DNA or RNA molecule. It is not something that happens without a lot of coaxing. The reactions sometimes occur more quickly if certain types of metal ions are present in the solution or if a solid surface, such as that of a clay crystal, is present to give the nucleotides something to stick to before they join together. The spontaneous replication of DNA and RNA is also a very slow and unreliable reaction without catalytic help.

In the last few years, however, a property of RNA has been discovered that could have profound implications for the origin of life (see, for example, Robertson and Joyce (1991)). Up until 1982, it was generally believed that there was a strict division of labour between the nucleic acids and the proteins: the nucleic acids stored the information required to produce proteins, and gave some assistance in their construction (as with tRNA and ribosomes). The proteins were the catalysts for a wide variety of biochemical reactions, including the replication of nucleic acids and the production of proteins.

In 1982, however, it was discovered that certain RNA molecules could also act as catalysts. The original discovery was made in the messenger RNA of a single-celled protozoan. Our discussion of the production of proteins earlier in this chapter omitted one feature that is common to most of the genes in organisms whose cells contain nuclei (the *eukaryotes*). In many cases, the code for a single protein does not occur as a single unbroken stretch of DNA or RNA. Rather, it is broken up by long stretches of DNA that do not appear to code for any protein and, in fact, do not seem to have any function at all. These stretches of inactive or 'junk' DNA are called *introns*. The sections of DNA that *do* code for part of the protein are called *exons*. In the manufacture of a protein molecule, the entire stretch of DNA, including all the introns, is transcribed into mRNA, but the introns are spliced out of the mRNA before it travels to the ribosome for translation into protein.

In most cases, this splicing is mediated by protein catalysts, as you might expect. However, in this protozoan, it was discovered that certain introns had the ability to catalyse their own removal. In other words, the RNA sequence in the intron was such that it spontaneously removed just the right amount of RNA and spliced together the two exons on either side of the intron. Such self-catalysing RNA sequences are known as *ribozymes*.

Since this initial discovery, several types of ribozymes have been found. They split into four broad categories. Two of these categories contain ribozymes that splice themselves out of an exon–intron sequence. The difference between these two groups is in the manner in which the splicing occurs. The third group of ribozymes aids in the production of tRNA molecules, while the fourth group, found in some viruses, simply cleaves RNA molecules into shorter segments.

Although the known catalytic abilities of ribozymes are still quite limited, the fact that RNA can act as a catalyst at all is big news. Experiments on the two intron ribozyme groups have shown that the catalytic ability is the result of specific RNA base sequences that cause the molecule to fold up into a precise three-dimensional shape which gives it its catalytic power. This is exactly the same mechanism which is responsible for the catalytic effects of the proteins. The few ribozymes that have been discovered may be remnants of a much greater repertoire that was present at the beginning of life on Earth. Experiments are currently underway to determine if other RNA sequences also possess catalytic properties. If they do, it is possible to envision an 'RNA world' in which strings of RNA could contain both the information required for propagation of the species and the catalytic abilities to speed the reactions along.

   Assuming the existence of the correct conditions for a self-replicating
DNA or RNA system, how can such a system evolve? That is, how can the
Darwinian principle of natural selection be applied to a molecular system?
Since the base sequence of a nucleic acid is arbitrary, we would expect that a
variety of different sequences would appear in a solution rich in nucleotides.
Because of intra-molecular interactions, some of these sequences will be
more stable than others, so they will last longer. The longer a molecule
'lives', the more chance it has of reproducing. Also, some molecules will
reproduce faster than others, so that, all other things being equal, they will
be able to use up the free nucleotides more quickly and starve the other
molecules of their reproductive material.

   If some sequences are 'fitter' than others, there will be a handful of
sequences that are the fittest for their particular environment. The closer a
molecule's sequence is to this 'best' sequence, the more it will dominate the
population. However, because the replication procedure will make errors,
the daughter sequences of one parent molecule will not all have sequences
identical to the parent. In some of the daughters, base substitutions will
occur, in others an extra base may have squeezed in between two others,
or a base may be left out. In all these cases, the daughter sequences will be
different from the parent in a few places. These alterations, or *mutations*,
may make the daughters more or less fit than their parent. If they lose
fitness, they will not fare as well as their parents and may eventually die
out. If they gain fitness, they will dominate the population even more
than the parent molecule. In such a way, the population can approach a
maximum fitness. This is evolution, or survival of the fittest, on a molecular
scale.

   We will examine a model in Chapter 2 which quantifies these ideas. This
model uses differential equations to examine the average behaviour of such
a system. The attraction of such a model is that differential equations can
always be solved (numerically, if necessary) to yield clean curves predicting
the numbers of the various molecular species as functions of time. The
difficulty with differential equations, however, is that they predict only the
average behaviour of a population. In any real system, there will always be
fluctuations around this average behaviour. If the number of molecules in
the system is large and the fluctuations relatively small, this randomness
may not be particularly important. However, in a system such as a prebiotic
soup, the population size of each of the individual species will not be large,
and fluctuations around these mean numbers will be important. For this
reason, we examine two other models which take account of the stochastic
nature of chemical reactions. In Chapter 3, a stochastic version of the
differential equation model in Chapter 2 is presented, introducing some
of the theory of stochastic processes used to deal with such situations.
In order for such a theory to be mathematically tractable, however, many

unrealistic assumptions are made about the variability of the system. Most of these assumptions are removed in Chapter 4, where we describe a fully stochastic model which relies entirely on simulating random processes on a computer.

The models presented in Chapters 2, 3 and 4 all deal with a system that contains only DNA or RNA. One of the consequences of the model in Chapter 2 is that, in a population where replication is inaccurate (as it always is) there is a limit on the size of molecule, and hence on the amount of genetic information, which can be maintained over many generations. To progress beyond this size, some new information processing system is required. This could be provided by the introduction of proteins as catalysts in the replication process, but for proteins to be introduced into the cycle, some means of producing them on demand is needed. This requires the introduction of the genetic code, which seems itself to be a rather unlikely event. In Chapter 5, we examine some estimates of just how likely it is that a genetic code could arise by chance, given a system of primitive transcription and translation molecules. In Chapter 6, we describe a differential equation model of a DNA-protein catalytic system called a hypercycle. Finally, in Chapter 7, we examine a few models from the area known as *artificial life*, which consist of computer-generated entities with many of the properties of real life.

If the selection of models given here appears biased in favour of the DNA-first arguments, that is because there are no detailed, quantitative models based on a proteins-first scenario, not because the author has any preference for a DNA-first model. Anyone who reads the books and papers referred to in this chapter and follows up the references contained in them will see that there is no consensus of opinion on what really happened to start inorganic molecules on the road to living organisms.

The models presented here have many gaps in their assumptions and reasoning, some of which their authors acknowledge and others which have been revealed by critical reviews. Such is the state of our knowledge of the origin of life. Perhaps readers of this book will be spurred on to improve on the state of affairs by constructing their own models.

2

Molecular evolution and quasi-species

2.1 Introduction

As our first model of a primitive biochemical system, we will examine a model originally proposed by Manfred Eigen in 1971, and developed further by Eigen in collaboration with Peter Schuster in 1977. The model assumes the existence of molecules of an indeterminate structure which have the ability to replicate themselves without the aid of catalysts. The reader may picture these molecules as DNA, but no details of the structure of the molecules are assumed or specified in the mathematics.

Each molecular species has its own rates of reproduction and decay, which will depend partly on its structure and partly on the environment in which the molecule is found. In addition, the replication mechanism is taken to be imperfect, so that some offspring of a parent molecule will not be faithful copies. This assumption allows mutations to occur, which in turn gives natural selection a chance to act. One species is 'fitter' than another if its net production of correctly copied offspring is larger.

The aim of the model is to see just how far such a simple system can evolve. We aim to answer such questions as: Will one species always dominate the population after sufficient time? Will the population survive at all or will all the molecules die out? How large an error rate in replication can be tolerated? With some assumptions about the internal structure of the molecules, we can also ask questions about how large a molecule can get and still be faithfully reproduced over many generations.

When modelling a system such as a collection of molecules, we must give careful consideration to the mathematical methods we use and the results we expect to obtain from them. We are building a model of a system in which we begin at some time $t = 0$ with precisely specified numbers of several molecular species (the initial conditions), and we want predictions of the numbers of these species at later times. The model in this chapter uses differential equations to predict the behaviour of the system as a function of time. The solutions to these equations give precise values for each population size at all times, that is, it provides a *deterministic model.*

Suppose we decide to test the model by conducting an experiment in which we begin with a solution containing the same number of each molecular species as specified in the initial conditions for the differential equation model. We then let the reactions proceed and measure the numbers of all species present as functions of time so that we compare our data with the solutions of the equations. If we repeated the experiment several times, we would not expect to get precisely the same numbers of molecules at the same times in each experimental run. Fluctuations in the environment will cause small variations in the molecular interactions which would result in different numbers and types of reactions taking place. If we repeated the experiment many (ideally, infinitely many) times and averaged the results at each time after $t = 0$ at which measurements were made, we would get a precise curve which, provided the differential equation model accurately represents the system, should agree with the theoretical solution. Thus, as a first approximation to the behaviour of the system, we may seek a theory which predicts only the *average* numbers of each species as functions of time. For such a theory, continuous functions are adequate.

Eigen and Schuster's model is just such an average theory. When using such a theory, we must always keep in mind that its predictions will probably not apply to any one experimental system. Such a theory should only be used as a first guide to the behaviour of such systems. To obtain a more accurate description, some account must be taken of the discreteness of the molecules and noisiness of the environment, as we will do in later chapters.

2.2   Construction of the model

Suppose we have n molecular species in some primordial soup as described in Chapter 1. We assume that each of these species has the ability to reproduce itself, but that errors in reproduction are common, so that mutant species can occur. We will also assume that the system is closed with respect to the number of different species, so that if a copy of molecule A, for example, is incorrect, the resulting mutant molecule must be one of the other molecular species, say species B.

Let x_i, $i = 1, \ldots, n$ be the number of molecules of type i present in the solution.

We suppose that molecules of type i reproduce at a constant average rate of A_i offspring per parent per unit time. The rate of production of offspring (of any sort) from all members of species i is therefore $A_i x_i$. Due to the inherent error in the reproduction process, not all of these molecules will be faithful copies of their parent. The parameter Q_i, $0 \leq Q_i \leq 1$, called a *quality factor*, specifies the fraction of copies of species i that are also of species i. The remainder of the offspring, amounting to a fraction $1 - Q_i$, will therefore be distributed among the other $n - 1$ species present. The net rate of production of species i children from species i parents is thus $A_i Q_i x_i$.

Molecules, like organisms, have a finite lifetime. Due to collisions with other molecules and interaction with light and other forms of radiation, there is always a chance that a molecule will disintegrate at any given time. The term which is to be added into the rate equations to account for molecular degradation depends on what we assume to be the dominant influence in the death of molecules. If external radiation is the main culprit, and if the strength of this radiation can be assumed roughly constant, we would expect the rate of death of any given molecular species to depend on the intensity of radiation, the susceptibility of that particular species to radiation and on the number of that species present. The first two effects will be constant, so that we may account for the degradation effect by adding in a term of form $-D_i x_i$ to the rate equation for species i, where D_i is a constant that describes the combined effects of radiation intensity and the vulnerability of species i to radiation. This is what Eigen and Schuster have chosen to do in their model.

It is worth pointing out, however, that this is not the only possibility for the death term in the rate equations. If intermolecular collisions account for a substantial fraction of the deaths, we would expect the death rate for species i to be proportional to not only x_i, but to the total molecular population, since the more molecules there are, the greater the chance of a collision with one of them. In such a case a term of the form $-D_i x_i \sum_{k=1}^{n} x_k$ would need to be included instead of the linear term $-D_i x_i$. We will follow Eigen and Schuster in assuming a death rate proportional only to the single species' population.

In addition to the contribution to the number of species i molecules from self-replication, there will be contributions from the erroneous copies of other species. If we define w_{ik} to be the rate at which a species k molecule produces a species i molecule because of incorrect replication, then the total rate of increase in the number of species i through mutation is $\sum_{k \neq i} w_{ik} x_k$. The sum is over all values of k from 1 to n except for $k = i$, since molecules do not make erroneous copies of themselves.

Combining all these effects, the system of rate equations so far has the form

$$\dot{x}_i = (A_i Q_i - D_i) x_i + \sum_{k \neq i} w_{ik} x_k \tag{2.1}$$

where a dot above a variable denotes a time derivative: $\dot{x} \equiv \frac{dx}{dt}$.

The model as it stands includes the effects of metabolism and mutation, but not selection. Selection of one species results from that species being better adapted to its environment than its competitors or, in other words, having a higher fitness. The only way we can measure biological fitness is by the number of offspring produced that, themselves, succeed in reproducing. In the modern world, organisms use many different strategies to improve their fitness. Most insects, for example, produce great numbers of offspring in the hope that only a few will survive long enough to reproduce themselves. Other organisms, such as humans, produce relatively few offspring, but care for them to such an extent that they are virtually certain to reach a reproductive age.

Selection comes about due to competition between species for resources. The model specified by the system (2.1) permits unlimited growth of all species (in the case where $A_i Q_i - D_i > 0$ for all i), and so cannot impose selection on the population as a whole. There are various ways in which we could impose some sort of constraint on the system, but the simplest seems to be to require that the population size remain constant. In this way, resources become limited, and any molecule wishing to reproduce must compete with other like-minded molecules for the raw materials to make a copy of itself.

To impose the constraint of constant size, we add a term ϕ_i to each equation in the system. This represents any non-chemical rate of change of number, for example, by means of a flow or diffusion of a particular species into or out of the system. This is a somewhat artificial construct, although Eigen and Schuster justify it by saying that it can be realized in laboratory experiments in which the numbers of the various species are adjusted manually to maintain a constant overall population level. It is, of course, unlikely that such an artificial constraint was present on the ancient Earth, but the main purpose of introducing such a term is to provide a constraint that will simulate the effect of natural selection. The flow term ϕ_i does this adequately.

We therefore arrive at the final form for the rate equations:

$$\dot{x}_i = (A_i Q_i - D_i)x_i + \sum_{k \neq i} w_{ik} x_k + \phi_i. \tag{2.2}$$

If we assume that the flow for each species is proportional to that species' population size, so that

$$\phi_i = \frac{\phi_t x_i}{\sum_k x_k} \tag{2.3}$$

where ϕ_t is the total net flow, and that

$$\sum_k x_k = c_0 \tag{2.4}$$

where c_0 is the constant total number of molecules, then we can put the rate equations into a somewhat simpler form. Since the total number is constant, we must have, by summing over the rate equations

$$\sum_i \dot{x}_i = 0 = \sum_i (A_i Q_i - D_i) x_i + \sum_i \sum_{k \neq i} w_{ik} x_k + \phi_t. \tag{2.5}$$

The term $\sum_i \sum_{k \neq i} w_{ik} x_k$ is the total rate at which error copies are made, so we have

$$\sum_i \sum_{k \neq i} w_{ik} x_k = \sum_i A_i (1 - Q_i) x_i. \tag{2.6}$$

In fact, we can write a version of this condition for a single species i by equating the two forms for expressing the total error rate for a single molecule of species i:

$$\sum_{k \neq i} w_{ki} = A_i (1 - Q_i) \tag{2.7}$$

This equation is useful for constructing specific quasi-species models.

Substituting eqn (2.6) into eqn (2.5), we obtain

$$\phi_t = -\sum_i (A_i - D_i) x_i \equiv -\sum_i E_i x_i \tag{2.8}$$

where $E_i \equiv A_i - D_i$ is the *excess productivity* of species i, that is, the excess of the reproductive rate over the death rate. The sum $\sum_i E_i x_i$ on the right of eqn (2.8), if positive (negative), is the net rate at which the population size would increase (decrease) in the absence of any constraint. This equation merely says that the total flow ϕ_t is equal and opposite to the rate at which the population size would change in an unconstrained system, thus it keeps the size constant.

We define two more terms:

$$W_{ii} \equiv A_i Q_i - D_i \tag{2.9}$$

$$\bar{E} \equiv \frac{\sum_k E_k x_k}{\sum_k x_k}. \tag{2.10}$$

W_{ii} is the net change in number of species i due to the actions of species i itself, and $\bar{E}$ is the weighted average value of E_i. With these definitions the rate equations become

$$\dot{x}_i = (W_{ii} - \bar{E})x_i + \sum_{k \neq i} w_{ik}x_k. \tag{2.11}$$

We see from the first term in eqn (2.11) that a species i can expect to increase in number if its net production of non-mutant offspring W_{ii} is greater than the average net production of offspring for the population as a whole ($\bar{E}$), even if no other species produces copies of species i by error (in which case the second term is zero).

We can simplify the notation used in eqn (2.11) by rewriting it as follows:

$$\dot{x}_m = \sum_k W_{mk}x_k - \bar{E}x_m \tag{2.12}$$

where the matrix W has the elements

$$W_{ij} = \begin{cases} W_{ii} = A_iQ_i - D_i & \text{if } i = j \\ w_{ij} & \text{if } i \neq j \end{cases} \tag{2.13}$$

These equations possess analytic solutions (Jones $et\ al.$, 1976). The result is

$$x_k(t) = c_0 \frac{\sum_l q_{kl}c_l e^{\lambda_l t}}{\sum_m \sum_l q_{ml}c_l e^{\lambda_l t}} \tag{2.14}$$

where λ_l and $\mathbf{q}_l$ are the eigenvalues and corresponding eigenvectors of W. The quantity q_{ml} is the mth component of $\mathbf{q}_l$. Alternatively, q_{ml} may be thought of as the element in row m and column l of a matrix Q with the eigenvectors of W as its columns. The c_l ($l = 1, \ldots, n$) are constants determined by the initial conditions. They are given by (Jones $et\ al.$, 1976)

$$c_i = \sum_{l=1}^n r_{il}x_l(0) \tag{2.15}$$

where r_{il} is an element from the inverse $R \equiv Q^{-1}$ of the matrix Q and $x_l(0)$ denotes the original numbers of each species.

2.3   The quasi-species

It is difficult to see the long-term behaviour of the various species directly from the solution (2.14). To get a better idea of what eqn (2.14) tells us about the ultimate population sizes x_i for large times we can use the following transformation of the population variables. Suppose we write

$$x_k = \sum_l q_{kl}b_l N_l; \qquad\qquad b_l \equiv \frac{1}{\sum_k q_{kl}} \tag{2.16}$$

where N_l is chosen (for reasons that will become apparent shortly) to satisfy the differential equation

$$\dot{N}_l = (\lambda_l - \bar{E})N_l. \tag{2.17}$$

Then

$$
\begin{aligned}
\dot{x}_k &= \sum_l q_{kl} b_l \dot{N}_l \\
&= \sum_l q_{kl} b_l (\lambda_l - \bar{E}) N_l \\
&= \sum_l \lambda_l q_{kl} b_l N_l - \bar{E} \sum_l q_{kl} b_l N_l \\
&= \sum_m W_{km} x_m - \bar{E} x_k
\end{aligned}
$$

The simplification of the first term in the last line uses the fact that λ_l is the eigenvalue of W corresponding to the eigenvector $\mathbf{q}_l$, so that $\lambda_l q_{kl} = \sum_m W_{km} q_{ml}$. The defining eqn (2.16) is then used to further simplify both terms.

The last form of this equation is identical to the original eqn (2.12) which we had for x_k, so the representation (2.16) and (2.17) is equivalent to the representation 2.12. This explains the requirement (2.17).

A further useful property of the N_ls is

$$\left(\sum_k x_k = \sum_k \sum_l q_{kl} b_l N_l = \sum_l N_l \right. \tag{2.18}$$

upon using the definition of b_l in eqn (2.16). Thus, if the total population size is a constant c_0, the sum of the variables N_l is also c_0.

It can be shown (Jones *et al.*, 1976) that

$$b_l N_l = c_0 \frac{c_l e^{\lambda_l t}}{\sum_m \sum_k q_{mk} c_k e^{\lambda_k t}} \tag{2.19}$$

From eqn (2.17), $\dot{N}_l$ is positive if $\lambda_l > \bar{E}$, and clearly the N_l corresponding to the largest eigenvalue[1] will grow the fastest. Suppose the

---

[1]It is possible for the largest eigenvalue to be repeated ($\lambda_1 = \lambda_2$, say), in which case the analysis here is not valid. Keep in mind that this model is dealing with a chemical system in which we do not know any of the rate parameters with a high precision. If a system is initially specified in such a way that the matrix W has a repeated eigenvalue, perturb the rate parameters slightly so that the eigenvalues are all different. There are those who will still worry about what happens if we should encounter a system where the two largest eigenvalues actually *were* precisely equal. In the context of this model, that is silly.

largest eigenvalue is λ_1. Then from eqn (2.19) and the definition of b_1 in eqn (2.16),

$$\lim_{t \to \infty} N_1 = c_0. \tag{2.20}$$

(To see this, multiply eqn (2.19) by $e^{-\lambda_1 t}/e^{-\lambda_1 t}$ and take the limit as $t \to \infty$.)

Now since we know that $\sum_l N_l = c_0$, N_1 must be the only non-zero value of all the N_l as $t \to \infty$. Further, since N_1 tends to a constant, $\dot{N}_1$ must tend to zero and, since $N_1 \neq 0$, we have from eqn (2.17),

$$\lim_{t \to \infty} \bar{E} = \lambda_1 \tag{2.21}$$

We can relate these conclusions to the population sizes x_i of the various species present by examining eqn (2.16) at large times:

$$\lim_{t \to \infty} x_i = \lim_{t \to \infty} b_1 N_1 q_{i1} = c_0 \frac{q_{i1}}{\sum_m q_{m1}}. \tag{2.22}$$

The prediction of the model is then that the populations of the various species will settle into fixed values. The relative numbers of each species depend entirely on the components of the eigenvector corresponding to the largest eigenvalue of the matrix W. Thus we expect that a combination of species in fixed proportions, rather than a single species, will dominate the molecular solution after the system has had a chance to settle down. This combination of species is referred to by Eigen and Schuster as a *quasi-species*, since it is a stable entity composed of more than one pure species.

Several species can coexist because of their crosslinking due to the error terms w_{ik}. If one species has a high reproductive rate but makes many errors in replication, other species that have lower birth rates will gain from these errors.

To illustrate the appearance of the solutions (2.14) we will consider two model systems, each with four species. To completely describe a system, we need values for A_i, Q_i and D_i, as well as the off-diagonal elements w_{ij}. By using the condition (2.7) we may choose a consistent set of values. We first state the values of A_i, Q_i and D_i:

Species i	A_i	Q_i	D_i
1	2.102	0.951	1.0
2	3.102	0.967	1.0
3	4.102	0.975	1.0
4	5.03	0.994	1.0

A matrix W consistent with these values is

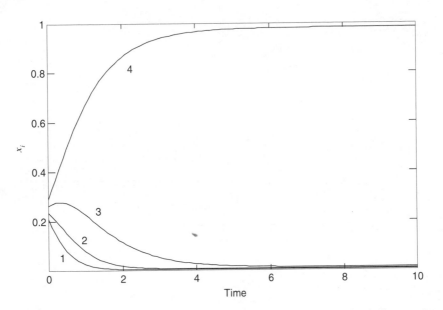

Figure 2.1   Behaviour of a system of 4 competing species when all mutation rates are low. Species 4, with the highest reproductive rate, eventually dominates the population.

$$W = \begin{bmatrix} 1 & .001 & .001 & .01 \\ .1 & 2 & .01 & .01 \\ .001 & .1 & 3 & .01 \\ .001 & .001 & .001 & 4 \end{bmatrix}. \tag{2.23}$$

Here the mutation terms w_{ij} are all small compared with the rate of correct reproduction W_{ii}. In such a case, as can be seen from Fig. 2.1, the species with the highest reproductive rate (species 4 in this case) dominates the population after transient fluctuations have died out. Species 4 does not make enough errors to support the other species with lower reproductive rates, so they cannot survive. The quasi-species here consists of just a single species.

As a second example, consider the following values:

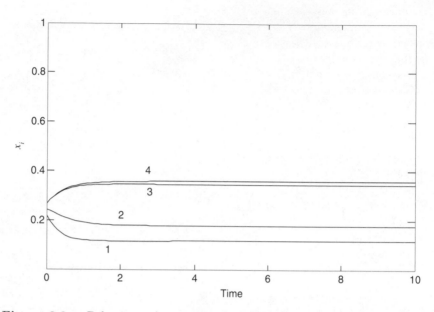

Figure 2.2   Behaviour of a system of 4 competing species when the species with the highest reproductive rate (species 4) also has high mutation rates to the other species. In this case, all four species co-exist as a quasi-species.

Species i	A_i	Q_i	D_i
1	2.102	0.951	1.0
2	3.102	0.967	1.0
3	4.102	0.975	1.0
4	8.0	0.625	1.0

$$W = \begin{bmatrix} 1 & 0.001 & 0.001 & 1 \\ 0.1 & 2 & 0.1 & 1 \\ 0.001 & 0.1 & 3 & 1 \\ 0.001 & 0.001 & 0.001 & 4 \end{bmatrix} \tag{2.24}$$

Here, species 4 still has the highest reproductive rate, but it also has very high mutation rates to the other three species. Because of this, it no longer dominates the population (Fig. 2.2). Rather, all four species coexist at large times, forming a quasi-species.

2.4 Limits on information transmission

One of the requirements of a biological system is an ability to pass on information from one generation to the next in such a way that the noise of the environment does not appreciably corrupt the message. Organisms store information in the base sequences of DNA molecules, so to store more information requires a longer molecule. The above model can be used to get a rough idea of how much information (that is, how large a molecule) can be retained intact over long periods of time. In order to do this, we must assume something about the internal structure of the molecule. Since the reader has probably had DNA in the back of their mind during this chapter, we will suppose that the molecule is composed of a number of units (for example, base pairs), each of which must be replicated correctly in order for a perfect copy to be made.

For the purposes of a crude estimate of the maximum molecular size that can be maintained over a large number of generations, suppose that one of the molecular species, say species m, in the above model is much more efficient than all the others at reproducing. That is, we have

$$W_{mm} \gg W_{kk} \qquad \text{if } k \neq m. \tag{2.25}$$

If the off-diagonal terms w_{ij} in W are also small, then the largest eigenvalue λ_m of W will be approximately

$$\lambda_m \approx W_{mm} \tag{2.26}$$

and the condition for selection derived from eqn (2.17) is roughly

$$W_{mm} > \bar{E}. \tag{2.27}$$

Using the definition of $W_{mm} \equiv A_m Q_m - D_m$ we have

$$Q_m > \frac{D_m + \bar{E}}{A_m} \equiv \frac{1}{\sigma_m} \tag{2.28}$$

where σ_m is a *superiority parameter*; a measure of how good a species is at replicating itself compared to other species in the solution. It is the ratio of the reproductive rate A_m of species m to the sum of the death rate D_m and the average productivity $\bar{E}$ of the population as a whole.

Now suppose that each unit of molecule m is replicated correctly with an average probability of $\bar{q}_m$. This probability is an average, since the probabilities of correctly replicating each unit will in general depend on the type of unit. For example, in DNA, GC pairs are replicated with considerably more accuracy than AT pairs, so that $prob\{$GC pair replicated correctly$\} \equiv q_{GC} > prob\{$ AT pair replicated correctly$\} \equiv q_{AT}$. In this case $\bar{q}_m = (q_{GC} + q_{AT})/2$. What we are concerned with here is an overall estimate of how accurately a particular molecule is replicated.

Assuming that the replication of each unit is an independent event, an entire molecule containing ν_m units will be replicated correctly with an average probability of $\bar{q}_m^{\nu_m} \equiv Q_m$. Inserting this into eqn (2.28) we obtain

$$\bar{q}_m^{\nu_m} > \frac{1}{\sigma_m} \tag{2.29}$$

or

$$\nu_m \ln \bar{q}_m > -\ln \sigma_m. \tag{2.30}$$

Since $\bar{q}_m$ is close to 1, we can approximate $\ln \bar{q}_m$ by its first degree Taylor polynomial: $\ln \bar{q}_m \approx \bar{q}_m - 1$. We therefore obtain a condition on the sequence length:

$$\nu_m < \frac{\ln \sigma_m}{1 - \bar{q}_m}. \tag{2.31}$$

This gives an estimate of the maximum sequence length that can survive over a large number of generations. As one would expect, the more efficient relative to its competitors the species is at reproducing (that is, the larger the value of σ_m), the longer the length that can be maintained, while the greater the error rate in reproduction, the shorter the length.

Since the superiority parameter enters only by way of a logarithm, it must change by a relatively large amount to affect the length of the sequence that can be maintained. The central effect comes from the error rate $\bar{q}_m$.

Experimentally, it is known that the replication of RNA without any enzymatic help is about 95 per cent accurate, so that a value of $\bar{q}_m = 0.95$ is reasonable.[2] Values of the superiority parameter are more difficult to estimate, but it is likely that the most efficient species would have a value of σ_m with an order of magnitude somewhere between 10^0 and 10^2. For values in the range $2 < \sigma_m < 200$, the corresponding sequence length lies in the range $14 < \nu_m < 106$ when $\bar{q}_m = 0.95$. It is perhaps dangerous to read too much into this result, but one cannot help noticing that most tRNA molecules are about 70 units in length. It is possible that some early version of a tRNA molecule was the first step on the road to the origin of life.

The amount of information that can be stored in a sequence of around 70 bases is, however, not great. In order to allow more complex systems to develop, we need some way of reliably increasing the amount information that can be transmitted from one generation to the next. As we have seen, this cannot be done by merely increasing the length of the molecule

---

[2]DNA in modern organisms is, of course, replicated much more accurately than this.

unless we have some way to reduce the rate of error in reproduction. This requires the introduction of proteins, with their enzymatic functions, into the picture. The theoretical picture becomes considerably hazier at this point.

2.5   Summary

We have explored a system of simple, self-replicating molecules and have discovered that, if the system is closed in the sense that any erroneous copy of one molecule is one of the other species present, a quasi-species, or stable collection of the various species, will result.

The model suffers from several drawbacks, however.

By using differential equations, we can deal only with averages of the behaviour of the system over many independent trials. This problem becomes acute when the number of any species drops to very low values (less than 10, say). In such cases, an average value may give little or no guidance to the actual behaviour in any one system. Some species may be extinct in certain systems and fairly numerous in others. Given the large number of different possible species in a collection of RNA and DNA molecules (remember every distinct sequence of bases is a different species), small numbers of many of the species are quite likely.

The molecules in the model are assumed to simply produce copies, accurate or otherwise, of themselves without any intermediary. If we believe that the original biomolecules were nucleic acid chains, they must have first produced complementary copies of themselves which in turn would produce a copy of the original molecule. Thus two steps are involved to produce an offspring, with twice the chance for errors to occur. In addition, the reproductive and death rates of the complement may be different from the original parent. See Eigen (1971) for more discussion of this point.

We will not have the space to fully explore the possibilities for solutions to these problems, but we will examine, in the next chapter, a method of determining the magnitude of the fluctuations in the average numbers of the molecules and, in Chapter 4, a fully stochastic model which deals with individual molecules reproducing by means of an intermediate complement.

3

Stochastic processes

3.1 Introduction

The model of the early stages in the origin of life presented in the last chapter is both deterministic and continuous. Neither of these properties is particularly suitable for a system, such as an evolving molecular soup, which consists of a relatively small number of molecules in random motion. A more realistic model of such a system must take account of both its discreteness and stochasticity.

To illustrate just how wrong a differential equation model can be, suppose we had a system of N molecules, each of a different species. Consider an ideal case, where $A_i = D_i$ and $Q_i = 1$, so that the birth and death rates are equal and there is no error in reproduction. In such a case, all the elements of the matrix W are zero, and the differential equation model predicts that nothing will ever change in the system. In reality, as we shall see, we should expect such a system to eventually die out due to fluctuations in the population number.

Even in a less extreme situation than that where all molecules are different, we would expect significant fluctuations in the individual species numbers that will not be predicted by a differential equation model. The progress of evolution can depend on both the nature and timing of random mutations.

Due to the complexity of such models, we will consider analytically only the case of a single molecular species in an unconstrained system. Analytic solutions for systems with constraints and/or with more than one species present are very difficult, if not impossible, to obtain. In such cases it is usually only possible to calculate such quantities as the means and variances of the numbers of each species as functions of time.

However, we will describe two methods whereby detailed computer simulations of systems with any number of species and constraints can be written. Although nothing general can be proved about such systems using computer simulations, such simulations allow us to watch the detailed behaviour of a population unfold with time. As well, if a large number of simulations is done, we can get a pretty good feel for the overall behaviour.

3.2 The Markov process

The sort of system we will consider is a very general one, which has applications in many fields other than theoretical biology. Consider a system which can occupy one of a number of states at any given time, and which, with a certain probability, makes transitions from one state to another as time progresses. For example, in a molecular solution, each state may correspond to a particular number of molecules being present. A transition from one state to another occurs when, for example, a molecule reproduces, thus changing the number of molecules present.

The set S of possible states may be finite or infinite, depending on the application. S consists of discrete elements S_i for $i = 0, 1, 2, \ldots$. Each element S_i is a possible state for the system at any time t. The probability $p_{ij}(t)$ of the system making a transition from state i to state j in a time interval t is a conditional probability defined as

$$p_{ij}(t) = Prob\{X_{t_0+t} = S_j | X_{t_0} = S_i\} \qquad (3.1)$$

where X_{t_0} is the state of the system at time t_0. The notation on the right-hand side of this definition is read as 'probability that the system is in state j at time $t_0 + t$ given that it was in state i at time t_0'.

We shall assume that our system is a *stationary Markov chain*, which means that p_{ij} is independent of t_0 in the above definition. The probability of the system making a particular transition depends only on the elapsed time interval, not on the absolute time. Another way of putting this is that the behaviour of the system between the times t_0 and $t_0 + t$ is independent of the history of the system before t_0. The details of the route taken for the system to arrive at the state S_i at time t_0 have no bearing on the events that occur after that time. For this reason, a Markov chain is said to be 'memoryless'.

We shall further require the transition probabilities to satisfy the following four conditions:

1.

$$0 \le p_{ij}(t) \le 1 \qquad (3.2)$$

for all i, j, and t. This is a standard condition imposed on any probability. Negative probabilities have no meaning. A probability of unity indicates the transition occurs with certainty.

2.

$$\sum_j p_{ij}(t) = 1 \qquad (3.3)$$

for all i and t. This is a completeness constraint which ensures that the system is always in one of the states defined in the set S.

3.

$$\sum_j p_{ij}(s)p_{jk}(t) = p_{ik}(s+t) \tag{3.4}$$

for all i, k, s and t. This condition is sometimes referred to as the Chapman–Kolmogorov relation. It states that the probability of going from state i to state j in time $s + t$ is the sum of the probabilities over all the different routes by which this transition can be achieved. This relation relies on the assumption that all the states S_i are mutually exclusive, so that if the system is in state i it cannot be simultaneously in state j if $j \neq i$.

4.

$$\lim_{t \to 0} p_{ij}(t) = \delta_{ij} \tag{3.5}$$

where δ_{ij} is the Kronecker delta symbol:

$$\delta_{ij} = \left\{ \begin{array}{ll} 1 & \text{if } i = j \\ 0 & \text{if } i \neq j \end{array} \right. \tag{3.6}$$

This condition simply states that the system cannot change state in zero time.

3.3   Poisson processes

We now turn our attention to how the idea of a Markov chain can be applied to a system such as an evolving collection of early biomolecules. As mentioned in the introduction, due to the complexity of systems with more than one species, we will consider only the analytic treatment of a single-species model in an unconstrained system.

Suppose we represent the average population level x of one of the molecular species by the simple rate equation

$$\dot{x} = (F - R)x \tag{3.7}$$

where F is the formation rate of x and R is the decay rate of x. Both F and R include contributions from all possible sources: F takes account of self-replication, mutation, and flow into the system, while R contains the effects of molecular decomposition and flux out of the system.

The deterministic solution to this equation is the exponential

$$x(t) = x_0 e^{(F-R)t} \tag{3.8}$$

where x_0 is the population level at time $t = 0$.

In order to reinterpret this equation as a stochastic process, we must consider x to be a discrete variable rather than a continuous one. Thus x

becomes the actual number of molecules present in the system at time t, rather than some average population level as in the continuous case. We can legitimately ask for two kinds of output from a stochastic model. We can require a prediction of the *probability* that the population will be a certain size at time t, or we can ask for a plot of the population size as a function of time for one particular system. This is a bit like making a prediction about the outcome of an experiment where someone tosses a coin repeatedly. We can ask for the probability, after 10 minutes say, that 57 heads and 43 tails have come up, or we can ask for a detailed plot of the numbers of heads and tails as functions of time. The prediction of the probability is something we can get from an analytic solution of a stochastic model, while to get a detailed list of results of the various tosses, we need to actually do the experiment.

In order to establish a connection with the concept of a Markov process, we must make some assumptions about how the population number can change from one instant to the next. The simplest such assumption is that all molecules in our system are independent, in the sense that the times at which each molecule gives birth or dies is independent of what all the other molecules are doing. If we also assume that births and deaths occur at random times, but with a constant average rate, we can model the birth and death events as *Poisson processes*.

In a Poisson process, independent events occur randomly in time with a constant rate. The assumption of independence is important: a system where events occur regularly at fixed time intervals, like the ticking of a clock, is not a Poisson process because the events are not independent. In such a clock-like system we can predict the time when the next event will occur if we know when the last event occurred.

A common example of a system that is approximately a Poisson process is that of cars crossing a bridge. For limited times during the day, the average number of cars per minute is roughly constant, and, if the bridge is far enough away from any ordering influence on the cars' distribution (like a traffic light), the times between successive cars leaving the bridge are more or less random. It would not be reasonable to use a single Poisson process to describe the traffic flow at all times of day, since we would expect the average number of cars to increase during morning aı evening rush hours and decrease in the early hours of the morning.

A single Poisson process deals with a single type of event, where that event occurs randomly and at a constant rate. We wish to use a Poisson process model to describe the evolution of a system of molecules which can both reproduce and die. Since we have two different types of events, we cannot use a single Poisson process to model the whole system. However, we shall assume that the birth and death processes are Poisson processes in their own right, each with their own constant rates. Such a process is known as a *linear birth–death process*.

To get some idea of how to analyse the birth-death process, we will start off by considering the birth process on its own. We suppose that each molecule can have only one offspring at a time. Let $b_i(t)$ be the probability that a single molecule has i births in time interval t. We will assume the transition probabilities can be expanded in Taylor series as follows:

$$
\begin{aligned}
b_0(\Delta t) &= 1 - F\Delta t + \mathcal{O}(\Delta t^2) & (3.9) \\
b_1(\Delta t) &= F\Delta t + \mathcal{O}(\Delta t^2) & (3.10) \\
b_j(\Delta t) &= \mathcal{O}(\Delta t^2); \qquad j > 1. & (3.11)
\end{aligned}
$$

Here Δt is a time interval that is small compared to $1/F$, where F is the constant average birth rate. The symbol $\mathcal{O}(\Delta t^2)$ means 'terms of order Δt^2 and higher', which, for small enough time intervals, should be negligible.

These three relations state that the probability of a single birth in time Δt is proportional to Δt, and that the probability of more than a single birth to one molecule in the time Δt is negligibly small. This proportionality of probability to time interval can only be true when the time interval is very small since probabilities must always lie between 0 and 1, and, for long enough time intervals, b_0 would eventually become negative and b_1 greater than one.

We can extend these results to a population of $N(t)$ identical, independent molecules at time t. Let $B_i(\Delta t)$ be the probability that there are i births in the entire population in time interval Δt. Extending our notation for probabilities of births to single molecules to $b_i^{(j)}(\Delta t)$, which stands for the probability that molecule j has i offspring in time interval Δt, we can use the assumption that all molecules are independent to obtain

$$
\begin{aligned}
B_0(\Delta t) &= \prod_{j=1}^{N(t)} b_0^{(j)} & (3.12) \\
&= \prod_{j=1}^{N(t)} [1 - F\Delta t + \mathcal{O}(\Delta t^2)] & (3.13) \\
&= 1 - N(t)F\Delta t + \mathcal{O}(\Delta t^2) & (3.14)
\end{aligned}
$$

and

$$
B_1(\Delta t) = \sum_{j=1}^{N(t)} b_1^{(j)} \prod_{k \neq j} b_0^{(k)} \qquad (3.15)
$$

$$= \sum_{j=1}^{N(t)} F\Delta t[1 - (N(t) - 1)F\Delta t] + \mathcal{O}(\Delta t^2) \qquad (3.16)$$

$$= FN(t)\Delta t + \mathcal{O}(\Delta t^2) \qquad (3.17)$$

All values of B_j for $j > 1$ are $\mathcal{O}(\Delta t^2)$. (The time t used in $N(t)$ is the time at the beginning of the time interval Δt.) Thus we see that births occur singly in the entire population as well.

The death process can be handled in exactly the same way. Defining $d_i(t)$ to be the probability of i deaths in time t we have

$$d_0(\Delta t) = 1 - R\Delta t + \mathcal{O}(\Delta t^2) \qquad (3.18)$$
$$d_1(\Delta t) = R\Delta t + \mathcal{O}(\Delta t^2) \qquad (3.19)$$

where R is the constant average death rate per molecule. Since a molecule can only die once, no equation is included for d_j when $j > 1$.

The death probabilities for the entire population can be worked out in the same way as the birth rates. We define $D_i(\Delta t)$ to be the probability of i deaths in the entire population in time interval Δt, and $d_i^{(j)}(\Delta t)$ to be the probability that molecule j will die (if $i = 1$) or not (if $i = 0$) in time interval Δt. Then we have

$$D_0(\Delta t) = \prod_{j=1}^{N(t)} d_0^{(j)} \qquad (3.20)$$

$$= \prod_{j=1}^{N(t)} [1 - R\Delta t + \mathcal{O}(\Delta t^2)] \qquad (3.21)$$

$$= 1 - N(t)R\Delta t + \mathcal{O}(\Delta t^2) \qquad (3.22)$$

and

$$D_1(\Delta t) = \sum_{j=1}^{N(t)} d_1^{(j)} \prod_{k \neq j} d_0^{(k)} \qquad (3.23)$$

$$= \sum_{j=1}^{N(t)} R\Delta t[1 - (N(t) - 1)R\Delta t] + \mathcal{O}(\Delta t^2) \qquad (3.24)$$

$$= RN(t)\Delta t + \mathcal{O}(\Delta t^2). \qquad (3.25)$$

Again, the probability of more than a single death in time interval Δt is $\mathcal{O}(\Delta t^2)$.

To combine birth and death in the same model, we must consider all possibilities for changes in the population number in a short time Δt. We

ΔN	Probability
0	$1 - N(t)(F + R)\Delta t + \mathcal{O}(\Delta t^2)$
+1	$N(t)F\Delta t + \mathcal{O}(\Delta t^2)$
−1	$N(t)R\Delta t + \mathcal{O}(\Delta t^2)$
other	$\mathcal{O}(\Delta t^2)$

Table 3.1   Probabilities of various changes in population number in a linear birth–death process.

define $\Delta N \equiv N(t+\Delta t) - N(t)$. To work out the probability of $\Delta N = 0$, for example, we list all the ways that there is no net change in the population level. We must have n births and n deaths, where $n \geq 0$. The probability for the case $n = 0$ is $B_0 D_0 = 1 - N(t)(F + R)\Delta t + \mathcal{O}(\Delta t^2)$, while for all $n > 0$ the probability is $\mathcal{O}(\Delta t^2)$. In a similar way, it can be seen that the only values of ΔN with probabilities containing first order terms in Δt are $\Delta N = 0, 1, -1$. A few simple calculations result in Table 3.1.

The probabilities in Table 3.1 are transition probabilities for the change in the state of the system over a small time interval Δt, that is, we may write them as $p_{ij}(\Delta t)$, where i is the state before the transition and j the state afterwards. In this simple model, the only thing distinguishing one state from another is the population size, so it is easiest to just label each state with its population number N. Thus the first entry in Table 3.1 is the transition probability from state N to state N, or $p_{NN}(\Delta t)$, the second line gives $p_{N,N+1}(\Delta t)$, and so on.

We can now attempt to determine values of the $p_{ij}(t)$ for all times and all population sizes i, j by constructing and solving differential equations for them.

First, we define the rates of change of the transition probabilities. Using the fact that $p_{ii}(0) = 1$, we have

$$q_{ii} \equiv \lim_{t \to 0} \frac{p_{ii}(t) - 1}{t} = \left. \frac{dp_{ii}}{dt} \right|_{t=0} \tag{3.26}$$

and for $i \neq j$, since $p_{ij}(0) = 0$ from eqn (3.5).

$$q_{ij} \equiv \lim_{t \to 0} \frac{p_{ij}(t)}{t} = \left. \frac{dp_{ij}}{dt} \right|_{t=0}. \tag{3.27}$$

For general t we have

$$\dot{p}_{ik}(t) = \lim_{s \to 0} \frac{p_{ik}(s+t) - p_{ik}(t)}{s} \tag{3.28}$$

$$= \lim_{s \to 0} \left[\sum_j p_{ij}(t) \frac{p_{jk}(s)}{s} - \sum_j p_{ij}(t) \frac{p_{jk}(0)}{s} \right] \qquad (3.29)$$

$$= \lim_{s \to 0} \left[\frac{p_{kk}(s) - 1}{s} p_{ik}(t) + \sum_{j \neq k} \frac{p_{jk}(s)}{s} p_{ij}(t) \right]. \qquad (3.30)$$

The second step uses the Chapman–Kolmogorov relation (eqn (3.4)) and the last line uses eqn (3.5). Taking the limit we obtain the differential equation for p_{ik}:

$$\dot{p}_{ik}(t) = q_{kk}p_{ik}(t) + \sum_{j \neq k} q_{jk}p_{ij}(t). \qquad (3.31)$$

We can use the expressions for the probabilities in Table 3.1 above to derive values for the q_{ij}. From the table we have

$$
\begin{align}
p_{ii}(\Delta t) &= 1 - i(F + R)\Delta t + \mathcal{O}(\Delta t^2) & (3.32) \\
p_{i-1,i}(\Delta t) &= (i - 1)F\Delta t + \mathcal{O}(\Delta t^2) & (3.33) \\
p_{i+1,i}(\Delta t) &= (i + 1)R\Delta t + \mathcal{O}(\Delta t^2). & (3.34)
\end{align}
$$

Using the definitions of the q_{ij} we have

$$
\begin{align}
q_{ii} &= \lim_{\Delta t \to 0} \frac{p_{ii}(\Delta t) - 1}{\Delta t} & (3.35) \\
&= -i(F + R) & (3.36) \\
q_{i-1,i} &= (i - 1)F & (3.37) \\
q_{i+1,i} &= (i + 1)R & (3.38)
\end{align}
$$

with $q_{ji} = 0$ if $|j - i| > 1$.

Substituting these values for q_{ji} into the differential equation (3.31) for the transition probabilities we obtain

$$\dot{p}_{ik} = -k(R + F)p_{ik} + (k - 1)Fp_{i,k-1} + (k + 1)Rp_{i,k+1} \qquad (3.39)$$

with the initial condition

$$p_{ik}(0) = \delta_{ik}. \qquad (3.40)$$

At first glance this may appear to be just a system of linear differential equations with constant coefficients, so that the usual techniques involving matrix algebra may be used to find a solution. The snag is that this is an infinite system of differential equations, so the matrix techniques, which are designed for finite systems, do not work here.

If we continue to assume that the rates of birth and death, F and R, are constant, there is a technique, using special functions called *generating functions* which can be used to solve this system of equations analytically.[1] The result is the hideous expression

$$
p_{ik}(t) \;=\; \sum_{r=0}^{\min(i,k)} (-1)^r \binom{i}{r} \binom{i+k-r-1}{k-r} F^{k-r} R^{i-r}
$$
$$
\times (e^{(F-R)t} - 1)^{i+k-2r} (Fe^{(F-R)t} - R)^{r-i-k}
$$
$$
\times (Re^{(F-R)t} - F)^r. \tag{3.41}
$$

In this formula, the quantity $\binom{i}{r}$ is a binomial coefficient: $\binom{i}{r} \equiv i!/r!(i-r)!$.

Now let us examine what this stochastic model predicts for the fate of a population of molecules. We can first calculate the mean population size at time t given that it is i at $t = 0$. The definition of this mean $\bar{k}$ is

$$
\bar{k}(t) \equiv \sum_{k=0}^{\infty} k p_{ik}(t). \tag{3.42}
$$

The sum may also be evaluated using generating functions, giving the result

$$
\bar{k}(t) = i e^{(F-R)t} \tag{3.43}
$$

which is just the deterministic solution, predicting exponential growth or decay depending on whether the birth rate is greater or less than the death rate.

The variance is

$$
\text{var } k(t) = i \frac{F+R}{F-R} e^{(F-R)t} [e^{(F-R)t} - 1]. \tag{3.44}
$$

The variance increases with time if $F > R$, becoming infinite at infinite time, and decreases to zero if $F < R$. Thus the stochastic model predicts that, if the birth rate is less than the death rate, the population will eventually die out with certainty. However if $F > R$, the behaviour of the population is predicted with much less precision. The average population size increases without limit, but this average is obtained by observing a large number of different populations and calculating the mean behaviour.

---

[1] The solution requires sophisticated methods, such as the aforementioned generating functions and solutions of partial differential equations, which are beyond the scope of this book. Readers who wish to pursue this topic should consult a textbook on stochastic processes, such as Cox and Miller (1977) or Karlin and Taylor (1980).

Since the variance of the population size also increases without limit, the actual behaviour of any one specific population is uncertain.

Before we investigate the behaviour of a particular population, we will state the results obtained when the birth and death rates are equal. The result for the transition probabilities is

$$p_{ik}(t) = \sum_{r=0}^{\min(i,k)} (-1)^r \binom{i}{r} \binom{i+k-r-1}{k-r} (Ft)^{i+k-2r} \quad (3.45)$$
$$\times (Ft-1)^r (Ft+1)^{r-i-k}.$$

The mean and variance in this case are

$$\bar{k}(t) = i; \qquad\qquad \mathrm{var}\, k(t) = 2iFt. \qquad\qquad (3.46)$$

The mean value again agrees with the deterministic case, as it predicts a constant population size equal to that at $t = 0$. However, the variance again increases without limit, so that the behaviour of any particular population is not known with any degree of certainty.

Now let us examine what can happen to a particular population. We will consider the case of equal birth and death rates so that $F = R$. The case $F \neq R$ is handled similarly.

First, let us consider the probability of extinction at time t. This is given by the transition probability $p_{i0}(t)$:

$$p_{i0}(t) = \left[\frac{Ft}{Ft+1} \right]^i. \qquad\qquad (3.47)$$

For large values of t this probability tends towards 1, indicating that extinction is ultimately certain even though the birth and death rates are equal.

This result may seem paradoxical, since we showed above that, in the case where $F = R$, the mean size stayed constant. However, the increasing variance for large times means that, very rarely, a population will grow very large and take a very long time to die out, thus maintaining the constant mean. The mean value is a weighted sum of terms of the form $k(t)p_{ik}(t)$. In the limit of very large values of population size k, the probability p_{ik} still tends to zero, but in such a way that the mean itself remains constant. This formula for the mean indicates the folly of trying to use intuition to deduce the behaviour of a system built on infinite series.

Now consider the probability that a species will undergo a k-fold increase in size in time t. The easiest way to calculate this is to start with a population of size 1, then find the probability of a transition from 1 to k molecules in time t. We have therefore,

$$p_{1k}(t) = \frac{(Ft)^{k-1}}{(1+Ft)^{k+1}} \qquad\qquad \text{if } k \geq 1. \qquad (3.48)$$

The maximum value of $p_{1k}(t)$, found by differentiating with respect to t and setting the result equal to zero, occurs when $t = t_m$, given by

$$Ft_m = \frac{k-1}{2}. \qquad\qquad (3.49)$$

The values of $p_{1k}(t_m)$ decrease monotonically with increasing k, with the highest probability (apart from that for $k = 1$) being $p_{1k}(t_m) = 0.15$, obtained when $k = 2$ and $Ft_m = 0.5$. Thus the chance of a population doubling its size is only 0.15 at best if $F = R$, and this occurs only at one time. For all times after this, the size will decrease on average.

The above analysis can give only a rough guide to the behaviour of a real stochastic system, since we have considered only a single species and have removed the constraint of constant population size, so that no selection is operating. This sort of model is certainly better than the differential equation version in the previous chapter because it gives us some idea of the degree of variability we can expect, but it still doesn't give us a feel for what a real evolving molecular system would look like.

A few attempts have been made to construct a birth–death process for a multi-species system incorporating the constraint of constant size. For example, Jones and Leung (1981) show that such a multi-species system with the constant size constraint is unstable in the sense that, although the mean population number remains constant, fluctuations in the population numbers grow with time so that there is a high probability of the system dying out, just as with the single-species model treated above. Not surprisingly, the stochastic equations for a multi-species system cannot be solved analytically (even with the aid of generating functions), and Jones and Leung's arguments are based on calculations of the various moments (means and variances) of the population numbers.

Rather than explore analytic models any further, we will turn now to computer simulations of stochastic processes. Such computer techniques have the disadvantage that they cannot be used to make general statements about the system. For example, we cannot say for certain what the precise mean and variance of the population number are, since such quantities are obtained only after an infinite number of runs have been made. However, if we do a fair number of computer runs, with different random number sequences on each run, we can get a representative sample of the sorts of behaviour we can expect. The computer simulation has the great advantage that we can actually see what a population looks like as a function of time, something even an analytic solution of the stochastic differential equations cannot give us. Such simulations can take a great deal of computer time, but the advent of the microcomputer means that cheap computer power is now available (or at least it should be) to anyone interested in exploring these questions.

3.4 Simple simulation of a stochastic process

To get the feel for the first method, we will consider initially a simulation procedure for the evolution of a single species. Refer back to the Taylor series approximation (3.11) for the probabilities of various numbers of births to a single molecule:

$$
\begin{align}
b_0(\Delta t) &= 1 - F\Delta t + \mathcal{O}(\Delta t^2) & (3.50) \\
b_1(\Delta t) &= F\Delta t + \mathcal{O}(\Delta t^2) & (3.51) \\
b_j(\Delta t) &= \mathcal{O}(\Delta t^2); \qquad j > 1. & (3.52)
\end{align}
$$

As was explained there, we may interpret $F\Delta t$ as the probability of a single birth in time Δt, provided we choose $\Delta t \ll 1/F$. We may construct a simulation algorithm as follows.

1. Set up the initial conditions by defining the number of molecules with which we start.

2. To determine the number of molecules present after an interval Δt, we check each molecule present at the beginning of the time interval to see if it (i) reproduces (with probability $F\Delta t$) or (ii) dies (with probability $R\Delta t$). We can do this check by having the computer 'roll dice'. Most programming languages contain a pseudo-random number generator which will provide a sequence of real numbers uniformly distributed on the interval [0,1) (including zero and excluding 1). To check whether a particular molecule reproduces, we generate a random number and compare it with the current value of $F\Delta t$ ('current' since we are allowing the possibility that F is a function of time). There is a probability of precisely $F\Delta t$ that the random number will be smaller than $F\Delta t$. If this happens we say that the molecule has reproduced, and increase the population size by 1. Similarly, we check each molecule to see if it dies by comparing a random number with the quantity $R\Delta t$.

3. We repeat the preceding step as many time steps as we wish, recording the population level at each step so that we may plot a graph of $N(t)$ vs time.

This technique is fairly easy to extend to the case where we have two or more interacting species. For example, consider the quasi-species system described by eqn (2.2) of Chapter 2. Let us consider a two-species example of this model, with the following parameters:

$$
\begin{array}{c|ccc}
i & A_i & Q_i & D_i \\
\hline
1 & 5 & 0.8 & 2 \\
2 & 6 & 0.5 & 1
\end{array}
\qquad
W = \left[\begin{array}{cc} w_{11} & 3 \\ 1 & w_{22} \end{array} \right]
\qquad (3.53)
$$

where $w_{ii} = A_i Q_i - D_i$.

Consider first species 1. Its reproduction rate is A_1 and its death rate is D_1. These correspond to F and R in the algorithm above. Thus we may determine whether or not a particular species 1 molecule reproduces using random numbers as before. However, we are now allowing for the possibility that, should a birth take place, the offspring may be a mutant and thus be a species 2 molecule. This will happen with probability $1 - Q_1$, so we generate another random number to see if this happens. If so, we increase the species 2 population by one, rather than the species 1 population. We check the behaviour of all species 2 molecules in the same way, allowing for the possibility that, should one reproduce, it may erroneously produce a species 1 molecule.

In this example, we do not actually need the values of w_{ij} as we can get all the information about the probabilities of the various types of births (whether they are mutants or not) from A_i and Q_i. If we have more than two species, however, we need the extra information in the w_{ij} coefficients.

For a given species i, the total rate of mutant births must be $A_i(1 - Q_i)$. This in turn must be equal to the total rate of production of erroneous copies, which is $\sum_{j \neq i} w_{ji}$. Therefore if a molecule of species i is found to give birth to a mutant, we know that the probability of this mutant being of species k is proportional to w_{ki} and, since the probabilities must sum to unity, must be equal to $w_{ki} / \sum_{j \neq i} w_{ji}$. We can therefore determine the identity of the mutant by generating a random number r and finding the value of k for which

$$
\frac{\sum_{m=1(\neq i)}^{k-1} w_{mi}}{\sum_{j \neq i} w_{ji}} < r < \frac{\sum_{m=1(\neq i)}^{k} w_{mi}}{\sum_{j \neq i} w_{ji}}. \qquad (3.54)
$$

In this expression the numerator of the term on the left is taken to be zero if $k = 1$. All sums exclude the term w_{ii}.

The procedure is equivalent to dividing the unit interval into segments of lengths $w_{ki} / \sum_{j \neq i} w_{ji}$ and labelling each segment with the corresponding value of k. A random number r is generated, and we observe in which segment r lies: that tells us which mutation occurs.

This procedure is straightforward, but rather inefficient, since if Δt is chosen to be very small, as it must be, there is a good chance that nothing will happen in most time intervals, and the program will spend most of its time generating random numbers that indicate that no births or deaths are occurring. In the next section, we examine a method that eliminates these problems.

3.5 Efficient simulation of a stochastic process

We would like a method in which every random number we generated told us something about an event which actually happened. The method we will develop here (due originally to Gillespie (1976, 1977)) generates only two random numbers for each event: one to determine the time of the next event and the other to determine the nature of the event. For our molecular soup, an 'event' can be a correct birth, a mutant birth, or a death.

To streamline the notation a bit, we will redefine some of the quantities used above. First, we will call every event a *reaction* in the chemical sense (since that's really what it is anyway). We suppose that there are M different reactions possible for a given set of N species of molecules. In the example in the previous section with two species ($N = 2$) there are 6 possible reactions, 3 for each species: each species can produce a correct copy of itself, a copy of the other species or die.

We define a set of rate constants k_i, $i = 1, \ldots, M$, so that there is one rate constant for each reaction. This rate constant can be interpreted on the molecular level as the probability per unit time (for very small times, as before) that one particular combination of molecules is realized so that a single reaction of a particular type occurs. Thus the probability that a reaction of type i occurs in time dt is (number of ways the particular combination of molecules can occur)$\times k_i$. All of the reactions we are considering here require only a single molecule to be present,[2] so the 'number of ways the particular combination of molecules can occur' is just the number of molecules x_j of the required species j. In other words, if a single molecule of species j is required for reaction i to take place, the probability that such a reaction will take place in a time dt is $k_i x_j dt$. This is just another way of stating the results for the transition probabilities derived in Table 3.1.

We will now derive an expression for $P(\tau, \mu)d\tau$, which is defined as the probability that the next reaction will be of type μ and will occur in time

---

[2]The birth process, of course, requires all the components of the daughter molecule to be present as well as the parent molecule, but we are assuming that these components are in plentiful supply so we may describe the process by means of the single parent molecule and the rate at which it makes use of the raw materials to create a daughter molecule.

interval $(t + \tau, t + \tau + d\tau)$, given that the population numbers at time t are $x_i(t)$, $i = 1, \ldots, N$. This probability can be expressed as follows:

$$
\begin{aligned}
P(\tau, \mu)d\tau &= prob(\text{nothing happens in interval } (t, t + \tau)) \quad &(3.55) \\
&\quad \times prob(\text{reaction } \mu \text{ occurs in interval } d\tau) \\
&\equiv P_0(\tau)P_\mu(d\tau) \quad &(3.56)
\end{aligned}
$$

The second factor, as we have already derived, is just

$$
P_\mu(d\tau) = x_j k_\mu d\tau \equiv a_\mu d\tau \tag{3.57}
$$

where a_μ is defined by this equation. Thus the probability that *any* of the M reactions occurs in that interval is

$$
\sum_{\mu=1}^{M} a_\mu d\tau \equiv a_0 d\tau \tag{3.58}
$$

where a_0 is defined by this equation. The probability that *no* reactions occur in the interval $d\tau$ is therefore $1 - a_0 d\tau$. Therefore

$$
P_0(\tau + d\tau) = P_0(\tau) \times (1 - a_0 d\tau) \tag{3.59}
$$

which can be rearranged to the differential equation

$$
\frac{dP_0}{d\tau} = -a_0 P_0 \tag{3.60}
$$

with solution[3]

$$
P_0(\tau) = e^{-a_0 \tau} \tag{3.61}
$$

which satisfies the initial condition $P_0(0) = 1$ (the probability of nothing happening in zero time is 1).

Finally, therefore, we have

$$
P(\tau, \mu)d\tau = a_\mu e^{-a_0 \tau} d\tau. \tag{3.62}
$$

From this, we have that the probability that the next reaction of any type will occur in the interval $(t + \tau, t + \tau + d\tau)$ is

---

[3]The reader may question this solution on the grounds that a_0 does not appear to be a constant, since it depends on the population variables $x_j(t)$ through equation 3.57. However, we are trying to find the probability that no reactions occur over a certain time interval. If no reaction occurs, the population sizes will remain constant, and a_0 is, in fact, constant for any time interval between reactions, although its value will change as soon as a reaction occurs.

$$P_1(\tau)d\tau \equiv \sum_\mu P(\tau, \mu)d\tau = a_0 e^{-a_0\tau} d\tau \qquad (3.63)$$

and the probability that, given that a reaction occurs in that interval, the reaction is of type μ is

$$P_2(\mu|\tau) = \frac{a_\mu d\tau}{a_0 d\tau} = \frac{a_\mu}{a_0}. \qquad (3.64)$$

Now in order to be able to use all of this in a stochastic simulation, we have to have some way of relating the random numbers generated by the computer to these probability distributions. Since random numbers are usually generated uniformly over the unit interval $[0, 1)$, we must relate the uniform, unit distribution to a general probability distribution.

Consider first the problem of how to generate randomly the time to the next reaction. The probability distribution function (pdf) for this time was given above, and is $P_1(x) = a_0 e^{-a_0 x}$. Consider the cumulative distribution function (cdf) $F(x)$, defined as

$$F(x) \equiv \int_{-\infty}^{x} P_1(y)dy. \qquad (3.65)$$

$F(x)$ gives the probability that a number chosen at random from the distribution given by P_1 will be less than x, and therefore must be a non-decreasing function, increasing from 0 to 1 as x increases from $-\infty$ to $+\infty$. For our particular P_1, we have

$$F(x) = a_0 \int_0^x e^{-a_0\tau} d\tau = 1 - e^{-a_0 x}. \qquad (3.66)$$

The lower limit in the integral is 0 since τ is a time *interval* and thus cannot be negative.

Now suppose we have chosen a random number r_1 from the unit interval. Then, for given numbers α, β satisfying $0 \le \alpha \le \beta \le 1$, we have $prob(\alpha \le r_1 \le \beta) = \beta - \alpha$. Since $0 \le F(x) \le F(x + dx) \le 1$ (remember $F(x)$ is non-decreasing), if we replace α and β by $F(x)$ and $F(x+dx)$ respectively, we obtain

$$prob(F(x) \le r_1 \le F(x + dx)) = F(x + dx) - F(x) = \frac{dF}{dx}dx = P_1(x)dx. \qquad (3.67)$$

In other words, if we choose a value x such that $F(x) = r_1$, the pdf of x will be P_1, which is what we want. Now because $F(x)$ in eqn (3.66) is monotonically increasing, the inverse function F^{-1} exists, and the random value of x can thus be obtained as $x = F^{-1}(r_1)$. In this case, we have

$$x = F^{-1}(r_1) = \frac{1}{a_0} \ln \left(\frac{1}{1-r_1} \right). \qquad (3.68)$$

Since r_1 is uniform on the unit interval, so is $1 - r_1$, so we can replace $1 - r_1$ by r_1 to obtain a random value for the time τ to the next reaction:

$$\tau = \frac{1}{a_0} \ln \left(\frac{1}{r_1} \right) = -\frac{1}{a_0} \ln r_1. \qquad (3.69)$$

To determine the nature of the reaction, we can apply similar reasoning to the discrete distribution function for the various reactions (exercise for the reader!). The result is that, if we choose a random number r_2 from the uniform unit interval, then the type of reaction that occurs at time τ corresponds to that value of μ satisfying the inequality

$$\sum_{j=1}^{\mu-1} (a_j/a_0) \leq r_2 \leq \sum_{j=1}^{\mu} (a_j/a_0). \qquad (3.70)$$

Going back to our 2-species example that we used in the last section, the 6 reactions are

$$X_1 \;\rightarrow\; 2X_1 \qquad\qquad (3.71)$$
$$X_1 \;\rightarrow\; X_1 + X_2 \qquad\qquad (3.72)$$
$$X_1 \;\rightarrow\; 0 \qquad\qquad (3.73)$$
$$X_2 \;\rightarrow\; 2X_2 \qquad\qquad (3.74)$$
$$X_2 \;\rightarrow\; X_1 + X_2 \qquad\qquad (3.75)$$
$$X_2 \;\rightarrow\; 0 \qquad\qquad (3.76)$$

The first 3 reactions correspond to, in the order given, species 1 produces a correct copy of itself, a mutant copy of species 2, and dies. The last 3 are the same for species 2. The rate constants (k_i) for the reactions are $A_1 Q_1$, $A_1(1 - Q_1)$, D_1, $A_2 Q_2$, $A_2(1 - Q_2)$, D_2 respectively.

Thus the algorithm proceeds as follows.

1. Define initial numbers of X_1 and X_2.

2. Determine time when next reaction occurs and increment time variable accordingly.

3. Determine nature of next reaction and adjust population numbers according to the reaction equation.

4. Repeat steps 2 and 3 until desired time is reached.

The above procedure will simulate an evolving molecular system without the flow term which was introduced in the previous chapter to allow the constraint of constant population size. The flow term can be included in the stochastic algorithm if we treat a flow event as just another reaction. However, the flow rate parameter is not quite as straightforward as those we have used in the algorithm so far.

A flow 'reaction' will be one of the form

$$X_i \to 0 \tag{3.77}$$

in the case where a molecule of type i flows out of the system, or

$$0 \to X_i \tag{3.78}$$

where one flows in. To determine the probability of a flow event occurring, we need the flow rate. This rate is a quantity analogous to A_i, the rate of reproduction, or D_i, the death rate. Unlike these quantities, though, the flow rate depends on the current population numbers, since the whole purpose of the flow is to keep the total number constant.

To see the form of the term we must use for the flow rate, let us backtrack a little and consider a reaction of the form

$$X_1 + X_2 \to X_3. \tag{3.79}$$

Suppose the reaction has a known constant rate of K. Now in this case, the number of distinct ways the reaction can occur, if there are x_i molecules of type i ($i = 1, 2$) present, is the number of ways of choosing one type 1 molecule and one type 2 molecule, which is $x_1 x_2$. The a_μ term for this reaction would therefore be $K x_1 x_2$. Using arguments from chemical kinetics, it can be shown that this is exactly the same term as would be present in a differential equation for x_3 to account for the production of species 3 through reaction (3.79):

$$\dot{x}_3 = \ldots + K x_1 x_2 + \ldots \tag{3.80}$$

where the omitted terms are those describing other ways of producing X_3. In other words, the a_μ term for a particular reaction is the same as the term that would appear in a differential equation describing the products of that reaction. This is known in physical chemistry as *the law of mass action*.

We can reverse the argument in the previous paragraph to obtain an a_μ term from the differential equation. The flow term for species i is

$$\phi_i = \frac{\phi_t x_i}{\sum_k x_k} \tag{3.81}$$

where the total flow is

$$\phi_t = \sum_i (D_i - A_i)x_i. \qquad (3.82)$$

Thus the a_μ term for the flow of a molecule of type i is just ϕ_i. The sign of ϕ_i indicates whether a molecule flows into (positive sign) or out of (negative sign) the system. Since a_μ is used in calculating probabilities, it must always be positive. We therefore take

$$a_\mu = |\phi_i| \qquad (3.83)$$

since $|\phi_i(t)|$ is the rate at which flow events (either in or out) are occurring at time t. Should the algorithm indicate that a flow event occurs at some point, we must check the sign of ϕ_i to see whether a molecule should be added or subtracted.

The rationale for handling flow events this way is that for each flow term, there is an equivalent chemical reaction which will have the same effects on the population numbers. Since the flow term for species i has the form $\phi_t x_i / c_0$, this reaction can be viewed as a birth (death) process if the sign of ϕ_t is positive (negative). The difference between this process and the birth (death) process governed by the parameter A_i (D_i), is that the birth and death rates are time-dependent in the flow case.

Adding in flow terms in the stochastic simulation will not, of course, result in the total number being held precisely constant as in the differential equation model. In fact, it is unlikely that the number will remain even approximately constant, since, as was shown above, for a stochastic population model where the overall birth and death rates are equal, it is certain that the population will eventually die out. A typical simulation of the 2-species system (3.53) (see Fig. 3.1) shows this happening.

One reason that the population dies out in the stochastic simulation is that, by defining the 'constant' total size c_0 in terms of the population numbers, we are making c_0 a stochastic variable, not a constant. Jones and Leung (1981) show analytically that the increasing fluctuations observed in the multi-species model can be eliminated if one replaces the constraint of constant total population size by a slightly different form of constraint. Rather than determine c_0 by $c_0 = \sum_i x_i(0)$, *specify c_0 in advance*, so that it is always the same, independent of the initial conditions. Then the total size should head towards c_0 in each run, no matter where it starts.

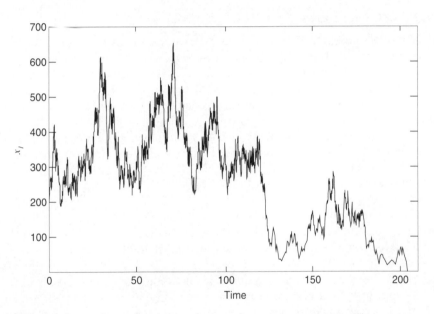

Figure 3.1   A stochastic simulation of a constant concentration system.

4

A spin glass model of the origin of life

4.1 The spin glass

The model presented in its deterministic and stochastic versions in the previous two chapters deals with primitive biomolecules in a general way. It says very little about their detailed structures, the methods by which they interact, and so on. The number of mutations allowed in the model is severely limited, and the fitness of each species must be specified in advance, by giving the rate parameters A, Q, and D.

We now consider a model in which all molecular interactions are explicitly performed as steps in a computer algorithm. There are no restrictions on the number of different species that may arise through mutation, and the fitness of a species is determined explicitly by its composition rather than imposed arbitrarily beforehand.

This model was proposed by P.W. Anderson, D.L. Stein and D.S. Rokhsar at Princeton University in the 1980s (see Anderson (1983), Stein (1984) and Rokhsar *et al.* (1986)). It is based on a mathematical model of a theoretical substance known as a *spin glass*, originally devised as a description of certain inanimate physical systems, such as magnetic materials.

A spin glass is a system of objects (you may think of them as atoms or molecules to make things definite, but the idea is more general than that), each of which can exist in one of several states. In the original model of a spin glass, each object was an atom which had a 'spin' whose 'axis' could point in one of two fixed directions: up or down. Such a spin is a purely quantum mechanical concept, and readers need not concern themselves with its physical properties. The term 'spin' is used here merely for conformity with the original work on the subject. The spin should be thought of in a purely abstract way as a quantity whose value will affect the energy of the system containing it.

In physics, the probability of a system of interacting objects being found in a certain configuration depends on the energy of that configuration. The energy depends on the interactions that occur between the components of the system. For example, in Newtonian physics, a system of objects (like the sun and its planets) that interact through the gravitational force have an energy that is composed of two terms: kinetic and potential energy. The kinetic energy is due to the relative motions of the objects, but the potential energy depends on the force law, which for the Newtonian gravitational force between two objects is directly proportional to the product of the two masses and inversely proportional to the square of the distance between them.

Systems that are left to themselves tend to take up configurations that minimize their energy. The 'normal' shapes of molecules, those they assume when they are in their ground (lowest) state of energy, are determined by finding the minimum energy of the system composed of the atoms in the molecule. If we have a mathematical expression for the energy of a system, sometimes called the *Hamiltonian*, we can determine the most likely state in which the system will be found by calculating the state or states that give local minima of the Hamiltonian. In the absence of any outside interference, a system will head towards the nearest minimum and stay there, but in any situation where external perturbations exist, there is always a chance that one such disturbance will cause the system to jump out of one local minimum and migrate toward another. In a 'noisy' system, then, we can speak of only a certain probability that it will be found in any given state.

Most of the physical systems that are studied in undergraduate physics courses have energy functions of a very simple form—ones that have only one or two minima. What distinguishes a spin glass from such systems is that its energy function often has a great many distinct minima, so that, in a noisy environment, the state in which a spin glass will be found is highly uncertain. To see this, consider the simplest kind of spin glass—one where each atom can exist in one of two states: spin up, represented by $S = 1$, and spin down, represented by $S = -1$. Consider a collection of such atoms, and define S_i to be the spin of atom i. The Hamiltonian of the collection is then defined to be

$$H = -\sum_{i<j} J_{ij} S_i S_j \qquad (4.1)$$

where the sum is taken over all distinct pairs of spins such that $i < j$, thus avoiding counting the pair ij twice (as ij and ji).

The quantities J_{ij} measure the strength and nature of the interaction between spins i and j. They can be positive or negative. For a given value of a J_{ij}, two spins S_i and S_j can be in a high or low energy state, depending on whether they are parallel (have the same sign) or antiparallel (have opposite signs). For example, if $J_{ij} > 0$ and the spins are parallel, then $J_{ij} S_i S_j > 0$, so the contribution to the Hamiltonian of the interaction between these two spins is negative (due to the negative sign in the definition of H). This is a low energy state. Antiparallel spins will reverse the sign of the term $J_{ij}S_iS_j$ so that the contribution to H is positive. This is the high energy state. The size of the contribution to the total energy depends, of course, on the magnitude of the interaction term J_{ij}.

In practice, the J_{ij} for all possible interactions are chosen randomly when the spin glass is set up, and then held constant for the duration of the simulation. The interaction terms may be thought of as a fixed environment in which the spins live. The spins adjust their behaviour so that they are best suited to the environment in which they find themselves. A spin's life is particularly simple, since it can only do one of two things: align itself so that its spin is either $+1$ or -1. Each spin will attempt to choose a value that will minimize the interaction energy with respect to all the other spins in the system. Since all spins are attempting to adapt to each other simultaneously, a considerable amount of toing and froing is necessary before the whole group of spins can find a configuration that is mutually satisfactory. In the presence of external noise (in the form of molecular or radiative bombardment, for example), several spins will be flipping from one state to the other during any time interval, so the system never really settles down. However, if it can find a configuration that matches a minimum in the Hamiltonian, it will tend to stay near that point unless a particularly large perturbation knocks the system away from that point by causing a lot of spins to flip in a short time.

If we think of the value of each spin S_i as a coordinate, we can define the state of a system of N spins as a point in an N-dimensional 'spin space' with coordinates given by the N values $S_1, S_2, \ldots, S_N$. The Hamiltonian is defined as a function over this spin space. The values chosen for the J_{ij} determine the specific form of the Hamiltonian and hence of the locations in spin space of the minima of H. For example, if we have a system of only two atoms and we choose a value of $J_{12} = 1$, then the energy is

$$H = -J_{12}S_1S_2 = -S_1S_2. \tag{4.2}$$

A minimum value of H occurs if $S_1 = S_2$ so that the spins are parallel. In this case there are two minima ($S_1 = S_2 = 1$ or $S_1 = S_2 = -1$).

To get an idea of how multiple minima arise in spin glasses with a large number of atoms, consider a system with four atoms (Fig. 4.1).

Suppose we choose the following values for the J_{ij}: $J_{12} = J_{13} = J_{24} = 1$, $J_{34} = -1$ and all other J_{ij} equal to zero. Since we wish to minimize the energy function, we should choose spin values to minimize each term in the sum, if we can. Suppose we choose $S_1 = 1$. Then we can minimize the interactions between spins 1 and 2, and between spins 2 and 4, by choosing $S_2 = S_4 = 1$. What do we choose for S_3? If we choose $S_3 = 1$, we minimize the interaction between spins 1 and 3, but maximize it between 3 and 4. If

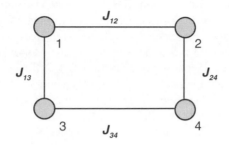

Figure 4.1 A spin glass with 4 atoms, showing the frustration effect.

we choose $S_3 = -1$, we do the exact opposite. In other words, no matter what we choose for S_3, we get the same value for H. In this case the spin glass has (at least) two configurations with the same energy minimum. Another two configurations can be found by starting with $S_1 = -1$. These configurations turn out to be just the same as the first two, but with all the spins reversed. There are thus four distinct spin states with the same minimum energy, out of a total of 16 ($= 2^4$) states possible for an array of 4 spins. The state to which the system will evolve depends on the initial conditions and the perturbations it receives from the environment.

Systems such as spin glasses in which some spins cannot be given a unique value which minimizes the Hamiltonian are said to be *frustrated* (for obvious reasons). It is this frustration which makes the spin glass a useful model for the origin of life. The number of minima for larger systems of spins diverges quite rapidly. Numerical simulations show that the number of minima in a system of N spins is of order $e^{\alpha N}$, with $\alpha \approx 0.2$. It turns out that the depth of a typical minimum also increases as N increases, which implies that the minima in larger systems are more stable than in small systems. The depth of the minimum is a measure of how large a perturbation is needed to disturb the system so that it will leave its location in spin space and possibly find another minimum.

4.2 From spin glass to origin of life

Recall from Chapter 1 that an evolving biosystem must have two properties: diversity and stability. There must be opportunities for new, possibly fitter, species to evolve, and these species must be resistant to minor environmental noise so that they can live long enough to reproduce.

A spin glass possesses both these qualities. The diversity is provided by the numerous locations in spin space at which a spin glass can live. The stability is provided by the fact that these locations are local minima of the Hamiltonian, so that minor disturbances will not push the spin glass away from its home for very long. However, we still have to show how we can map the origin of life problem onto a spin glass model.

To begin, we draw an analogy between a system of atoms with a discrete set of spins and a linear molecule, such as RNA or DNA, composed of units, each of which can take on one of a discrete set of forms (as in RNA, where each unit is a base which can be one of four types).

The interactions between the spins which are used to calculate the energy function H have their analogy in the chemical interactions between the bases in the RNA chain. We would expect the strongest interactions to be those between nearest neighbour bases, but longer-range interactions among RNA bases are known to exist as well. Because of the flexibility of RNA molecules, some long-range interactions can be fairly strong if two distant bases come into contact with each other due to a bend in the molecule, but in general there will be a decrease of interaction strength with distance.

So far, so good. However, one problem arises when we try to decide how to interpret the energy function in the case of an RNA molecule. In the spin glass, H is a measure of the stability of a given spin configuration, which in turn is a measure of how likely it is for the spin glass to be found in that state. A spin glass in an unstable state will adjust its structure by flipping a few spins, acquiring a more stable configuration.

An RNA molecule with an unstable value of H cannot respond quite so readily, however, as the base sequence of the molecule is not easy to change once it is formed—you can't just 'flip' a few of the bases from one form to another. An alternative interpretation which is in better accord with the way biomolecules behave is to assume that the value of H is a measure of the probability of survival of the molecule (higher H means lower probability of survival), and that molecules that do not survive are broken down into their component parts. That is, the energy function is reinterpreted as a 'death function' (to use Anderson and Stein's graphic term) which determines whether an RNA molecule lives or dies. Because of the inverse relation between H and probability of survival, the death function D is defined as

$$D \equiv -H \qquad (4.3)$$

so that a higher value of D means a higher probability of survival.

Since the death function D_N for an N-spin system

$$D_N = \sum_{i<j} J_{ij} S_i S_j \qquad (4.4)$$

can in principle be any quantity from $-\infty$ to ∞, it cannot be used as it stands as a probability, which must lie between 0 and 1. The transformation from values of D_N to a probability measure is somewhat arbitrary, since any monotonic mapping of the interval $[-\infty, \infty]$ to the interval $[0, 1]$ can serve as a probability function. One such formula is

$$d_N = \frac{\exp[D_N + \mu(N)]}{1 + \exp[D_N + \mu(N)]}. \tag{4.5}$$

The quantity $\mu(N)$ is a scaling factor. It determines what value of D_N corresponds to a probability of survival of 0.5, since this occurs when $D_N = -\mu(N)$.

A primitive molecular soup is envisaged in which we start with a collection of fairly short RNA molecules. By means of complementary base pairing, the complementary strands of the existing RNA molecules are formed, and by repeating the complementary strand formation from these new molecules, new copies of the original RNA molecules are created. At each stage in this process, each molecule has a chance of survival which depends on its energy value—the energy or death function is used as a probability of survival. Also, each time a complementary strand is formed, mutations (changes in the base sequences due to incorrect complement formation) or strand elongations may occur, resulting in an ever-changing collection of RNA sequences. A mutation may create a new sequence which has a lower energy and consequently higher chance of survival.

How can we justify using a spin glass type energy function to describe an RNA molecule? Those readers accustomed to a rigorous justification for every step taken will be disappointed here. There is no step-by-step derivation which will take us from an atomic spin system to an evolving collection of nucleotides. The purpose behind the model is best stated using Stein's own words (Stein, 1984): '...we would like to be able to construct a mathematical model that contains the *essential* features of such a transition [from a system with no biological information to one with a great deal of information], features that might be called "universal" in the sense that a large number of biochemical models specifying molecules and reaction pathways leading to information growth would be expected to exhibit them, independently of chemical details. (Of course, no such model may in fact exist, but that doesn't stop us from trying.)' We may state the goal behind this model as one of attempting to discover if a system with the properties of a spin glass will spontaneously evolve the way we would expect a primitive biosystem to evolve. That is, will it exhibit the principle of mutation and natural selection: will new species be generated and only the fittest survive? If so (and it does, otherwise this chapter would never have been written), then we can dig deeper to try to find a specific chemical system which exhibits the spin glass properties.

Having said this, however, we can get some idea of how a spin glass type Hamiltonian may arise for a system of molecules that replicate using complementary pairing. Suppose we consider the death function D as a function of the set of spins $\mathcal{S} = \{S_1, S_2, ..., S_N\}$: $D = D(\mathcal{S})$. Then we can write D as a sum of terms which depend on successively higher-order interactions between the spins. There will be a term that depends on single spins which will have the form $\sum_i h_i S_i$, a term that involves pairwise spin–spin interactions (this will be the spin glass term), and higher-order terms involving interactions between three or more spins. Thus D will have the form

$$D = \sum_i h_i S_i + \sum_{i \neq j} J_{ij} S_i S_j + \sum_{i \neq j \neq k} C_{ijk} S_i S_j S_k + ... \qquad (4.6)$$

Now if we define the 'spins' corresponding to complementary bases to be the negative of each other (for example, we could assign $S_C = 1$ and $S_G = -1$, where C, G stand for cytosine and guanine respectively), then, since the survival of one RNA sequence from one generation to the next requires the existence of its complement, any sequence must have the same probability of survival as its complement. That is, D must be the same if we replace all S_i by their negatives. This immediately tells us that all terms in the expansion with an odd number of S_i factors must be zero. The first non-zero term in the expansion of D is therefore the spin glass energy function. If we make the assumption that all higher order terms are negligible compared to this term, we have our spin glass–RNA analogy.

We are perfectly at liberty to make the assignment of spin values to bases that we made in the last paragraph. If we had chosen some other assignment (for example $S_C = 1$, $S_G = 2$, and so on) we would get a different model, but we could not make the simplifying assumption that all terms with an odd number of S_i factors are zero.

The elimination of the first term in the expansion turns out to be vital to the argument, since if this term *is* present and has a significant magnitude relative to the spin glass term, it turns out that D usually has only one stable minimum. Thus in the absence of complementarity, the diversity and adaptability required of an origin of life model disappear. For further discussion of this point see Anderson (1983).

4.3   The model

Assuming we have now convinced the reader of the motivation and plausibility of the spin glass approach, we will now proceed to describe the implementation of the model.

The molecules which we will consider are similar to RNA strands, except that only two bases are used rather than four. This is done merely for the sake of computational ease, since there is nothing in the formulation of the model that prohibits higher numbers of bases, though if we are going to use complementary base pairing we must, of course, always have an even number. If we were to use four bases, for example, we define four different

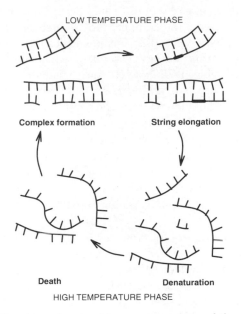

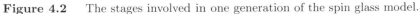

Figure 4.2   The stages involved in one generation of the spin glass model.

spin values, say $-2, -1, 1, 2$. In order for the argument used above to eliminate those terms with an odd number of spin factors in the expansion of D, we should ensure that the spins of complementary base pairs are always the negative of each other.

Before the simulation starts, we generate the 'environment' by randomly producing the J values. The only other environmental influence is a high-temperature/low-temperature cycle simulating day and night (see Fig. 4.2).

We start in the low-temperature part of the cycle with a soup of small molecules, mainly short fragments of one or two bases (*monomers* and *dimers*, respectively). The low temperature allows the fragments to form complementary base pairs. Each pair of molecules that meet have a probability of binding to each other, depending on their relative alignment and the nature of the bases opposite each other. This pairing is allowed to proceed until no more pairs can be formed within some reasonable time. During the pair formation stage, two or more fragments may have paired with the same complement in such a way that their free ends abut each other. At these points, covalent bonds may form joining the two fragments together, creating a longer molecule (see Fig. 4.2).

It is also possible that, due to mismatches in some of the complements, some mutations may occur.

After all the pairing and bonding has occurred, we enter the high-temperature stage. Here, the temperature is high enough to break the complementary bonds between different molecules (though not, of course, the covalent bonds within a single strand) so that the solution contains only single stranded molecules. Now the death function is applied to each molecule in turn, to see if it will survive this part of the cycle. Those molecules that die are eliminated from the soup; those that survive are left untouched.

In the next low-temperature phase, an influx of monomers and dimers is allowed to provide raw materials for string building, and also to simulate the debris left behind by those molecules that have just died. Those molecules surviving the last high-temperature phase are allowed to form complementary pairs and covalent bonds as before, and the cycle repeats itself.

The process is allowed to continue for a large number of temperature cycles (several hundred being a typical number), during which time the population levels are recorded. What we hope to see are (i) a steady increase in the average molecular length in the soup, showing accumulation of information and (ii) the clustering of the longer molecules into 'families' of molecules whose sequences are broadly similar. These clusters should correspond to minima of H in the spin space, that is, they should be close to those sequences that have maximum survival probability. The families of strings may also be thought of as a quasi-species in the sense of Chapter 2.

There are many practical problems in writing a program to simulate this model. Some of these problems are discussed in Rokhsar *et al.* (1986).

A typical simulation obtained using a program which implements the model[1] are shown in Figs 4.3 – 4.5. In these figures, the environment is held constant until generation 500, where it is changed and then held constant until generation 1000. The J_{ij} are chosen randomly from the interval $[-10, 10]$ and $\mu = -6$.

Fig. 4.3 shows the mean length of all 'long' molecules (those containing 5 or more bases), Figure 4.4 shows the fate of two selected quasi-species of lengths 6 and 7 bases, and Fig. 4.5 shows the actual number of long molecules present.

It can be seen that the model exhibits many of the features expected of an evolutionary system. The mean length of the molecules tends to increase in most simulations, corresponding to an increased capacity for storing genetic information. The long molecules tend to be grouped into quasi-species, of which several are present at any time. Varying the environment

---

[1]The author is indebted to Michael Pullen for writing a Pascal version of the spin glass model, which was used to produce the graphs in this chapter.

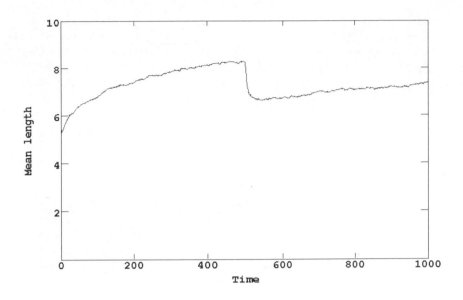

Figure 4.3   Mean length of long molecules (more than 5 bases).

can drastically alter the characteristics of the environment in some cases and barely affect them in others. Note in Fig. 4.4 that the environment change causes the quasi-species of length 6 to increase while that of length 7 fares less well. In other simulations, sizes of quasi-species may not change much at all when the environment changes.

In the simulations shown, the environmental change causes a drastic drop in the overall population, but the numbers rapidly recover. This sort of phenomenon has been observed many times in the fossil record: mass extinctions (the most famous being the extinction of the dinosaurs) of species occur fairly regularly.

4.4   Other adaptive landscape models

The spin glass model is one example of a general class of models in which the mutation/selection cycle central to the theory of evolution by natural selection is modelled by a walk on an *adaptive landscape*. There is not enough space to go into a detailed discussion of other adaptive landscape models of the origin of life here, but the interested reader may consult some of the following papers.

A study of the general properties of spin glass models of molecular evolution may be found in Amitrano *et al.* (1989).

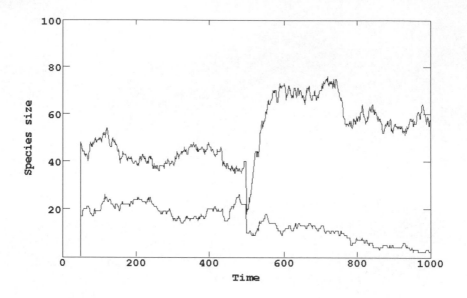

Figure 4.4   The numbers of two quasi-species of lengths 6 (top curve for entire plot) and 7 (bottom curve).

Abbott (1988) uses the spin glass Hamiltonian in a somewhat different way than Anderson and his colleagues and shows that chemical evolution is possible even in a system where no explicit template-complement matching occurs, though he is vague about the chemical details. Abbott's model has the virtue that it is considerably simpler than Anderson's, though the lack of detail in the model leaves some doubts as to its applicability to any specific prebiotic system.

A comprehensive computer model of evolution is described by Conrad and Strizich (1985). Although it is designed more as a model of an evolving ecosystem on the modern Earth, many of the techniques used could be applied to an origin-of-life scenario.

Finally, a more general approach to the theory of adaptive landscapes is undertaken by Kauffman and collaborators. See Kauffman and Levin (1987), Kauffman (1988), and Kauffman (1989) for more details. We will examine Kauffman's adaptive landscape as a model for maturation of the immune response in Chapter 10.

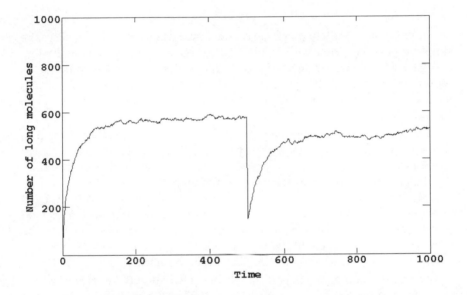

Figure 4.5   The total number of long molecules present.

5

The origin of the genetic code

5.1   Introduction

The preceding three chapters have concerned themselves only with the simplest possible primitive biochemical systems. The only constituents of such systems are nucleic acid type molecules whose only function is reproduction, either with or without a complementary intermediary. No mention has yet been made of the other half of the modern genetic cycle: the proteins.

There is no convincing theoretical model of the transition from the simple reproducing systems of the previous chapters to the present-day system of DNA–protein–DNA–protein cycles. Eigen and Schuster have developed their hypercycle theory (see Chapter 6) which goes some way towards a model of cyclic chemical systems but still relies heavily on much of the machinery being in place to begin with. Also, Stein and Anderson (1984) have extended their stochastic spin-glass model described in the previous chapter to include the beginnings of a catalytic cycle, but again, much that goes into the model must be taken on faith.

Before we examine the hypercycle theory in Chapter 6, let us have a look at a theory proposed by Hoffmann (1974, 1975a) to study the likelihood of a genetic code arising spontaneously given the existence of molecules with some 'adaptor' properties that allow the translation of a DNA or RNA sequence into an amino acid sequence.

5.2   Theories

The reader will recall from Chapter 1 that the translation of the base sequence of DNA into protein is done by treating each triplet of bases, or codon, on the DNA as a code word for one of the 20 amino acids commonly used in the construction of a protein. In present-day organisms, the translation involves a complex series of steps beginning with the transcription of the master sequence on the DNA into messenger RNA, which is subsequently translated into a protein by being passed through a ribosome and visited by a succession of transfer RNA molecules which can match each codon on the mRNA with its corresponding amino acid.

One of the more mysterious aspects of this translation process is the latter step: the association of a triplet of RNA bases with a specific amino acid. How did such an association ever arise? There are two competing theories that attempt to explain this.

5.2.1 The stereochemical theory

The *stereochemical* theory proposes that an amino acid such as glycine has a particular affinity for either the codon or codons which code for it (in glycine's case, the codons are GGX, where X is any of the four bases) or to the tRNA which serves as the translator. If such affinities do exist, it would not be difficult to envisage a scenario on the early Earth where, once a few nucleic acid molecules of appreciable length had managed to form, the natural attraction of particular amino acids for either the codon or the tRNA would cause the amino acids to link up in the same order as their codons to form a primitive protein.

Unfortunately for the adherents to the stereochemical theory, very little evidence exists to support their claims. For example, it has been possible to artificially alter the anti-codon loop in a tRNA molecule so that the tRNA would no longer recognize the codon on the mRNA to which it should bind. Even with this alteration, the tRNA will still bind the same amino acid that it would have before the change. Thus there cannot be a direct link between the codon or anti-codon and the amino acid. The assignment of an amino acid to a tRNA molecule must be done on the basis of the overall shapes of the tRNA and the amino acid, not on the basis of the composition of one small part of the tRNA molecule.

Direct measurements of the affinities of amino acids to the four bases present in mRNA have also yielded no significant correlations between an amino acid and the bases that are present in its codons. It thus seems unlikely that any direct chemical preference of an amino acid for a codon played a significant role in the determination of the present genetic code.

5.2.2 The frozen accident theory

In the absence of any particular attraction between an amino acid and its codon, how could a code have arisen? If there really is no direct connection between a codon and an amino acid, there must have been intermediary molecules, even at the earliest stages of molecular evolution. These molecules must have been similar to modern tRNA, in the sense that they must have had an affinity for particular codons at one location, and an affinity for a particular amino acid somewhere else on the same molecule. In present-day organisms, the activation of a tRNA, that is, the attachment of an amino acid to it, is done by means of a helper protein which can recognize a tRNA and its corresponding amino acid and provide a favourable chemical environment for the two to join. Since we have seen that no direct connection seems to exist between a tRNA and an amino acid, the actual 'choice' as to which codon corresponds to which amino acid is made not by the tRNA, but by the protein which causes the two to join. The frozen accident theory states that it was largely a matter of luck which proteins happened to be around when the code was still being sorted out, so that the determination of which codon ended up coding for which amino acid was also to a large extent random. If a protein that paired a tRNA which matched the codon GGG with a glycine molecule happened to be present, then that particular tRNA would find itself with a glycine attached to it, which would subsequently be inserted into a protein chain when a GGG codon was encountered.

At first glance, this scheme may appear to be unworkable. After all, it is unlikely that early proteins had a specificity that was tuned finely enough so that they would match one particular tRNA with one particular amino acid all the time, and completely ignore all other molecules. The key to the success of the model lies in the fact that nucleic acids and proteins are locked into an auto-catalytic loop: the nucleic acids contain the code for the proteins which in turn act on the nucleic acids to produce more protein. Consider a stretch of mRNA which contains the code for one of the proteins that serves as an adaptor in the translation process. If that protein makes the same assignment of a codon to an amino acid as was used when the protein itself was made, then the same nucleic acid sequence will give rise to the same amino acid sequence when the next generation of proteins starts to do the translations. If, however, the protein produced by the nucleic acid sequence makes *different* assignments of codons to nucleic acids than those that were used in its own production, a different amino acid sequence will result from the same stretch of mRNA. It is highly unlikely that this new protein will have similar (or even any) translation properties.

We see, therefore, that in order for such a translation system to evolve in an auto-catalytic system, the codon assignments must be consistent from one generation to the next. Any system which constantly changes the code is highly unlikely to survive, since the probability of a random sequence of amino acids producing a protein with a useful function is very small. The principle of natural selection enters again at this stage, as only those molecular systems that give rise to a consistent code over several generations will be selected, with all other systems being eliminated.

The major difference between the frozen accident model and the stereochemical model is that no particular affinity between amino acid and nucleic acid is assumed here. It is assumed that a wide variety of codon–amino acid assignments are possible, depending on which proteins are present.

The choice of which protein is ultimately selected is determined partly by the requirement that the codon assignments made in the next generation be the same as in the present generation. If more than one such selection is possible, the final choice must be a matter of luck. Clearly we cannot have more than one set of codon assignments in operation at any one time, since that would result in the same stretch of mRNA being translated into different proteins at different times. Thus one of the possible codes must be ultimately selected, resulting in a freezing of the possibilities—a frozen accident. We now investigate just how likely it is for such an 'accident' to occur.

5.3 The probability of a consistent genetic code

We will consider a system of nucleic acids and proteins in which we have λ different codons which are translated into λ different amino acids by means of λ protein adaptors. In order for a particular genetic code to 'freeze' out of such a system, the set of proteins that is produced by the first generation must make the same assignments of codons to amino acids as those made by the first set of proteins[1].

Suppose we start with a simple system, in which $\lambda = 2$. We have two codons, which we shall refer to as A and B, which must be translated into two amino acids a and b. If the first-generation adaptors make the assignments $A \rightarrow a$ and $B \rightarrow b$, then the adaptors synthesized in this generation must make the same assignments when their turn comes to translate codons to amino acids.

Any one adaptor could make one of four assignments of codon to amino acid: $A \rightarrow a$, $A \rightarrow b$, $B \rightarrow a$ or $B \rightarrow b$. We assume that any particular adaptor has a probability of $\frac{1}{4}$ of making any one of these assignments. Since there are four possible assignments and two adaptors there are $4^2 = 16$ possible combinations of assignments. The only pairs of assignments that are acceptable if we wish both codons and both amino acids to be used in an unambiguous way are: (first assignment, second assignment) = (Aa, Bb), (Ab, Ba), (Bb, Aa), or (Ba, Ab). The probability of one of these 4 pairs occurring is then $\frac{4}{4^2} = 0.25$. Now the probability of the second-generation adaptors making the *same* assignments is only half as great since, if the first-generation adaptors make the assignments (Aa, Bb), say, then the second-generation adaptors must make one of the two assignments (Aa, Bb) or (Bb, Aa). Thus the probability of the second-generation giving rise to the same unambiguous assignments is $\frac{1}{8}$. The overall probability of the first- and second-generation adaptors making the same assignments

---

[1] We are assuming that molecules with adaptor properties already exist, and that they will still exist in the next generation. This assumption will be dealt with in Section 5.4

is thus (assuming the properties of the two generations are independent) $\frac{1}{4} \times \frac{1}{8} = \frac{1}{32}$.

In the general case of λ codons, amino acids, and adaptors, there are λ^2 possible codon–amino acid assignments. We assume that each of the adaptors has a probability of $\frac{1}{\lambda^2}$ of making any one of these assignments. We will only consider a combination of such assignments such that each of the λ adaptors makes a different assignment from all the others. To find the probability of such a combination, consider the adaptors in order. For the first adaptor there are λ^2 assignments available and the adaptor has probability of $\frac{1}{\lambda^2}$ of making any one of them, so the net chance of the first adaptor making an acceptable assignment is $\lambda^2 \times \frac{1}{\lambda^2} (= 1)$. For the second adaptor, there are $(\lambda - 1)$ unassigned codons and $(\lambda - 1)$ available amino acids, so there are $(\lambda - 1)^2$ acceptable assignments, each of which has a probability of $\frac{1}{\lambda^2}$. The net probability of one of these assignments being made is then $\frac{(\lambda-1)^2}{\lambda^2}$. Continuing in this way we see that the probability of the nth adaptor making an acceptable assignment is $\frac{(\lambda-(n-1))^2}{\lambda^2}$. The overall probability of all λ adaptors making acceptable assignments is the product of all these terms:

$$\text{overall probability} = \prod_{n=1}^{\lambda} \frac{(\lambda - (n-1))^2}{\lambda^2} = \frac{(\lambda!)^2}{\lambda^{2\lambda}}. \tag{5.1}$$

Having found how likely it is that the first generation will produce an acceptable set of adaptors we must now work out the probability of the second set of adaptors making the same assignments. Since there are $\lambda!$ distinct ways of assigning λ different amino acids to λ different codons, and we have decided on one of these ways in choosing the set of adaptors in the first generation, the probability of the second generation making the same assignments will be only $\frac{1}{\lambda!}$ times that of the first generation making an acceptable set of assignments, so we have for this probability $\frac{\lambda!}{\lambda^{2\lambda}}$. The total probability P_{adapt} of a system of λ adaptors giving the same unambiguous assignments in two consecutive generations is the product of these two factors:

$$P_{adapt} = \frac{(\lambda!)^3}{\lambda^{4\lambda}}. \tag{5.2}$$

Some of the values of this probability are shown for various values of λ in the following table:

λ	2	3	4	5	20
P_{adapt}	0.031	4.1×10^{-4}	3.2×10^{-6}	1.8×10^{-8}	1.2×10^{-49}

Considering that the present day-translation system uses 20 amino acids with some 60 codons and a comparable number of adaptors, these probabilities look depressingly small. But when one considers that an early translation system would most likely have used considerably fewer amino acids and codons, things don't look so bad, especially when one remembers how much time was available for a code to arise. The age of the Earth is estimated at about 4×10^9 years, or about 10^{17} seconds. The earliest fossils are dated at about one tenth the age of the Earth, or about 10^{16} seconds. A translation event driven by an adaptor can take less than one second, and in any primordial soup, many such reactions would be taking place simultaneously, so it is possible that more than 10^{16} trials could have been performed before the code nucleation event actually took place. Given these orders of magnitude, the probability of a reliable translation mechanism with around 5 or fewer adaptors arising randomly is not so low. From a biochemical point of view, the 20 amino acids in modern organisms tend to fall naturally into about 5 groups within each of which the chemical structure is fairly similar, so that it is possible that early life used only 5 or so different amino acids.

Of course this analysis has avoided any consideration of how likely it is that any molecule with translation properties would arise in the first place—we have merely assumed that some such molecules could arise spontaneously. We also leave open the question of how the translation apparatus evolved from an early 5-adaptor code to the modern 20 amino acid one, but once a code was started it is not too difficult to envisage successive refinements to include more amino acids which would, in turn, fine tune the proteins of which they became a part.

5.4 The probability of a full catalytic system

This sort of probabilistic estimation can be extended to get some idea of how likely it is for a full-blown biological system to appear. In the absence of suitable enzymes to speed things along, most biochemical reactions proceed at an agonizingly slow rate. It therefore seems essential that, in any primitive biosystem, a certain number of proteins must have been present that had such catalytic activities. The adaptors which attach amino acids to tRNA molecules are just one example of proteins with catalytic abilities. Many other functions not directly related to protein production would also require enzymatic assistance. Suppose that a minimum of ν such catalysts are required in order that a self-sustaining system can become established.

Certain proteins, however, also have negative effects. Some may bind to sites on nucleic acids or other molecules and inhibit any further reactions, while others may actively degrade the very proteins or nucleic acids we are trying to construct. Many of these functions have a place in a more advanced organism but could not be tolerated in a primitive biosystem. Suppose there are μ negative activities that are absolutely prohibited in our early environment.

Now assume that any protein has a probability p of possessing one of the activities, either good or bad. It is possible for a single molecule to possess more than one activity, but if we assume all activities are independent, the probability of one molecule possessing two activities is p^2. Since the possession of even one activity is extremely unlikely ($p \ll 1$), the probability that a single molecule will have more than one activity is very small.

In a collection of N proteins, the probability of a particular activity *not* being present is $(1-p)^N$, making the probability of the same activity being present $1 - (1-p)^N$. The probability of our environment containing the ν desirable activities and not containing the μ deleterious ones is therefore

$$P(p, N; \mu, \nu) = [1 - (1 - p)^N]^\nu (1 - p)^{N\mu}. \tag{5.3}$$

This probability has a maximum with respect to p when

$$\frac{\partial P(p, N; \mu, \nu)}{\partial p} = \nu(1 - p)^N - \mu + (1 - p)^N \mu = 0 \tag{5.4}$$

or

$$(1 - p)^N = \frac{\mu}{\nu + \mu}. \tag{5.5}$$

Taking natural logarithms and using the fact that $p \ll 1$ so that we may use the approximation $\ln(1 - p) \approx -p$ we obtain

$$N \approx -\frac{1}{p} \ln\left(\frac{\mu}{\nu + \mu}\right) = \frac{1}{p} \ln\left(1 + \frac{\nu}{\mu}\right). \tag{5.6}$$

Using this expression to eliminate N we obtain for the maximum probability P_{max} of an acceptable set of activities

$$P_{max} = \frac{\nu^\nu \mu^\mu}{(\nu + \mu)^{\nu+\mu}}. \tag{5.7}$$

The maximum value is quite a sharp one, in the sense that if the relation (5.6) between N and p at the maximum is violated more than slightly, the probability drops quite rapidly. If N is much larger than the optimum, it becomes very likely that one of the disruptive activities is present, while if N is smaller than the optimum, it is unlikely that all the essential activities will be present.

Since we require all these activities to be present for two successive generations for a catalytic system to become established, we must square the above probability to get the chance P_{cat} that a minimal catalytic system will nucleate. We therefore obtain

$$P_{cat} = P_{max}^2 = \left[\frac{\nu^\nu \mu^\mu}{(\nu + \mu)^{\nu + \mu}} \right]^2 . \tag{5.8}$$

The values of P_{cat} are not quite as frighteningly small as those for the genesis of the genetic code. For $\mu = 2$ and $\nu = 5$, for example, $P_{cat} = 2 \times 10^{-4}$, while for $\mu = 4$ and $\nu = 20$ we have $P_{cat} = 4 \times 10^{-10}$.

We can get an overall estimate of how likely it is for a system that has both the required catalytic properties *and* a set of λ adaptors for setting up a primitive genetic code. If we assume that the adaptor property has the same probability p of occurrence as any other catalytic activity, then the probability P_λ of precisely λ molecules out of a total population of N having an adaptor property for two generations in a row is given by the square of a term from the binomial distribution:

$$P_\lambda = \left[\binom{N}{\lambda} p^\lambda (1-p)^{N-\lambda} \right]^2 . \tag{5.9}$$

Since $N \gg \lambda$ and $p \ll 1$, we can obtain an order of magnitude estimate of P_λ by using the approximation $\frac{N!}{(N-\lambda)!} \approx N^\lambda$. We obtain

$$P_\lambda \approx \left[\frac{N^\lambda p^\lambda (1-p)^N}{\lambda!} \right]^2 . \tag{5.10}$$

If N and p are related according to eqn (5.6) we obtain

$$P_\lambda \approx \left\{ \frac{\mu}{\lambda!(\mu + \nu)} \left[\ln\left(1 + \frac{\nu}{\mu}\right) \right]^\lambda \right\}^2 . \tag{5.11}$$

The probability of an appropriate genetic code forming is given by the product of the probability P_λ of there being λ adaptor properties present in the environment and the conditional probability P_{adapt} in eqn (5.2) that, given λ adaptors, they form a correct genetic code. The overall probability P_{total} that a complete system consisting of a genetic code with λ adaptors and a catalytic system with ν essential activities present and all μ deleterious activities absent is thus the product of P_λ, P_{adapt}, and P_{cat}:

$$P_{total} = \left\{ \frac{\mu}{\lambda!(\mu + \nu)} \left[\ln\left(1 + \frac{\nu}{\mu}\right) \right]^\lambda \right\}^2 \frac{(\lambda!)^3}{\lambda^{4\lambda}} \left[\frac{\nu^\nu \mu^\mu}{(\nu + \mu)^{\nu + \mu}} \right]^2 \tag{5.12}$$

For a system with 5 adaptors, 3 deleterious activities that must be avoided, and 10 activities that must be present, so that $\lambda = 5$, $\mu = 3$, and $\nu = 10$, $P_{total} \approx 2 \times 10^{-18}$. Again, given the enormous time available for the development of such a system, such a probability is not outside the realm of credibility. Of course, all these calculations are only order of magnitude estimates and, as Hoffmann himself points out, must not be taken too seriously. Still, they are useful guidelines. For example, if the probability of any one of the stages we have considered turned out to be something like 10^{-50} or less for even a simple system of, say 3 or 4 adaptors and a comparable number of good and bad catalytic activities, we would have to abandon any hope that such a system could evolve by chance. The fact that the probability of a primitive biochemical system arising largely through chance events is *not* vanishingly small indicates that attempts to build theoretical models of how it may have happened that way are not a waste of time.

5.5   Stability of a primitive genetic code

We now suppose that we have struck it lucky and that a catalytic system as envisaged in the last section has in fact arisen. Since these early molecules have not had the advantage of millions of years of evolution to fine tune their properties, we expect that they will be fairly error prone. Even though an adaptor may make the same assignment of amino acid to codon in two successive generations, it will do so with only a limited accuracy. How poor can this accuracy be before the whole system breaks down?

For the purposes of a sample calculation, we will again simplify the system with which we deal. Suppose we have a single gene which codes for the protein that is needed to translate the DNA into that protein. Further, suppose that protein production occurs in discrete generations. In generation i, the proteins produced in generation $i-1$ are used to translate the DNA to produce the proteins of generation i. Suppose the probability that a codon is translated correctly by a generation i protein is q_i. Then the average rate A_i (in units of, for example, codons per second) at which the DNA is translated correctly in the production of generation i proteins is a function of q_{i-1}:

$$A_i = A_i(q_{i-1}) \tag{5.13}$$

as is the rate of incorrect translation B_i:

$$B_i = B_i(q_{i-1}). \tag{5.14}$$

The probability q_i that a codon will be correctly translated in generation i is the ratio of the correct translation rate to the total translation rate:

$$q_i = \frac{A_i(q_{i-1})}{A_i(q_{i-1}) + B_i(q_{i-1})}. \tag{5.15}$$

Our goal is to get some idea of the behaviour of q_i as $i \to \infty$. If q_i tends to a value reasonably close to 1, we will have a stable system, in the sense that the proteins in successive generations will retain a high accuracy in translation and can therefore be relied upon to produce accurate copies of themselves. If, on the other hand, q_i degenerates to a value near zero, we expect the system to decay into a random collection of non-functional molecules.

To explore this model further, we need to find explicit forms for A_i and B_i in terms of q_{i-1}. To this end, we make a couple of assumptions about the structure of the protein. First of all, we assume that, of all the amino acid sites in the protein, m of them must be correctly assigned for the protein to have any activity at all. In other words, if any of these m amino acids is incorrect, the protein will not be able to act as an adaptor from codons to amino acids. Further, we assume that an additional n amino acids must be correctly assigned in order for the protein to assign the correct amino acid. Thus, if all of the m amino acids are correct, but one or more of the n is incorrect, the protein will act as an adaptor, but will assign an amino acid at random, rather than the one specified by the codon which it is currently translating.

For simplicity we are assuming that a single, correctly functioning protein is capable of translating all codons into their respective amino acids. This is equivalent to assuming that, in the case where we have a different adaptor for each amino acid, all the adaptors have the same general structure, that is, that each has m sites which must be correct for the protein to have activity at all and a further n which must be correct to ensure specificity. In the latter case, if we had λ different adaptors, each would have its own gene and all λ adaptors would be required to translate each gene. If all the adaptors have the same general properties, however, such a system is identical to the one we are considering. (We are ignoring here minor differences due to slightly varying compositions of the different adaptors—again we are after a rough model.)

With these assumptions, we see that a protein produced in generation $i - 1$ has a probability of q_{i-1}^m of having any activity at all. Thus a fraction $1 - q_{i-1}^m$ of the proteins will be inactive, and we may ignore them from here on.

Of the active proteins, a fraction q_{i-1}^n will be specific, with the remaining $1 - q_{i-1}^n$ being active but non-specific.

We now define the *activities* or rates at which each type of protein incorporates amino acids correctly and incorrectly, as follows.

	specific	non-specific
correct	α	α/S
incorrect	$(\lambda - 1)\alpha/S$	$(\lambda - 1)\alpha/S$

A fully specific protein correctly translates codons at a rate of α per second, and will incorporate each incorrect amino acid at a rate α/S, where S is a parameter we shall call the *specificity*. S defines the relative accuracy of a correctly functioning adaptor. The larger it is, the more accurate is the protein. Since there are λ amino acids available, the total rate at which a specific adaptor will incorporate an incorrect amino acid is $(\lambda - 1)\alpha/S$.

The non-specific protein incorporates all amino acids with the same reduced rate, so that it has the same rate of incorporating an incorrect amino acid as the specific protein, but a rate of only α/S of incorporating the correct amino acid[2].

The overall rate of incorporating correct amino acids is

$$A_i = q_{i-1}^m [q_{i-1}^n \alpha + (1 - q_{i-1}^n)\alpha/S] \tag{5.16}$$

and the rate of incorrect translation is

$$B_i = q_{i-1}^m [q_{i-1}^n (\lambda-1)\alpha/S + (1-q_{i-1}^n)(\lambda-1)\alpha/S] = q_{i-1}^m (\lambda-1)\alpha/S \tag{5.17}$$

The probability that the protein correctly translates a codon is then

$$q_i = \frac{A_i}{A_i + B_i} = \frac{(S - 1)q_{i-1}^n + 1}{(S - 1)q_{i-1}^n + \lambda}. \tag{5.18}$$

This is a recursion relation for q_i. We can find the equilibrium points (that is, the points where $q_i = q_{i-1}$) by plotting q_i versus q_{i-1} and finding the intersection of this curve with the line $q_i = q_{i-1}$. Such a plot for $\lambda = 4$, $n = 8$, and $S = 80$ is shown in Fig. 5.1. We see there are 3 intersection points, labelled A, B, and C, so there are 3 equilibrium points. Points A and C are stable while B is unstable. To see this, consider point A. Starting at A, we decrease q_{i-1} slightly. Then, since the point on the curve at this new value of q_{i-1} lies above the line $q_i = q_{i-1}$, we must have $q_i > q_{i-1}$ so that the accuracy increases back to the value it had at point A. Similarly, if we start at A and increase q_{i-1} slightly, the point on the curve at this new value of q_{i-1} lies below the line, so the accuracy decreases back towards A. The same reasoning applies at point C.

---

[2]The assumption that loss of specificity always leads to loss of activity has been criticized. See Section 5.5.1

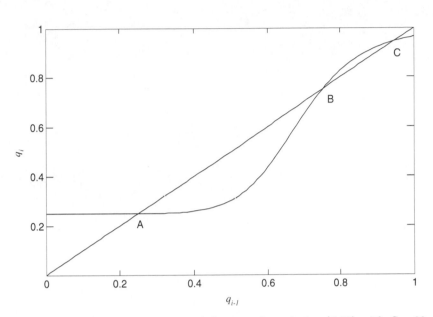

Figure 5.1   Equilibrium points of the recursion relation (5.18) with $S = 80$.

Just the opposite situation occurs at point B. Here, any slight motion away from B results in accuracy values in succeeding generations lying even further away. Thus, A and C are *stable* equilibria and B is *unstable*. For this particular choice of parameters we have a stable point corresponding to an ordered state (point C) and another corresponding to a disordered state (point A). Because B is unstable, it can never be attained in practice, so we need not consider it as a state in which we expect to find the system. However, it does act as a threshold value. If the system starts with any value of q greater than that at point B, it will ultimately converge on the ordered state C, while if it starts at any point below B, it will converge on the disordered state A. The threshold is an absolute barrier: once the system finds itself on one side, it cannot cross over to the other. (Of course, in a real situation, fluctuations would be present which would allow a transition over the barrier, but we are assuming such fluctuations to be negligible here.)

If we change the parameters, however, the situation can change quite drastically. Taking $\lambda = 4$ and $n = 8$ as before, but reducing the specificity to $S = 40$, we arrive at the situation shown in Fig. 5.2. Now there is

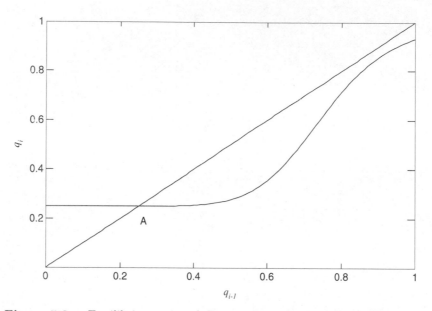

Figure 5.2   Equilibrium point of the recursion relation (5.18) with $S = 40$.

only one equilibrium point, corresponding to a disordered state. Both the unstable point and the stable, ordered state have disappeared. This is not very surprising, since we would expect that, if we decreased the specificity S, there should come a point at which the ordered state is no longer viable.

  This observation leads us naturally to the question: What is the minimum value S_T of S, for fixed values of λ and n, at which there is a stable, ordered state? This will occur when the line $q_i = q_{i-1}$ is tangent to the curve and so we must satisfy the two conditions

$$\left.\frac{\partial q_i}{\partial q_{i-1}}\right|_{q_{i-1}=q_T} = 1 \qquad\qquad (5.19)$$

and

$$q_i = q_{i-1} \equiv q_T \qquad\qquad (5.20)$$

where q_T is the value of q at which the curves are tangent.

  We apply these conditions to eqn (5.18). The first condition yields

$$\frac{n(S_T - 1)q_T^n(\lambda - 1)}{q_T[(S_T - 1)q_T^n + \lambda]^2} = 1 \qquad (5.21)$$

and the second gives

$$(S_T - 1)q_T^n = \frac{\lambda q_T - 1}{1 - q_T}. \qquad (5.22)$$

Combining these two equations gives a quadratic in q_T:

$$n\lambda q_T^2 - (n\lambda - \lambda + n + 1)q_T + n = 0. \qquad (5.23)$$

The two possibilities for q_T are therefore

$$q_T = \frac{1}{2n\lambda}[n\lambda - \lambda + n + 1 \pm \sqrt{[\lambda(n-1) + (n+1)]^2 - 4n^2\lambda}]. \qquad (5.24)$$

Using the identity

$$[\lambda(n-1) + (n+1)]^2 = [\lambda(n-1) - (n+1)]^2 + 4n^2\lambda - 4\lambda \qquad (5.25)$$

we can express the roots in the form

$$q_T = \frac{1}{2}\left(1 - \frac{1}{n} + \frac{1}{\lambda} + \frac{1}{n\lambda}\right) \pm \frac{1}{2n\lambda}\sqrt{[\lambda(n-1) - (n+1)]^2 - 4\lambda}. \qquad (5.26)$$

Now, if $[\lambda(n-1) - (n+1)]^2 \gg 4\lambda$ (reasonable, since both λ and n are likely to be around 10), and we choose the $+$ sign in the above equation, we may use the approximation

$$\sqrt{1 - x} \approx 1 - \frac{1}{2}x \qquad (5.27)$$

to obtain

$$q_T \approx 1 - \frac{1}{n} - \frac{1}{(\lambda - 1)n^2} \qquad (5.28)$$

and

$$S_T \approx [n(\lambda - 1) - \frac{1}{2}(\lambda + 1)]e + 1. \qquad (5.29)$$

The last equation uses the approximation

$$\left(1 - \frac{1}{n}\right)^n \approx \frac{1}{e}\left(1 - \frac{1}{2n}\right) \qquad (5.30)$$

where e is the base of natural logarithms. The approximation may be verified by taking logarithms of both sides and expanding in a Taylor series.

We have ignored the value of q_T obtained if one takes the negative sign in eqn (5.26), as its meaning is something quite different than what we are interested in at the moment. This value of q_T gives the condition for the smallest specificity for which the disordered equilibrium state exists.

When $n = 8$ and $\lambda = 5$, we find that the minimum value of the specificity for which there exists an ordered state is $S_T \approx 80$, with a corresponding $q_T \approx 0.87$. Such a specificity is not difficult to imagine in a primitive system. Differences in specificity can be due to various causes, but the most likely is a difference in the strength with which the correct and incorrect amino acids are bound. If one assumes that this is the only effect giving rise to the specificity, it is possible to show, using arguments from thermodynamics, that a specificity of 80 can arise from binding energy differences equivalent to only one or two of the weaker types of chemical bond. (See Hoffmann (1974) for a more complete discussion.) In other words, a relatively crude molecular system can give rise to the sort of discrimination between amino acids necessary to construct a stable translation system.

5.5.1   The specificity and activity of the adaptors

Hoffmann's assumption of a much lower activity for the non-specific adaptors and his resulting recursion relation (5.18) has come in for some criticism. Kirkwood *et al.* (1975) have listed several enzymes whose non-specific forms have activities approaching those of their specific forms. They proposed a revised version of Hoffmann's model in which the total activity of a non-specific protein is a fraction R, $0 \leq R \leq 1$, of the activity of the specific proteins. That is, given that the total activity (the total rate at which an adaptor molecule incorporates amino acids, both correctly and incorrectly) of the specific adaptor is $\alpha + (\lambda - 1)\alpha/S$, we simply define the total activity rate of the non-specific adaptor to be $R[\alpha + (\lambda - 1)\alpha/S]$. Doing this results in the following revised formula for q_i:

$$q_i = \frac{q_{i-1}^n[\lambda S - (S + \lambda - 1)R] + (S + \lambda - 1)R}{q_{i-1}^n \lambda(S + \lambda - 1)(1 - R) + \lambda(S + \lambda - 1)R}. \tag{5.31}$$

This equation is equivalent to eqn (5.18) if $R = \lambda/(S+\lambda-1)$. For typical values of λ and S, R in Hoffmann's model is of the order of 0.05 or less (that is, the non-specific adaptors have activities $1/20$ or less than those of the specific adaptors). Kirkwood *et al.* point out that, if R is much higher than this, Hoffmann's conclusions cease to be valid. However, Kirkwood *et al.* are primarily concerned with an application of Hoffmann's model as an explanation of the effects of ageing. Hoffmann had claimed that, contrary to what some workers had proposed, it is not possible for a slight increase in the error rate in protein production (as might occur when an organism ages) to lead to an 'error catastrophe' (a rapid rise in the error rate) because his model showed that once a protein production system converges on the upper stable point in his model, it will tend to stay there so that any slight increase in the error rate will be damped out. Kirkwood *et al.* mention several proteins, some of which are found in the RNA/DNA to protein translation system, which retain most of their activity even when they lose their specificity. In such cases, R is considerably larger than what Hoffmann has assumed with the result that no stable point exists in the model. However, the enzymes cited by Kirkwood *et al.* are all highly evolved molecules found in present-day organisms and it is not clear whether such efficient molecules would have been present in the primitive environment.

6

Hypercycles

6.1 Introduction

We now return to the problem last mentioned in Chapter 2: how can we devise a model in which more information than that contained in single 100-base RNA molecules can be maintained over many generations?

There are two main approaches that have been taken to this problem. The first is that of the proteins-first advocates: in order to give an information system a chance to develop, we must provide semi-isolated compartments in which molecular evolution can proceed relatively unmolested by the outside world. The second is that of the nucleic acids-first group: some sort of chemical reaction scheme must be found which is self-perpetuating, even in relatively dilute solutions.

Both of these arguments have their merits, but unfortunately, there is no quantitative theoretical model based on the compartmentation approach. As a result, the model which is presented in this chapter will give an un-intended bias towards the RNA/DNA-first approach, although we will see that the theory leaves many problems unsolved and many questions and criticisms unanswered.

The hypercycle model is developed in three large papers by Eigen and Schuster (1977, 1978a, 1978b). Its starting point is the observation that *catalytic chains* and *catalytic cycles* are common in all modern organisms, and therefore must have evolved at some stage near the origin of life. A catalytic chain is a sequence of chemical reactions where the product of one reaction is needed as a reactant in the next. A cycle is merely a closed chain: if there are n separate reactions, the product of the nth reaction is needed as a reactant in the first. Although Eigen and Schuster include a peripheral discussion of chemical cycles in general and a review of current ideas on such things as the origin of the genetic code, the actual quantitative theory concentrates entirely on the analysis of the systems of differential equations used to describe such catalytic cycles. The goal of this analysis is to show that such cycles allow many quasi-species (in the sense of Chapter 2) of molecules to co-exist in such a way that all quasi-species will be maintained over many generations. It is also postulated that a catalytic cycle can enlarge itself by including extra species within itself and, by so doing, increase its capacity for storing and transmitting information.

In order for the reader to make a more informed judgement on the applicability of the hypercycle model to the origin of life, we will first present the theory and defer until later a discussion of how Eigen and Schuster have interpreted their results. A sampling of the criticisms that have been levelled at this interpretation will follow as well.

6.2 The rate equations

The differential equations studied in the hypercycle model apply to any cyclical chemical reaction system, biological or otherwise. In anticipation of the biological application, however, the reader should picture each chemical species as either one of the quasi-species discussed in Chapter 2, or as one of the successful sequence families in the spin glass model of Anderson and Stein discussed in Chapter 4. The hypercycle model assumes that a collection of such species has accumulated and that some sort of cyclic connection has been established between two or more of these species. We will consider a system of n such species, where the population level or concentration of species i is given by $x_i(t)$, with $i = 1, \ldots, n$. In general, the time dependence of the collection of species is given by a system of first-order ordinary differential equations (ODEs):

$$\dot{x}_i = \Lambda_i(x_1, \ldots, x_n; k_1, \ldots, k_m; t) \qquad\qquad i = 1, \ldots, n \qquad (6.1)$$

where Λ_i is some, in general non-linear, function of its arguments, the k_is are parameters and t is the time.

As we mentioned in Chapter 3 and reinforced in Chapter 4, a model of the prebiotic soup based purely on differential equations can make predictions only about the average behaviour of the system. In a system consisting of a large number of species, each representing a fairly small fraction of the total population, such average predictions are not likely to be particularly accurate for any single system. After studying the results obtained from the hypercycle model, it would therefore be useful to extend one of the stochastic treatments given in Chapters 3 and 4 to deal with catalytic cycles. In fact, Anderson and Stein have extended their original model to do just that (see Stein and Anderson (1984)).

In all the cases with which we shall be concerned, the ODEs will be autonomous, that is, there is no explicit dependence on the time t. If we define the vectors

$$\mathbf{x} = \begin{bmatrix} x_1 \\ x_2 \\ \vdots \\ x_n \end{bmatrix}; \qquad\qquad \mathbf{k} = \begin{bmatrix} k_1 \\ k_2 \\ \vdots \\ k_m \end{bmatrix} \qquad (6.2)$$

then such an autonomous system can be written as

$$\dot{x}_i = \Lambda_i(\mathbf{x}, \mathbf{k}) \qquad (6.3)$$

We may split the contributions to each function Λ_i into two parts: those arising from chemical processes such as reactions or degradation of the molecules, and those arising from fluxes or flows into or out of the system. We shall represent the first part by the symbol Γ_i and the second by ϕ_i, so that we have

$$\dot{x}_i = \Gamma_i + \phi_i. \qquad (6.4)$$

At this point we must make some decision as to what sort of system we are going to study. This involves choosing forms for the reaction terms Γ_i and the flux terms ϕ_i. We will suppose, as in Chapter 2, that the flux of species i is proportional to some overall flux $\phi(t)$ and to the fraction of the total population represented by that species. That is, we assume

$$\phi_i(t) = \frac{x_i(t)}{c(t)}\phi(t) \qquad (6.5)$$

where $c(t)$ is the total population or concentration of all species:

$$c(t) = \sum_{i=1}^{n} x_i(t). \qquad (6.6)$$

The rate of change of the total concentration is then

$$\dot{c} = \sum_i \dot{x}_i = \sum_i \Gamma_i + \phi \qquad (6.7)$$

We see, therefore, that we may constrain the system by specifying either a condition on the total concentration c or on the overall flux ϕ, but not both, since one is determined by the other. For example, we may decide to impose the constraint that the total concentration remains constant, so that $\dot{c} = 0$ and $c(t) = c_0 = \text{constant}$. In this case,

$$\sum_i \Gamma_i = -\phi \qquad (6.8)$$

and

$$\dot{x}_i = \Gamma_i - \frac{x_i}{c_0} \sum_j \Gamma_j. \tag{6.9}$$

In the general case, the total concentration need not be constant, so that

$$\dot{x}_i = \Gamma_i + \frac{x_i}{c}\phi = \Gamma_i - \frac{x_i}{c} \sum_j \Gamma_j + \frac{x_i}{c}\dot{c} \tag{6.10}$$

We now introduce normalized coordinates

$$\xi_i \equiv \frac{x_i}{c} \tag{6.11}$$

so that

$$\dot{\xi}_i = \frac{\dot{x}_i}{c} - \frac{x_i}{c^2}\dot{c}. \tag{6.12}$$

Then, from eqn (6.10) we have

$$\dot{\xi}_i = \frac{1}{c}\left[\Gamma_i(\mathbf{x}) - \xi_i \sum_j \Gamma_j(\mathbf{x})\right]. \tag{6.13}$$

We must now convert Γ_i from a function of $\mathbf{x}$ to a function of ξ. To do this, we may recall the discussion from Section 3.5 on constructing terms in differential equations describing chemical reactions (the law of mass action). If one way of producing of a new molecule of species i is by means of an interaction between a molecule of species i and another of species j, then a term $k_l x_i x_j$ is present in the differential equation for x_i. The parameter k_l is the rate constant, which describes how fast the reaction proceeds.

For example, suppose we have a system with 3 molecular species. If the production of a molecule of species 1 can occur either when a molecule of species 1 and another of species 2 meet and interact, or when a molecule of type 1 reproduces itself without outside help, the form of Γ_1 would be

$$\Gamma_1 = k_1 x_1 x_2 + k_2 x_1 \tag{6.14}$$

where k_1 is the rate at which the (species 1)–(species 2) reaction takes place, and k_2 is the rate at which species 1 can reproduce itself.

Obviously, many possibilities exist for the various Γ_is, depending on what we assume about the various chemical pathways for producing each species. A particularly simple form for the equations is obtained if we assume that all the Γ_is are *homogeneous* polynomials of degree p of the x_is. By homogeneous of degree p, we mean that all terms in each Γ_i have precisely p factors of x_i. The example in eqn (6.14) is not homogeneous, since one term has two x_is in it while the other has only one. A homogeneous polynomial of degree $p = 2$ is, for example,

$$\Gamma_i = k_1 x_1 x_2 + k_2 x_2 x_3. \tag{6.15}$$

This condition is equivalent to assuming that all reactions that produce molecules of any species require the same number of reactants to come together. While this is certainly not true in higher organisms, it is probably not a bad approximation in a primitive situation where solutions of such molecules would be very dilute. In such cases, it is unlikely that any reaction requiring more than two reactants would progress very far, since the chance of 3 or more molecules arriving at the same place within a reasonably short time span would be very small.

If we assume that all the Γ_is are homogeneous polynomials of degree p, the conversion from x_i to ξ_i becomes

$$\Gamma_i(\mathbf{x}) = c^p \Gamma_i(\xi) \tag{6.16}$$

and the differential equations become

$$\dot{\xi}_i = c^{p-1} \left[\Gamma_i(\xi) - \xi_i \sum_j \Gamma_j(\xi) \right]. \tag{6.17}$$

The dependence on the total concentration is now restricted to the single factor of c^{p-1}. Provided that the concentration remains finite and non-zero, the fixed points (the points at which all the concentrations remain constant, so that $\dot{\xi}_i = 0$ for all i) of this system are the same whether the concentration remains constant or not.

6.3   The concentration simplex

The concentration variables x_i, $i = 1, \ldots, n$ are all non-negative quantities: $0 \leq x_i < \infty$. Thus the normalized variables ξ_i satisfy the two conditions

$$0 \leq \xi_i \leq 1, \qquad i = 1, \ldots, n \qquad \sum_{i=1}^{n} \xi_i = 1. \tag{6.18}$$

The region spanned by the set of ξ values is called a *simplex*. Geometrically, a simplex is an $n - 1$ dimensional regular polyhedron with n vertices. For example, if $n = 3$, the corresponding simplex is an equilateral triangle (Fig. 6.1).

The simplex is always embedded in an n-dimensional space corresponding to the true concentration variables x_i. For $n = 3$, the triangular simplex rests in a 3-dimensional space with its vertices lying on the three coordinate axes (Fig. 6.2). To find the point on the simplex corresponding to a particular set of concentrations x_i, draw a line from the origin to the

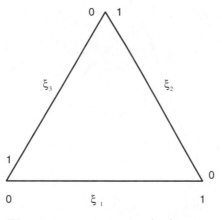

Figure 6.1   A simplex for 3 species.

point representing the concentration configuration. The point where this line intersects the simplex gives the corresponding values of the ξ_i variables (Fig. 6.2).

Representing the location of a system on a simplex rather than in the full n-dimensional space has the advantage of allowing us to follow the evolution of a 3 species system on a two-dimensional diagram. In those cases where the behaviour of the system is independent of the total concentration c (that is, when the functions Γ_i are homogeneous) the fixed points in the normalized coordinates do not change when c is changed. Thus the actual location of a fixed point in x_i space can be obtained for any size system by finding the vector in ξ_i space extending from the origin to the fixed point on the simplex and simply multiplying it by c.

However, we know from the previous section that, if the functions Γ_i are not homogeneous polynomials in the concentration variables x_i, the locations of the fixed points when the system is represented in the normalized coordinates ξ_i are not independent of the total concentration c. In other words, if we locate a fixed point on the simplex by working with the ξ_i variables, we cannot obtain the corresponding fixed point in the x_i variables by just multiplying by c. In those cases where Γ_i is not homogeneous, it is often easier to work directly with the x_i variables.

Plotting a point in a triangular simplex is easy enough if you remember that the coordinate axes are not orthogonal. Lines of constant ξ_i are parallel to the ξ_{i-1} axis, where the subscripts are cyclic, so that lines of constant ξ_1 are parallel to the ξ_3 axis.

For example, to plot the point $[0.25, 0.25, 0.5]$ in the simplex where the

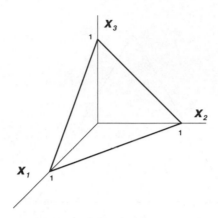

Figure 6.2   The 3-species simplex embedded in three-dimensional space.

base of the triangle corresponds to the ξ_1 axis, the right side to the ξ_2 axis and the left side to the ξ_3 axis, we draw lines corresponding to $\xi_1 = 0.25 =$ constant and $\xi_2 = 0.25 =$ constant, which are parallel to the ξ_3 and ξ_1 axes respectively (Fig. 6.3).

The point where these two lines intersect is the required position. Notice that it is not necessary to draw in the third line corresponding to $\xi_3 = 0.5$, since the summation condition $\sum_i \xi_i = 1$ determines the value of ξ_3 automatically once ξ_1 and ξ_2 have been specified.

6.4   An example: The linear growth rate

As a simple example of the above theory we will consider the case of a system where all the molecules obey a linear growth law, that is, each species' growth rate depends only on how many of that species are present at time t. In this case, we have

$$\Gamma_i = k_i x_i \tag{6.19}$$

so that $p = 1$ in eqn (6.17):

$$\dot{\xi}_i = k_i \xi_i - \xi_i \sum_j k_j \xi_j. \tag{6.20}$$

We must first find the fixed points, which occur at those values $\bar{\xi}_i$ of ξ_i such that $\dot{\xi}_i = 0$ for all i. This condition results in

$$\bar{\xi}_i \left(k_i - \sum_j k_j \bar{\xi}_j \right) = 0. \tag{6.21}$$

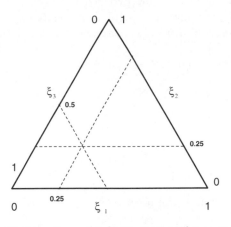

Figure 6.3   Plotting the point $[0.25, 0.25, 0.5]$ in a 3-species simplex.

For any set of values of $\bar{\xi}_j$, $j = 1, \ldots, n$, the sum $\sum_j k_j \bar{\xi}_j$ can, of course, take only one value. Thus if eqn (6.21) is to be satisfied for all values of i, and all the rate constants k_i are different, we can have $\bar{\xi}_i \neq 0$ for at most one value of i, say $i = l$. Recalling that the ξ_j coordinates are normalized so that their sum is unity, we must have

$$\bar{\xi}_i = \delta_{il} \tag{6.22}$$

for some value of l, where δ_{il} is the Kronecker delta. There are therefore n different equilibria, each consisting of a pure state, that is, one in which there is only one species present.

To check the local stability (see appendix A for the mathematical details of the technique we are about to use) of each of these fixed points, we can perform a perturbation. We replace $\bar{\xi}_i$ by $\bar{\xi}_i + z_i$ in eqn (6.20), where z_i is the small perturbation. We obtain, after multiplying out terms and rearranging:

$$\dot{z}_i = \left[k_i \bar{\xi}_i - \bar{\xi}_i \sum_j k_j \bar{\xi}_j \right] + z_i \left(k_i - \sum_j k_j \bar{\xi}_j \right) - \bar{\xi}_i \sum_j k_j z_j + \mathcal{O}(z^2). \tag{6.23}$$

The term in square brackets is zero, since it is merely the condition for equilibrium (see eqn (6.21)). The linearized equation for the perturbations is then

$$\dot{z}_i = z_i(k_i - \sum_j k_j \bar{\xi}_j) - \bar{\xi}_i \sum_j k_j z_j. \tag{6.24}$$

In the general case we would now proceed to check the stability of each equilibrium in turn by substituting the appropriate expression in place of $\bar{\xi}_i$. In this case, the equilibria have particularly simple forms, so we can check all of them at once.

Using the condition that $\bar{\xi}_i = \delta_{il}$ we have

$$\dot{z}_i = k_i z_i - z_i \sum_j k_j \delta_{jl} - \delta_{il} \sum_j k_j z_j \qquad (6.25)$$

or

$$\dot{z}_i = \begin{cases} -\sum_j k_j z_j & \text{if } i = l \\ z_i(k_i - k_l) & \text{if } i \neq l \end{cases} \qquad (6.26)$$

which can be written in the form (see appendix A)

$$\dot{\mathbf{z}} = B\mathbf{z} \qquad (6.27)$$

where the matrix B is

$$B = \begin{bmatrix} (k_1 - k_l) & 0 & 0 & \cdots & 0 \\ 0 & (k_2 - k_l) & 0 & \cdots & 0 \\ & & \vdots & & \\ -k_1 & -k_2 & -k_3 & \cdots & -k_n \\ & & \vdots & & \\ 0 & 0 & 0 & \cdots & (k_n - k_l) \end{bmatrix} \qquad (6.28)$$

where the row with the non-zero off-diagonal elements is the lth row. The eigenvalues of B are thus the $n - 1$ quantities $k_i - k_l$ for $i \neq l$, and $-k_l$.

Since rate constants are necessarily positive, and we have assumed them to be all different, we see that if k_l is the largest rate constant, all the eigenvalues are negative. If k_l is the smallest rate constant, all the eigenvalues (except $-k_l$) are positive. For this and all other cases where k_l is not the largest constant, there is a mixture of positive and negative eigenvalues. There is therefore only one stable equilibrium consisting of a population containing only the species with the highest rate constant. The other equilibria are all unstable to varying degrees. The common sense chemical explanation of these results is simply that the species that can reproduce itself the fastest eventually takes over the population, so that all other species become insignificant in comparison.

6.5   Catalytic chains

The above example would not serve as a model of the beginnings of catalysis, since it permits the survival of only one species, regardless of how many arc present to begin with. Of course, no catalytic links were built into the model, so we should not be surprised that its behaviour is rather sterile. It seems to be a general feature of models lacking any sort of cyclic link that only one of the original species survives, even if some of the molecules depend on others for their creation. For example, consider a chain of n molecular species where the rate of change of species i depends on both the concentrations of species i and $i-1$ (except for species 1, which is entirely autocatalytic).

The rate equation for species 1 is then

$$\dot{x}_1 = k_1 x_1 + \phi_1 \tag{6.29}$$

where ϕ_1 is a flow term. The remaining $n-1$ species can reproduce either autocatalytically, or with the help of one other species in the set. We therefore have

$$\dot{x}_i = k_i x_i + k'_i x_i x_{i-1} + \phi_i \qquad i = 2, \ldots, n \tag{6.30}$$

where the k_i and k'_i are rate constants.

The forms of the flow terms ϕ_i depend on what constraints we impose on the system. If we choose the usual constraint of constant total concentration c_0 and assume, as we did when discussing the quasi-species model in Chapter 2, that the flow term for each species is proportional to its concentration, we have the two conditions

$$\sum_i x_i = c_0; \qquad\qquad \phi_i = x_i \Phi \tag{6.31}$$

where Φ is a function of the concentration vector $\mathbf{x}$ which is the same for all species.

The constant concentration constraint can be used to derive the form of Φ:

$$\sum_j \dot{x}_j = 0 = \sum_{j=1}^{n} k_j x_j + \sum_{j=2}^{n} k'_j x_j x_{j-1} + \Phi \sum_{j=1}^{n} x_j \tag{6.32}$$

so

$$\Phi = -\frac{1}{c_0}\left[\sum_{j=1}^{n} k_j x_j + \sum_{j=2}^{n} k'_j x_j x_{j-1}\right]. \tag{6.33}$$

The system of differential equations thus becomes

$$\dot{x}_1 = k_1 x_1 - \frac{x_1}{c_0}\left[\sum_{j=1}^{n} k_j x_j + \sum_{j=2}^{n} k'_j x_j x_{j-1}\right] \tag{6.34}$$

and, for $i = 2, \ldots, n$:

$$\dot{x}_i = k_i x_i + k'_i x_i x_{i-1} - \frac{x_i}{c_0} \left[\sum_{j=1}^{n} k_j x_j + \sum_{j=2}^{n} k'_j x_j x_{j-1} \right]. \qquad (6.35)$$

These equations are *not* homogeneous, so we cannot ignore the total concentration in the fixed point analysis, as we did in the preceding example.

There turn out to be a fair number of fixed points for this system, but there is only one where all n species are present. The components of this point are

$$\bar{x}_i = \frac{k_1 - k_{i+1}}{k'_{i+1}} \qquad i = 1, \ldots, n-1 \qquad (6.36)$$

$$\bar{x}_n = c_0 - \sum_{j=1}^{n-1} \bar{x}_j. \qquad (6.37)$$

In order for this fixed point to even exist in the system, k_1 must be the largest rate constant (otherwise some of the equilibrium concentration values will be negative), and c_0 must be large enough for $\bar{x}_n$ to be positive. The first condition is reasonable, since species 1 must support the synthesis of itself and all other species in the chain.

As might be imagined by looking at the form of the equations, the linearization procedure is very tedious here. The matrix B has no simple form, but it can be seen, either by constructing B directly, or by numerical solution of the equations, that in any case where this fixed point exists, it is stable, while all the other fixed points containing fewer than n species are unstable to some degree.

Although such a situation looks encouraging, there are a number of worrying aspects. We would like the equilibrium point to be fairly robust against environmental changes, that is, if the rate constants or total concentration value should change, we would like the equilibrium to remain in existence. That will not happen here. What is particularly worrying is that, should c_0 drop below a certain critical level, the equilibrium disappears. It is likely that primitive solutions would have been fairly dilute, so we would like processes that can proceed even in 'thin' solutions.

Another problem is that, as the concentration becomes richer so that c_0 increases, only the nth species will increase its representation. We would prefer a system where all species increased in population size together.

6.6   Catalytic cycles

The hypercycle is suggested by the cyclic property of the DNA–protein synthesis reactions in modern organisms. DNA contains the information

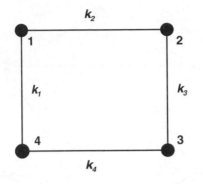

Figure 6.4   A 4-species hypercycle.

for constructing proteins, which are in turn necessary to construct more DNA. The flaw in the linear catalytic chain studied in the last section is that there is no feedback from the last species in the chain to the first. To correct this problem, we take the simple step of closing the loop by requiring the last species as a catalyst for the production of the first.

The actual chemical system envisaged by Eigen and Schuster is as follows. We suppose we have n different species of 'information molecules' I_i (such as RNA or DNA sequences), each of which contains the instructions for manufacturing one protein E_i. This protein is assumed to be a 'replicase' whose function is to recognize and translate the next information molecule I_{i+1} into its replicase E_{i+1}. Thus the rate of change of species i depends on how many replicases E_{i-1} and how many information molecules I_i are present.

There are various ways in which this can be done, but to keep things reasonably simple at this stage, we will assume homogeneous rate terms. For example, in a hypercycle with four species, the interactions may be as shown in Fig. 6.4.

In this case, each species relies on itself and one other species in the chain for its own reproduction. The rate term for species 1, for example, is

$$\Gamma_1 = k_1 x_1 x_4 \tag{6.38}$$

since species 1 requires one of its own molecules and one of species 4 to produce another copy of a species 1 molecule.

A more complicated example would be as shown in Fig. 6.5. Here, we have 6 species, and each species requires 2 other species besides itself for reproduction. In this case, the rate terms are all of degree 3. A typical rate term is that for species 1:

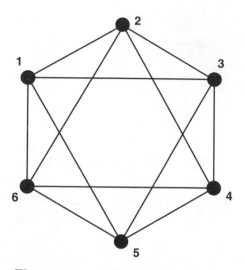

Figure 6.5   A 6-species hypercycle.

$$\Gamma_1 = k_1 x_1 x_5 x_6. \tag{6.39}$$

A general hypercyclic system will have n species in the loop, with p species participating in each reaction. (Of course, in an even more general system, we need not restrict ourselves to having the same number of species in each reaction, but in such cases the rate equations are no longer homogeneous.) The rate term in such a system will have the general form

$$\Gamma_i = k_i \underbrace{x_i x_j x_k \ldots x_r}_{p \text{ factors}} \qquad i = 1, \ldots, n \tag{6.40}$$

where the indices j, k, ..., r denote all the other species participating in the reaction that produces a copy of species i.

If we impose the constraint of constant concentration, then the system of ODEs obeyed by the species in a hypercycle becomes, using eqn (6.10)

$$\dot{x}_i = k_i x_i x_j \ldots x_l - \frac{x_i}{c_0} \sum k_r x_r x_s \ldots x_t \tag{6.41}$$

where the sum is taken over all sets of indices $\{r, s, \ldots, t\}$ such that the resulting product of factors is one of the rate terms Γ_i. In general, there will be n such terms in the sum.

The general fixed point analysis is very difficult to do analytically. In the special case where all the rate constants are equal, that is, $k_1 = k_2 =$

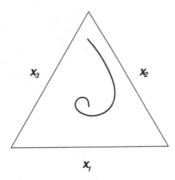

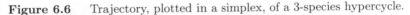

Figure 6.6   Trajectory, plotted in a simplex, of a 3-species hypercycle.

$\cdots = k_n \equiv k$, the analysis is somewhat easier. This is a very artificial case, however, and for any proper understanding of hypercycle behaviour, a wide variety of numerical simulations should be carried out.

The fixed point analysis of the equal rate constants case is carried out by methods given in appendix A. We find that when n (the number of species) is 2, 3, or 4, there is one fixed point with all species present, and this fixed point is asymptotically stable. For $n \geq 5$, a stable limit cycle appears in which all species participate. That is, all species remain present for all times, but they oscillate in quantity.

See Figs. 6.6–6.8 for some sample plots of the trajectories for $n = 3, 4, 5$.

The theory of the hypercycle equations is given in much more detail in Eigen and Schuster's papers, especially Eigen and Schuster (1978a). In them can be found, for example, analytic proofs that the fixed points are asymptotically stable for $n = 2, 3, 4$. In addition, many examples of numerical solution of the equations for cases where not all rate constants are equal are given. The general conclusion from these studies is that the hypercycle equations virtually always have either a stable fixed point or a stable limit cycle in which all species are present, so that they provide a chemical system in which all the information present in a set of molecules can be maintained over long times. One can envisage hypercycles encompassing more and more information by inserting extra links in the chain as more information-carrying molecules evolve.

6.7   Hypercycles and the origin of life

We now examine in more detail Eigen and Schuster's application of the hypercycle model to the origin of life.

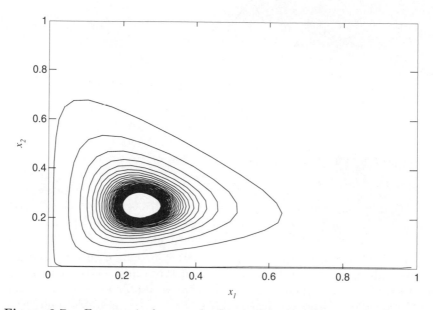

Figure 6.7   Four species hypercycle. Species 2 is plotted vs. species 1, showing the slow convergence to the stable equilibrium. The 'hole' in the plot would eventually be filled in as the trajectory approached the equilibrium.

The catalytic cycle envisaged as a primitive information processing system is shown schematically in Fig. 6.10.

Each information storing molecule I_i is assumed to store the code required to synthesize a catalytic molecule E_i. The catalyst E_i is then assumed to have a strong chemical affinity for the next information molecule I_{i+1}, which in turn contains the code for the next catalyst E_{i+1}.

There are several problems with this interpretation. Perhaps the most obvious is that this is not the way in which modern organisms deal with information in the DNA sequence. Rather than having a separate catalyst for each gene, there is one set of catalysts that serve as translators for all genes. Of course, there are many proteins other than those that assign amino acids to tRNA molecules, some of which are required to activate a particular region of DNA so that it can be translated to produce a specific protein, so it could be argued that the modern organism actually does have a cyclic loop with more than just two members (the DNA and the proteins). Still, if hypercycles actually were present during the early evolution of

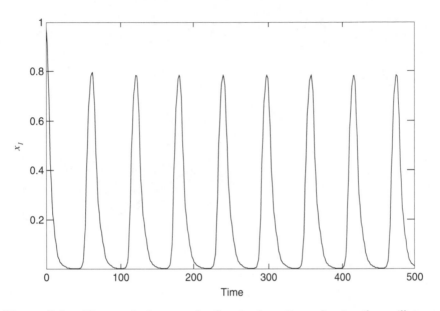

Figure 6.8 Five species hypercycle. Species 1 vs. time, showing the oscillatory behaviour.

life, there is a large conceptual gap between the hypercyclic stage and the current information processing system.

One other problem is that the only molecules that are actually being replicated in the above scenario are the proteins. The information molecules (DNA or RNA) are just sitting there as reference books that are consulted but not replicated themselves. In order to allow the hypercycle model above to be interpreted accurately, we need to assume that the information molecules are replicated each time they are translated, and therefore that the same protein that translates the RNA also is a catalyst for its replication. Eigen and Schuster (1978a) get around this by proposing that 'polynucleotides [DNA or RNA] and polypeptides [proteins] form specific complexes that are also catalytically active in the synthesis of polynucleotide copies'. In other words, they propose that proteins and DNA can associate in some way so that they form an enzyme that replicates the information molecules I_i. They briefly consider some kinetic equations to analyse this case, but they do not present a strong case for it.

The hypercycle theory has come in for a great deal of criticism from

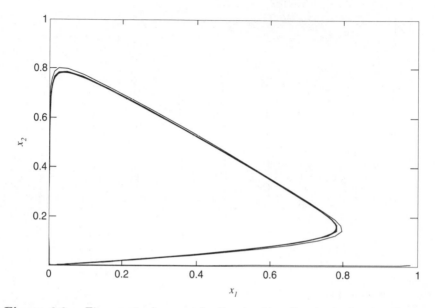

Figure 6.9   Five species hypercycle. Species 2 vs. Species 1, showing the limit cycle.

other authors, perhaps partly because of the way the theory was originally presented. The trilogy of papers by Eigen and Schuster in which the theory is laid out are written in a rather grandiose style, and it is easy to come away from them with the impression that the question of the origin of life has been settled once and for all.

In addition to the problems mentioned above, several others have been raised in the literature. A good summary of the critiques can be found in Bresch *et al.* (1980) and Wicken (1985). We will discuss a few of these problems here.

The hypercycle differential equations implicitly assume that replicase E_i has an affinity only for molecule I_i, or at least a much higher affinity for I_i than for any other information molecule. This is inherent in the fact that only rate terms of the form $k_i X_i X_{i+1}$ are present in the equations, and not terms of the form $k_i X_i X_{i+2}$, $k_i X_i X_{i+3}$, and so on. Eigen and Schuster have shown that such a structure is stable against fluctuations in population number, but this sort of strict interdependence makes the hypercycle quite vulnerable to mutations. For example, if replicase E_i

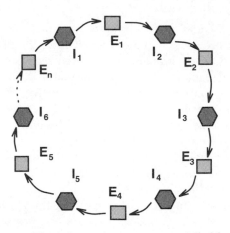

Figure 6.10   The information system modelled by hypercycles.

mutated so that it now has a high affinity for I_{i+2}, say, instead of I_i, the cycle has been effectively short-circuited, since molecules I_i and I_{i+1} have been excluded from the loop and the information they contain is lost.

It is also possible for an information molecule I_i to mutate into a so-called parasite which still has an affinity for its replicase E_i but no longer produces the correct code for the next replicase in the cycle E_{i+1}. In such a case, the cycle is broken and the whole loop collapses. Of course, it is also possible for a mutation to cause a replicase E_i to cease having an affinity for any of the information molecules, in which case the loop also collapses.

The technique of loop growth is seen as highly improbable by many people. In order for a hypercycle of size n species to increase its size by one species, an information molecule I_{n+1} and its corresponding replicase E_{n+1} must simultaneously appear in such a way that replicase E_n has a higher affinity for I_{n+1} than for I_1 (the molecule it used to translate) and that replicase E_{n+1} has a higher affinity for I_1 than for any other information molecule in the loop. The larger the cycle gets, the more difficult it is to convince oneself that molecules with such precise affinities will appear.

There are several other problems of a biochemical nature that are discussed by Wicken (for example, the likelihood of such a limited set of molecules having so many biochemical properties—replication of the DNA, translation of the DNA, implementation of a genetic code, and so on), but unfortunately no one has yet produced a quantitative alternative theory to compete with the hypercycle model.

6.8   Stochastic simulation

Since the hypercycle equations are non-linear, analysing them using the theory of stochastic processes is more difficult than the linear case considered in Chapter 3. One such attempt has been made by Ishida in 1986, who uses a similar technique to that of Jones and Leung (1981) referred to in Chapter 3. He finds that hypercycles can give rise to increasingly large fluctuations in population sizes. Rather than explore this analytic treatment which can only give information on the means and variances of the population, we will examine a detailed computer simulation.

The hypercycle equations represent chemical reactions, so we can apply Gillespie's method (described in Section 3.5) to generate a stochastic simulation of a hypercycle.

For a two-species system with equal rate constants (chosen here to be $k = 0.0001$), the stochastic simulation roughly agrees with the solution to the differential equation model: the two species converge on a stable equilibrium point where both are present.

For a five-species system with equal rate constants (still using $k = 0.0001$) we see the beginnings of a limit cycle in the simulation, but soon one of the species dies out. When this happens, of course, the hypercycle is broken and all other species die out, since each species depends on the one preceding it in the cycle to survive. Some inkling that this sort of thing would happen should have been gleaned from examining the limit cycle solutions to the differential equations, since on one part of the cycle the population levels of some species approach perilously close to zero (see Fig. 6.8). In practice, every time the simulation of a five species cycle was run (with different random number seeds and varying initial conditions) the system died out after less than one circuit around the limit cycle (Fig. 6.11).

The moral: there is still a long way to go before we have a good theory of the origin of life.

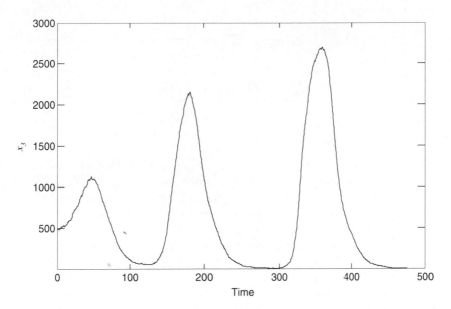

Figure 6.11 A stochastic simulation of a 5 species hypercycle, showing species 1 as a function of time.

7
Artificial life

7.1 Introduction

One of the problems in the study of the origin of life is that we have only one example of a biosystem to study. There may be other examples of life elsewhere in the universe (despite the negative findings of the Viking mission to Mars, scientists have not totally ruled out the possibility of life there) but, discounting some of the more inventive reports of UFOs, the only system available to us for direct study is that of which we are a part.

The uniqueness of life has naturally led to such questions as 'How probable is life?', 'What conditions are necessary for life to arise?' and 'What is the most general definition of life?'. Recent attempts to answer these questions have led to the field of *artificial life.*

Although the ideas behind artificial life can be traced back to the mathematician and originator of much of computer science, John von Neumann, in the 1940s and 1950s, interest in the field has only become more widespread with the advent of fast, powerful computers in the 1980s and 1990s. The first major conference on artificial life was held in 1988 at the Sante Fe Institute in New Mexico. Since that time, interest in the field has been growing steadily.

One of the aims of artificial life is to provide new and different systems which display the properties we commonly associate with life, but without the underlying carbon chemistry of 'real' life. If we can construct such new life forms inside the computer's memory, we can study the conditions necessary for its creation and evolution. The more 'living' systems of this sort we can study, the better will be our understanding of the principles behind the origin and evolution of carbon-based life, or so the proponents of artificial life will have us believe.

In its attempts to create new life forms, artificial life uses the so-called *bottom-up* approach. We assume the existence of small, simple components which interact with each other according to simple, local rules.[1] If we

---

[1] Although the goal of artificial life is to create new forms of life, it may help the reader to think of components such as nucleotides and amino acids interacting through local chemical bonds. It must be remembered, however, that the components in artificial

have constructed our components properly and specified the right local interactions, we should see some sort of 'life' arise out of initial chaos if we release some of these components and let them interact over time.

For such an experiment to be successful, we need to know what we are looking for as a result. In other words, if we are hoping to create life in a silicon chip, how will we know when we have done it?

This is a surprisingly difficult question. Although we may think we understand what we mean by 'life', trying to formulate a precise definition is not easy. Even when we settle on a definition, we are still faced with the problem of applying the definition to our computer model.

As a start, let us cast our minds back to Chapter 1 of this book, where we attempted to summarize the important properties of living systems. We observed then that there are three main features of any living system.

1. **Metabolism.** A living system must be able to extract energy from its environment and use that energy to maintain itself.

2. **Reproduction.** Since the lifespan of any organism is finite, it must be able to make a copy of itself if the species is to survive.

3. **Evolution.** In order to adapt to a changing environment, a species increases its fitness over several generations through the processes of mutation (or other methods of generating diversity) and selection.

We must look for these features arising in any computer-generated artificial life. How this is done depends on the specific model, so we will leave this point until we consider some artificial life systems later in the chapter.

7.2 Simulations, realizations, and theories

The traditional scientific community may have been slow to embrace the merit of theoretical biology, but the response to artificial life has, at times, verged on hostility. Before we proceed to examine some of the models in detail, it is worthwhile examining the causes of this reaction.

Part of the problem has been the tendency of those who work on artificial life to make sweeping claims about how the field will revolutionize our view of biology. Scientists who have spent decades doing painstaking and conscientious research in traditional biology do not take kindly to what they view as a few computer whiz-kids claiming that they can now explain life using a few simple computer programs and some flashy graphics. Perhaps the claim that has caused the most controversy is that the models generated inside a computer are not just simulations of life; rather they *are* life.

life are not assumed to be molecules, nor are their interactions necessarily chemical.

The modellers have made this claim based on the three-point definition of life given in the last section. From their point of view, they have designed a system which performs all three functions (as we will see in the following sections) using only simple components and local rules, so the resulting process should be called 'alive'.

The problems in interpreting the results of an artificial life experiment have been discussed in an article by Pattee (1989). Some of his points are worth making here.

Pattee draws a distinction between *simulations, realizations*, and *theories*. These three concepts derive from the *scientific method*, which is a tried-and-true method for obtaining objective information about the world.

In its simplest form, the scientific method begins with an observation of some phenomenon. As an example, suppose we observe that objects fall to the ground when we drop them. From the observation, we formulate a theory to explain the observation. Newton's theory of gravitation proposes that there is an attractive force between any two massive objects, and goes on to give a formula for the force. We now need to test the theory by performing an experiment. Newton's theory gives us precise numerical predictions as to how long it should take for an object to fall a given distance. We can attempt to measure this time in our experiment and, if the measurement agrees with the prediction, we feel that our theory now has some support. However, if we do an experiment and find that the result disagrees with the theory (we may test Newton's theory of gravity by dropping a piece of paper, for example, and find a major disagreement) we must revise our theory to take account of the new observation.

In the case of artificial life, however, all our observations and experiments are performed on a computer. We may start our investigation by proposing a set of objects and some interaction rules, writing a computer program which implements this system, and sitting back and watching what happens. Ideally, we would then formulate a theory of the system's behaviour, which we could then test by doing some more experiments with our computer model. If the theory is designed to be a general theory of how such computer models should work, we could check the theory by designing other models and seeing if they behave in a similar manner.

All this may seem to be standard science. However, there is one big difference between these computer experiments and all other science that has gone before. When we tested Newton's theories, we resorted to making measurements on the natural world—we did not create our world inside the computer, impose Newton's laws on it and do the experiment on a silicon chip. We *could* have done this, of course. Most calculations on Newtonian systems are done on computers, simply because the calculations are too complicated and lengthy to be done by hand. But all we are doing here is speeding up the process—if we had the time and patience to do the calculations on paper, we would end up with the same result. We are *simulating* what we would expect a real-world system to do.

Simulations make no claim to actually *be* the systems they describe. We can simulate the motions of the planets in our solar system in a computer, and by so doing, produce highly accurate predictions of where the planets will be at some given time. However, no one would seriously propose that we actually have a planetary system inside our computer. A simulation is useful as a test for a theory, since it can generate specific predictions based on the theory which can then be checked by comparison with a real system.

A *realization* of a theory or a simulation is an actual, physically present instance of a phenomenon. For example, we may use the theory of aerodynamics to predict the optimum shape for an aircraft wing. We may then simulate the behaviour of this wing on a computer by feeding in the equations produced by the theory and observe the predictions. However, to actually *realize* an aircraft wing, we must actually build one out of real materials, such as metal or fibreglass.

If we now return to the claims of artificial life, we can examine four categories (Pattee, 1989):

1. Computer-dependent realizations of living systems. This class of objects would correspond to the *strong* claims of artificial life: that the systems created inside a computer actually are alive.

2. Computer simulations of living behaviour. Here we assume that the computer has been programmed with some theory of how life should behave and is producing a specific instance of this theory as its output.

3. Theories of life that derive from simulations. Here we start with a simulation which is constructed by specifying the components and interactions. The simulation runs and produces certain behaviour patterns. We attempt to construct a theory based on the output of the simulation.

4. Theories of life that are testable only by computer simulation. Any theory of life that claims to apply to *any* living system, whether carbon-based or not, can, at the moment, only be tested by computer simulation. As well, most theories of the origin of life, whether they restrict themselves to the carbon-based form or not, can only be tested by simulation, simply because the real event occurred so long ago, and took so long to happen.

Pattee proposes that there are only two ways that an artificial life system could satisfy the first condition: (1) the artificial life is some form of robot which exists within the natural environment, and is capable of metabolism, reproduction, and evolution within that environment; (2) the artificial life is computer code, which satisfies the three conditions of life within an environment defined by the host computer.

The important point to be gleaned from all this is that if we choose to define life as satisfying the three conditions of metabolism, reproduction and evolution, then, yes, we can consider the sorts of computer models that have been produced under the heading of artificial life to actually be alive. However, we must not claim that, simply because such computer programs can produce results that satisfy those conditions, the same principles used in constructing these programs must also have applied in the origin of carbon life. As Pattee puts it: 'There is nothing wrong with a good illusion as long as one does not claim it is reality...the field of artificial life should pay attention to the enormous knowledge base of biology. In particular, artificial life should not ignore the universals of cell structure, behaviour, and evolution without explicit reasons for doing so. These presently include the genotype, phenotype, environment relations, the mutability of the gene, and the constructability of the phenotype under genetic constraints, and the natural selection of populations by the environment.'

We will examine some artificial life systems to give the reader a taste of what they can do. We will examine models from two main areas: cellular automata and 'living' computer code. A readable popular survey of artificial life is given in the book by Levy (1992). More detailed information with contributions by the original authors can be found in the two volumes of Santa Fe Institute conference proceedings (Langton, 1989; Langton *et al.*, 1992).

7.3   Cellular automata

An *automaton* is any object which can exist in one of a set of states and makes transitions between these states based on a set of rules. Automata can be *deterministic*, which means that if an object is in a particular state and its neighbours are also in particular states, then it will always make the same transition to the same state. On the other hand, a *non-deterministic* automaton is one where the rules allow one of several transitions to occur for any given initial state. Many processes in everyday life can be interpreted as automata. For example, a car approaching an intersection controlled by a traffic light should be a deterministic automaton. If the light is green, the car should remain in the same state (moving at constant speed). If the light turns yellow and the car's speed and distance from the intersection are such that it can stop safely, or the light is red, the car should make a transition from its initial state (moving towards the intersection) to another state (stopped at the intersection). If the light is yellow and the car cannot stop safely, then it should continue in the same state (moving).

However, as we are all aware, cars tend to act more like non-deterministic automata when confronted with a traffic light, especially of the yellow variety. Some cars will stop on a yellow light, but others make a different transition: they speed up. Occasionally, a car that cannot stop safely for a yellow light will still attempt to do so, making a transition from steady motion to uncontrolled deceleration, often accompanied by screeching tyres. As well, an occasional car will not change its state when it encounters a red light, but will continue moving through the intersection, often with disastrous consequences.

Although any system which makes transitions based on its current state and a set of rules can be called an automaton, most artificial life models based on automata use a particular kind called a *cellular automaton* or CA for short. A CA consists of a set of objects usually arranged in a regular grid, such as the squares on a sheet of graph paper. Each of these objects is a *cell*, hence the adjective *cellular*. Each cell can exist in one of a set of (usually discrete) states, and transitions between states depend on a cell's current state, on the states of its neighbours, and on a set of rules telling the cell what to do in each case. The rules may be deterministic or non-deterministic, depending on the model. With the right choice of states and rules, CA models can give rise to some surprisingly lifelike behaviour.

7.3.1 The Game of Life

One of the simplest CA models that could be called artificial life was invented by the mathematician John Horton Conway in 1968 (see Gardner, 1970 and Gardner, 1983 for readable accounts). The rules for the Game of Life, as it became known, are quite simple:

1. Life is played on a (ideally infinite) rectangular grid of cells.

2. Each cell can be in one of two states: alive (occupied) or dead (unoccupied).

3. Begin by seeding a selection of cells with live occupants. The seeding may be done randomly, or else a certain pattern may be specified in order to examine some particular behaviour.

4. Generations are discrete. In each generation, the rules for altering the state of a cell depend on the state of the cell and the states of its 8 nearest neighbours.

5. A live cell remains alive if it has either 2 or 3 living neighbours.

6. A live cell dies if it has fewer than 2 or more than 3 living neighbours.

7. An unoccupied cell becomes occupied ('gives birth') if it has exactly 3 living neighbours.

Although the connection with biology may seem very tenuous at this point, the 'biological' interpretation of these rules was as follows. A live cell needs at least 2 other living neighbours if it is to survive because life requires other life from which to derive its sustenance or to reproduce. However, if a live cell has more than 3 living neighbours, it dies of overcrowding—too much competition for the available resources. If an unoccupied cell has just the right number of living neighbours, life will appear in that cell either through birth or migration.

In order for the Game of Life to qualify as true artificial life, however, it must satisfy our three-point test specified in the introduction to this chapter. The model does indeed metabolize because it uses the power provided by the computer to perpetuate itself. In fact, all computer models satisfy the metabolism condition trivially, since any such model must, by definition, consume some of the power used to run the computer's processor. For this reason, we will not explicitly consider metabolism any further in any of the models described here.

How about reproduction? It turns out that certain configurations of cells can in fact 'give birth' to an infinite number of offspring. One of the simplest forms in Life is the *glider*, so called because in a cycle of 4 generations it displaces itself one square to the right and one square down. A structure called the *glider gun* was discovered that gave birth to an infinite series of gliders by 'shooting' them off one at a time. Even more elaborate structures were devised that actually gave birth to glider guns, which in turn, of course, gave birth to more gliders.

Because the rules for Life are deterministic, there is no scope for random mutation or, therefore, for the selection that could act on it. Once the initial configuration of a game has been defined, all its future history is contained in the rules. As such, it is certainly not a candidate for a computer simulation (or even realization) of the behaviour of a 'real' living system. Despite its limitations, however, Conway himself sees great things for his Life system. As quoted by Levy (1992), Conway says 'On a large enough scale you would really see living configurations. Genuinely living, whatever reasonable definition you care to give to it. Evolving reproducing, squabbling over territory. Getting cleverer and cleverer. Writing learned Ph.D. theses. On a large enough board, there's no doubt in my mind this sort of thing would happen.' This is certainly a *strong* claim for artificial life, though it is unlikely to convince many main-stream biologists.

7.3.2 Cellular automata in general

Although the Game of Life considered in the last section is useful for illustrating the idea of a cellular automaton in a simple context, its behaviour is not sufficiently 'life-like' for it to qualify as a full member of the artificial life club. Since the time of Conway's model, much more work has been done on cellular automata as models for many natural systems, both inside and outside the field of biology. In the remainder of this section, we will survey some of the work of Chris Langton, who was one of the pioneers in applying CAs to artificial life (Langton, 1984, 1986).

As a prelude to Langton's work, we need to take note of a thorough study of cellular automata by Stephen Wolfram (1984). Wolfram was interested in the dynamical properties of CAs in general, without any special regard for their use as biological models. In all cases, we begin by specifying the allowable states, the transition rules, and the initial configuration of the CA. We then let it evolve and examine the behaviour. Wolfram studied the behaviour of many different CAs, obtained by varying the number of states allowed to each cell and the set of rules for determining transitions over successive generations. After much experimentation, Wolfram devised four classes into which all CAs can be divided.

- The CA evolves to a homogeneous state, in the sense that the pattern of the cells converges to a stable state, in which all cells remain in the same state for all time. We can draw analogies between the dynamics of a CA and those of a continuous system, which are described by a system of differential equations. This first class of CA behaviour would then be analogous to a system of differential equations whose solution curves converge to a stable limit point.

- The CA falls into a periodic cycle of patterns. The periods may be of various lengths, but in general are not too long (for example, 2 alternating patterns). The analogue in the differential equation system would be a trajectory converging to a limit cycle.

- The CA behaviour becomes chaotic. No obvious periodicity is present, and the succession of patterns appears random, with no internal or persistent structure over time. This behaviour is, of course, analogous to chaotic behaviour in the solutions of systems of non-linear differential equations.

- The fourth class of CA behaviour is that of complex patterns with no obvious periodicity, but exhibiting localized and persistent structures that are not present in class 3. In particular, some of these structures have the ability to propagate through the CA's grid. (One example of such a structure is the glider in the Game of Life.) Although some differential equations show structures that crudely match this behaviour (such as solitons, which are wave-like features that can propagate for long distances in the solution of certain differential equations), there are no known differential equations that can provide the richness of localized structure and long-term behaviour of class 4 CAs.

CAs of classes 1 and 2 produce behaviour that is far too tame to be of interest in biological modelling. Although class 3 CAs produce a rich catalogue of patterns, there is no *emergent behaviour*, that is, no coherent, long-lasting structure above the single-cell level appears. We therefore cannot consider class 3 CAs to be reasonable candidates for biological models either.

We are left, therefore, with class 4. Here we do find emergent behaviour. The important point about these class 4 CAs is that this emergent structure arises from a system that is defined only in terms of *local* interactions: CA transition rules are defined only in terms of the current state of a cell and its nearest neighbours.[2] Thus one of the goals of artificial life that we discussed in the introduction is realized by class 4 CAs: the emergence of order from purely local interaction rules.

In order to do some experiments with class 4 CAs, we need some way of generating systems that have the required behaviour. To this end, let us define a few quantities.

Let the number of allowed states for each cell be k, and suppose that each cell has a *neighbourhood* of n cells. Here, a neighbourhood is defined as the set of all cells that affect the transition rule for the cell concerned. Thus n is the number of nearest neighbours of a cell, plus 1 for the cell itself (n is usually 5 or 9, depending on whether the definition of 'nearest neighbours' include the diagonally adjacent cells or not). Then any cell may find itself in one of k^n states, and we must define a transition rule for each of these states.

For example, in the Game of Life, $k = 2$ and $n = 9$, so each cell could exist in one of $2^9 = 512$ states. The transition rules for Life, however, depend only on the number of neighbouring cells in each of the two states and not on their positions, so the actual number of distinct transition rules required is considerably fewer than 512. In principle, however, we could define a CA with 512 different rules.

In order to classify the large number of possible sets of rules for a given architecture of CA (that is, given values of k and n), Langton defines a

---

[2]There are two main types of transition rules: those that depend on the cell itself and its four neighbours (up, down, left and right); and those that include the four diagonally adjacent neighbours as well. These two types of rules are known as the *five-cell* and *nine-cell* neighbourhoods, respectively.

parameter λ which may be thought of as a measure of the activity in the CA. In any set of CA states, it is customary to reserve one of the states as a 'quiescent' or 'inactive' state. In the Game of Life, one of the two states was interpreted as an unoccupied or dead cell, for example. The parameter λ is defined as the fraction of all possible states (k^n) that will cause a transition to a *non*-quiescent state. Thus, the higher the value of λ, the fewer rules there are that will cause a cell to become inactive.

As an example, let us calculate λ for the Game of Life. According to the rules given in the previous section, a living cell remains alive if it has either 2 or 3 living neighbours. The number of ways that 2 cells out of the 8 nearest neighbours of a living cell could be chosen is the binomial coefficient $\begin{pmatrix} 8 \\ 2 \end{pmatrix} = 28$. Similarly, the number of ways of choosing 3 nearest neighbours is $\begin{pmatrix} 8 \\ 3 \end{pmatrix} = 56$. The total number of transitions where a cell initially in the live state remains in the live state is therefore $28 + 56 = 84$. The only other rule that results in a transition to a living state is that which allows a birth to occur in an unoccupied cell if exactly 3 of its neighbours are alive. The number of ways this can happen is 56 (as calculated above), so the total number of transitions resulting in a transition to a living state is $84 + 56 = 140$. Thus, the activity parameter for Life is $\lambda = 140/512 = 0.273$.

In the more general case, we will have k allowable states for each cell. Let us number the states from 0 to $k - 1$ (in the Life case, the two states would be called 0 and 1), and call the 0 state the inactive or quiescent state. Rather than trying to specify a deterministic set of rules which gives a particular value of λ, we can treat λ as a *probability* (since it always in the interval [0,1]) that a transition to an active state will occur. If we have k possible states, the probability that a cell will become inactive in the next generation is then $1 - \lambda$, and the probability that it will assume any one of the $k - 1$ active states is $\lambda/(k - 1)$.

Langton has done a series of experiments using different values of λ and classifying the types of CA that result. He finds that Wolfram's four classes of CAs tend to fall neatly into certain domains for the parameter λ. He finds that class 1 CAs occur when $0.0 \leq \lambda < 0.2$; class 2 and class 4 CAs occur when $0.2 < \lambda < 0.4$ and class 3 CAs occur when $0.4 < \lambda < 1.0$. Broadly speaking, these results show that when the activity level is very low (small λ), the system tends to converge to single, stable pattern. If the activity is high, unstructured, chaotic behaviour occurs. It is only for intermediate levels of activity that localized structure and periodic behaviour (classes 2 and 4) occur. The main difference between classes 2 and 4 is that the localized, periodic structures in class 2 do not move in space, while the localized structures in a class 4 CA propagate through the grid (as the glider does in Life), and thus can transmit the effects of one localized structure to another.

Langton speculates that the difference in complexity of class 2 and class 4 automata is due to this travelling interaction. As he says: 'Without the possibility of interaction, the localized periodic structures of class 2 give rise to global limit-cycle behaviour. In class 4, however, the existence of propagating structures means that there can be arbitrarily complex interactions between localized periodic structures and propagating periodic structures. This means that the global behaviour of a class 4 cellular automaton is potentially in the chaotic regime.'

Langton therefore refers to class 4 CAs as expressing *partially* developed chaotic behaviour, while those in class 3 show *fully* developed chaotic behaviour. He goes on to propose that the only types of CA in which artificial life can arise are those in class 4. For this reason, artificial life models based on class 4 CAs have been referred to as 'life on the edge of chaos'.

Langton has constructed several specific class 4 CAs which mimic some of the aspects of 'real' life. In one simulation with $\lambda = 0.218$, two interacting species form a sort of 'catalytic cycle' in which both species conspire to maintain each other's population levels. Langton calls this an example of artificial biochemistry.

In another simulation, a population of 'virtual ants', or *vants*, for short, exhibits some of the aspects of social insect behaviour.

7.4   Tierra

7.4.1   Introduction

Tierra is unusual among the zoo of artificial life programs in that it was designed and written by a biologist. Most of the other artificial life projects were designed by people whose primary interest was computers. The author of Tierra, Thomas Ray, however, wanted to see if artificial life could be used to model some specific biological problems (see Ray, 1992). The problem with the origin of life and evolutionary simulations that had been written up to that time was that they did not allow the computer organisms much leeway in their evolution. The replication mechanisms are programmed into the simulation, as is the fitness function, which determines which organisms live and die. In nature, organisms evolve by interaction with each other and their environment: the fitness function is determined by this interaction and not imposed externally by some guiding hand. Ray wanted to write a simulation where natural evolution could take place within a computer.

As mentioned in the introduction, a general definition of life requires the abilities to reproduce, metabolize, and evolve. In nature, organisms are constrained by limited food supplies and limited space in which to live. The less efficient an organism is at gathering food and reproducing, the less fit it is, and the less chance it has of passing on offspring to the next generation.

These considerations apply equally well to molecular scenarios and to full-sized contemporary organisms. In order for molecules to reproduce, they must find the components of which they are made and assemble these components to produce a daughter molecule.

Tierra models this process by representing an organism by a string of machine code instructions in a computer. These instructions are modelled after the instructions found in most low-level assembler languages used in all computers, although Tierra uses its own machine language rather than adopting one of the 'real' ones.[3] A block of space in the computer's RAM (random access memory) is reserved as the experimental field, and a single 'ancestor organism' is placed upon the field. By following the instructions contained in its assembler code, an organism can attempt to reproduce and pass along to its daughter the code essential to survive and reproduce in turn. As the number of organisms increases, the available space on the field decreases, so that organisms find themselves competing for living space.

In order to process the instructions contained in its assembler code, an organism requires some time from the computer's central processing unit (CPU time). Ideally, since each organism is supposed to be an independent entity, each organism would have access to its own private CPU. This would be possible on a parallel processor but, since most computers are still serial processors (that is, they have only a single CPU), a compromise is necessary. The solution used by Tierra is to allocate each organism in turn a 'slice' of time on the single processor. This is the same method used by any computer running a so-called *multi-tasking operating system*, which allows the user to run several jobs at once on the one machine. The jobs are not really running simultaneously; rather, one job is given a certain amount of time (say 1 second) during which it progresses a certain amount. If it does not finish in that time, it is suspended and some time is given to the next job. The process continues until all jobs have had a share of the time, after which the first job is restarted for another slice, and so on.

In Tierra, therefore, an organism will get a time slice during which it can execute a fixed number of instructions before it must become dormant and let another organism have a chance. This introduces another form of competition into the simulation. An organism that can carry out its functions in fewer time steps (by using fewer instructions) will be at an

---

[3]The main reason for doing this is that a program similar to Tierra written in 'real' machine languages could turn out be a *computer virus*. Such viruses can cause serious damage to data stored on computer disks. Many such viruses have been written by persons with malicious intent, and have become a serious problem all over the world. The computer virus' ability to replicate and propagate has given rise to the speculation that they, too, may be a form of computer life. See Levy (1992) and Clough and Mungo (1992).

advantage, since it will be able to reproduce faster than its neighbours and therefore be able to claim the vacant space before anyone else can.

The competition for CPU time and memory space therefore results in an implied fitness for any organism. Those organisms that use time efficiently will, presumably, be fitter than those that dawdle and take a long time to do anything. The important point is that Tierra does not have an *imposed* fitness function: the fitness of an organism arises naturally as a consequence of its actions and the current state of the environment, just as in nature.

The ancestor organism (designed by Ray) contained 80 assembler instructions, including a stretch of code which contained the recipe for producing a daughter organism. The replication mechanism is therefore built in, at least at the start. Evolution is possible because each of the actions encoded by an assembler instruction has a certain probability of being executed incorrectly. In addition, there is a small background mutation rate, in which one bit of the code can be altered at random. Thus the generation of diversity is also built in.

If this system were left to its own devices, it would quickly fill up all the space available. To prevent this, and to simulate natural death, Tierra contains a 'reaper' function, which begins to kill off organisms once the population reaches a certain critical level. As soon as an organism is born, it enters the reaper queue. When the reaper function decides it is time to claim a victim, it always removes the organism at the front of the queue. Organisms that make errors (we will see how this can happen in the next section) are advanced in the queue, while organisms that perform actions efficiently are pulled back, thus prolonging their lives.

7.4.2   The Tierran model

In order to understand how an organism is represented in Tierra, we must explain a bit about how a computer's machine code works. All computer languages (such as Pascal, C, Fortran, and so on) must be translated into machine code before their instructions can be executed. The actual form of machine code depends on the type of computer you are using, but most codes share similar characteristics. An assembler language is a set of mnemonics for the actions that can be carried out in machine code. Typical actions are simple arithmetic operations such as addition and subtraction, branching instructions that tell the controller to jump to a different location in the code, and so on.

The data in a computer are stored in discrete locations in RAM, but to process the data, the computer makes use of several active storage locations called *registers*. If a number is to be added to another number, for example, each number will be moved into a register, the addition carried out, and the result stored back in the RAM location allocated to it.

In Tierra, each organism has allocated to it a *virtual CPU* (although recall that only one organism at a time can do anything on a serial machine). The virtual CPU for each organism contains the following items:

- 2 address registers, used for storing addresses of locations in RAM.

- 2 numerical registers, used for storing numbers.

- a flag, using for indicating the state of some calculation.

- a *stack*, which is a set of 10 memory locations used for storing data. A stack works on the last-in, first-out principle. A number is pushed in at the top of the stack, and pushes all the other numbers already on the stack down to make room for the new number. When a number is retrieved from the stack, it is popped off the top; hence last-in, first-out.

- an instruction pointer, which points to the location in the organism's code currently being executed.

The instruction set consists of 32 commands. Each of these commands is stored as a sequence of 5 bits.[4] The instructions can do simple bit manipulations such as incrementing or decrementing registers, pushing or popping registers onto or off the stack, redirecting the instruction pointer so that some code at a different location is executed, and so on.

Two of the 32 instructions are 'no-ops' or null operations. These are instructions 0 and 1, represented in 5-bit binary by 00000 and 00001. They are used to form templates or markers in the code on which other instructions act.

We will illustrate the effects of these instructions by considering the actions of Ray's ancestor organism, which contains 80 instructions. The beginning of the ancestor's code in RAM is marked by four no-ops in the pattern 1,1,1,1; and the end of the code by the four no-ops 1,1,1,0. Within the 80 instructions is a section of code which will copy the ancestor's code to a new location in memory. The beginning of the copy code is marked by 4 no-ops as well: 1,1,0,0. There are several instructions that can search for templates in the code, provided that the templates are within a certain distance of the search instruction. The first action performed by the ancestor is to locate its beginning and end using search instructions, and calculate its size by subtracting the two addresses. It will then attempt to reserve enough memory to create a daughter organism of the same size. In order for this to occur, there must be enough free memory in the allocated

---

[4]A *bit*, or binary digit, is a digit in base two and can therefore take on one of two values: 0 or 1. All computer data is ultimately stored as bit sequences.

section of RAM within a certain distance. If there is not, the attempt at reproduction will fail.

If sufficient memory exists, it is reserved by the ancestor. The next instruction searches for the beginning of the copy procedure by looking for the template 1,1,0,0. Again, the search is limited to a certain distance. If a copy procedure is found, the code between the begin and end addresses (found at the beginning of the cycle) is copied into the new location in memory, thus producing a new organism. After copying the code, the DIVIDE instruction severs all links between parent and child by creating a virtual CPU for the daughter cell and entering it into the time slicer and reaper queues.

As the number of organisms grows, competition for available CPU time begins to be felt. As well, due to inbuilt mutation and copying errors during replication, several different species will arise. Some of these species will contain fatal mutations which, for example, remove their ability to determine their start and end points, or remove the ability to replicate. Such organisms will quickly rise to the top of the reaper queue and be eliminated.

However, certain types of mutations can give rise to different species that are perfectly viable. One species that appears within a few million instructions[5] is a parasite, which is formed by a single mutation from the 80-instruction ancestor. Recall that the end of an organism is marked by the four no-ops 1,1,1,0 and the beginning of the copy procedure by the no-ops 1,1,0,0. The third no-op in the end marker, in 5-bit notation, is therefore 00001, while the corresponding no-op in the copy code marker is 00000. A single bit mutation in the copy code marker could therefore convert the third no-op from instruction 0 to instruction 1, which would convert the copy code marker to an end-of-organism marker. This means that an ancestor with such a mutation would be shorter than the standard 80-bit ancestor (due to the location of the copy code, the mutant organism has length 45), and would be missing its own version of the copy procedure.

However, when the instruction to search for a block of code to perform the copy is encountered in the 45-bit organism, it searches within its allowed distance in an attempt to find the correct template (1,1,0,0). Although it cannot find the code within its own section of memory, it may find that section of code within another organism, if that organism is close enough in memory for the search to include it. Although organisms are only allowed to change their own code, they are allowed to read other organisms' code, so if the search locates the copy procedure in another organism, it can use it to copy its own code into the newly allocated memory location,

---

[5] A few million instructions may seem a huge number, but in an actual computer simulation of Tierra, it takes under an hour.

and therefore reproduce. Because the 45-bit organism is using someone else's code to reproduce, it is acting like a parasite. It gets the ability to reproduce without having to maintain the code to do so. Providing there are enough 80-bit (or similar) organisms around to provide copy codes that can be accessed by the parasites, they will do quite well, since they require less CPU time to complete a reproduction. However, if they proliferate too much, they will occupy so much of the available space that many of the parasites will not be near an organism that contains the copy procedure, so they will not be able to reproduce and will die out.

The response of the system to parasitic invasion is quite remarkable. A 79-bit variant of the ancestor frequently evolves which appears to block the parasite's attempts to use its copy procedure, so that although the 45-bit parasites make repeated attempts to invade a system populated with these 79-bit mutants, they never make any headway. New parasites have been observed that can live off the 79-bit mutants, however.

More complex behaviour, such as hyper-parasites (parasites that live off other parasites) and even hyper-hyper-parasites evolve. Over long runs (2 or 3 billion instructions) some of the features of long-term evolution as deduced from the fossil record seem to appear. The phenomenon of punctuated equilibrium (the idea that evolution proceeds very slowly for long periods of time, but every so often a period of rapid evolution occurs, giving rise to many new species in a comparatively short time) has been observed in Tierran simulations. The initial population is dominated by organisms with sizes of under 100 instructions, and this continues until after more than one billion instructions a series of large (400 to 800 instructions) organisms appear which take over the population.

Although the Tierran simulation does not simulate the earliest stages in the origin of life,[6] since the population begins with a pre-formed ancestor containing enough information to reproduce itself, it certainly demonstrates all three of the properties of life we listed in the introduction to this chapter. It would be interesting to see a similar simulation of the events leading to the first organism.

7.5   Conclusion

The artificial life models discussed in this chapter, and many more discussed elsewhere in the literature, show that many of the features of 'natural' life can arise in relatively simple computer-generated models with nothing more than local interactions. Although we are certainly not yet in a position

---

[6]Ray actually intended Tierra to be a simulation of the events in the *Cambrian explosion*, a period around 600 million years ago in which many new forms of life appeared in a very short period of time. Many of these life forms appear bizarre to our modern eyes, and did not last long. Others gave rise to the species presently on the Earth.

to claim that these models simulate the events actually occurred in the origin of life on Earth (or that do occur in life today), they are thought-provoking experiments because they show that the general principles on which life is based may actually be inevitable consequences of the way in which molecules are constructed and interact with each other. The field of artificial life is still in its infancy, and it will be fascinating to watch it grow up.

Part II

The Immune System

8

The immune system

8.1 Introduction

The immune system is popularly conceived as the body's defence system which valiantly fights off attacks from hordes of parasites, such as bacteria and viruses. To a certain extent, this is true, but the immune system is much more than this. It is a complex cellular and molecular system which is capable of recognizing and eliminating virtually any substance which is foreign to the organism in which it resides, while at the same time ignoring cells and molecules produced by its own body. When one considers the enormous variety of molecules in both categories, foreign and 'self', one begins to understand the sophistication of such a biochemical system.

The immune system is not totally successful in its attempts to distinguish foreign cells from local cells. If it were, such medical breakthroughs as blood transfusions, skin grafts, and organ transplants would not be possible. Still, great care must be taken to match blood types in a transfusion or match tissue types in skin grafts and organ transplants to prevent the host's immune system from rejecting these foreign objects and, quite probably, kill the host in the process.

Up to now, most of our understanding of the immune system has come from a series of ingenious experiments, primarily on mice, during the course of the late nineteenth and twentieth centuries. Once a sufficient body of knowledge was accumulated from these experiments, it became clear that certain aspects of the immune system's organization and dynamics could benefit from theoretical modelling. In order to see where a theorist could make a useful contribution, we must retrace the discoveries of the experimentalists. The summary presented in this chapter will hopefully allow the reader with no prior knowledge of immunology to understand the basics of the field, although in a book of this size we cannot do full justice to the many intricate and beautiful experiments from which this understanding arose. The reader interested in a more thorough understanding of the development of immunology is advised to consult an introductory textbook. An excellent, up-to-date book is *Immunology: A Synthesis* (second edition) by Edward S. Golub and Douglas R. Green. This is a readable, comprehensive and at times humorous account of the key experiments in the field which should be accessible to readers with little biological background. Once this book, or a similar one, has been consulted, the book *Immunology* edited by Ivan Roitt, Jonathan Brostoff, and David Male is worth a browse. This book is more concise than that by Golub and Green, but is filled with superb multi-coloured figures, photographs, and diagrams which illustrate the main points.

8.2   Components of the immune system

The immune system mounts a multi-pronged attack against foreign matter. The various cell types can attack invaders directly, and they can also secrete molecules with a variety of functions, including attacking foreign cells and signalling other immune cells to proliferate.

All of these cells develop from so-called *stem cells* which are found in the bone marrow. A stem cell is an undifferentiated parent cell which, depending on various factors, can develop into one of several mature cell types. Stem cells give rise to red blood cells by following one developmental pathway to one of the several types of immune cells (white blood cells) known as *lymphocytes* by following other pathways and to various other types of cells by still other pathways. The two main types of cells with which we shall be concerned here are called *B cells* and *T cells*.

The B cell, so called because it not only originates in the bone marrow, but matures there as well, is the cell that manufactures the main molecular component of the immune system: the *antibody*. B cells synthesize antibodies (using the DNA to protein pathway described in Chapter 1) and then display them on the surface of the cell by projecting them through the cell membrane. A B cell thus resembles a pin-cushion where the protruding pins are the antibody molecules. These B cells drift around the body until they encounter some foreign object such as a bacterial cell or any other cell or molecule that does not 'belong' in the body. Such foreign objects are collectively known as *antigens*. If the antibody molecules displayed on the surface of the B cell 'fit' the antigen (in much the same way as a key fits a lock), a chain of events (which we will consider in more detail below) is set in motion that results in the proliferation of the B cell and the destruction of the antigen, and others like it.

The astute reader will have noticed that this chain of events resulting in the destruction of the antigen will only occur if the original B cell recognizes the antigen. If the antibody on the surface of the B cell is not sufficiently close in form to the antigen for any interaction to occur, the antigen and B cell ignore each other and nothing happens. However, a remarkable property of the immune system is that antibody molecules come in such an enormous variety of forms that it is virtually certain that *some* B cell somewhere in the body will be carrying antibodies that will match *any* antigen (except, of course, cells and molecules from the host organism). Once this B cell encounters its antigen, the process leading to proliferation and destruction of antigen begins.

What of the T cells? T cells, like B cells, originate in the bone marrow, but travel to the thymus (hence the name T cell) to mature. (The thymus is a small organ just over the heart.) Unlike B cells, however, T cells do not produce or use antibody and, as we shall see, they cannot recognize free antigen. In order for a T cell to respond to antigen, the antigen must be associated with a host cell.

T cells come in several forms—there is still some controversy over just how many distinct forms of T cell there are. Two forms about which there is no doubt, however, are the *helper T cell* and the *killer T cell*.

Killer T cells (or, to use their technical name, *cytotoxic cells*), can recognize infected host cells, bind to them and, through a complex series of reactions, kill them.

Helper T cells, as their name implies, help other immune cells, usually B cells, to respond to antigen. A helper T cell on its own cannot eliminate antigen; rather when a helper T cell and a B cell encounter antigen together, the helper cell produces several proteins which trigger the B cell to proliferate.

One of the controversial forms of the T cell is the *suppressor T cell*, which is alleged to have the ability to dampen certain immune reactions. There is no doubt that some form of T cell can suppress immunological responses to certain specific antigens. What is in doubt is whether there is a separate form of T cell whose only job is that of suppressor, or whether the suppression is being carried out by other T cells in disguise.

The scenario just described occurs in an immune system which has never seen the antigen before. Typically, the initial response to an antigen takes a few days to mature. The lifetime of a lymphocyte is also several days, even in the absence of antigen, so the immune response is a dynamic process, constantly being renewed by input from the bone marrow.

This initial exposure to an antigen, though, has a long-lasting effect on the immune system. If, after the initial infection has been repelled, the same antigen should appear again, the immune system mounts what is known as the *secondary response*. This consists of a much faster and stronger response to the antigen, providing a much improved defence the second time round. In many cases, this feature of the immune system is sufficient to provide complete immunity from attack by the antigen. This, of course, is the property of which a vaccination takes advantage—a mild case of the disease, or sometimes an inactive version of the antigen, such as heat-killed bacterial cells, is injected into the person, which provides just enough antigen to cause a primary response in the immune system. If the person should be exposed to the antigen again, the immune system has been primed so that it will respond vigorously and repel the invasion.[1]

The method by which the immune system 'memorizes' encounters with antigen is still unknown, but several theories have been proposed, which we will consider in Section 8.5.1.

This section has provided an overview of some of the components of the immune system and their abilities, without going into any of the details of how the various functions work. In the following sections, we will examine each of these properties in a little more detail, beginning with the question of how the immune system can recognize such a variety of antigens without reacting to itself.

8.3   The genetics of antibody diversity

The number of antigens with which an organism could make contact in its lifetime is almost limitless, yet the immune system seems capable of generating antibody against almost anything that is thrown at it. Researchers have injected mice with such things as camel red blood cells, various exotic organic molecules, and other substances which an average mouse would never expect to meet if it were not unfortunate enough to be a laboratory animal, yet the mice seemed able to generate antibody responses to all these substances. It is simply not plausible that an animal would possess a gene which encoded an antibody molecule for every conceivable antigen—the entire genome in most animals is just not big enough.

To see how the immune system does manage to cope with the plethora of antigens, we must first examine the structure of the antibody molecule. An antibody is a Y-shaped molecule consisting of four subunits: two *heavy chains* and two *light chains* (see Fig. 8.1). The heavy chains (so called because they are larger than light chains and therefore weigh more) are bonded together in the base of the Y, but separate so that each heavy chain forms one of the two wings at the top of the Y. The light chain is equal in length to one of the wings in the top of the Y, and there is one light chain bonded to the top of each heavy chain.

The base of the Y is a *constant region* in that its amino acid sequence is essentially the same for all antibody molecules in a given organism. It is this base region that remains inserted in the cell membrane of a B cell, while the top section of the Y protrudes through the membrane and is capable of binding to antigen (see Fig. 8.2). The top sections of both the

---

[1]You may wonder why this principle doesn't work against all diseases. For example, why do many people get colds every winter? This is not a deficiency in your immune system; rather it is due to the fact that the cold virus has a high mutation rate, so that although you *have* become immune to the virus you caught last winter, you can be sure that next winter's cold virus will be of a different strain.

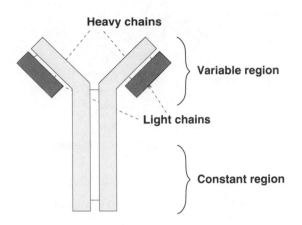

Figure 8.1   An antibody molecule.

light and heavy chains (that is, the parts of the antibody nearest the top of the Y) are *variable regions*: the amino acid sequences of these areas will be the same for all antibodies in a given B cell, but will vary from one B cell to another.

The variation is produced by using some elementary combinatorics on the genes coding for antibody. The section of DNA coding for the variable regions of the heavy and light chains consists of several segments. To form a complete heavy chain variable region, for example, there are three segments: V (for variable), D (for diversity), and J (for joining, since it is the segment which connects the variable and constant regions together). The corresponding region in the light chain contains only the V and J regions. For each of these segments, there are a number of gene fragments occurring in tandem in the DNA. For example, in human DNA, there are between 100 and 200 different gene fragments coding for the V segment of the heavy chain, so that when an antibody molecule is being made up the cell has a 'free choice' of any one of these fragments. Similarly, several choices exist for the D (about 30) and J (6) regions in the heavy chain and for V (around 100) and J (5) regions in the light chain. The total number of possible antibody molecules is therefore the product of the numbers of possible choices for each segment. For humans, this gives a total of around 10^7 possibilities. Thus, by using combinations of genes, the immune system is able to provide a repertoire of some ten million different antibody species using only a few hundred genes. In addition to the variation obtained from different combinations of gene fragments, the locations on each fragment where the joins with neighbouring fragments

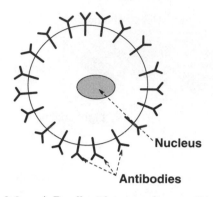

Figure 8.2   A B cell with protruding antibodies.

occur vary from one antibody to another, yielding yet more possible end
products. This additional variability may raise the number of possible
antibodies produced by purely genetic means up to 10^9 or 10^{10}.

Now, 10^{10} is a large number, but you may well wonder if it is large
enough. It is certainly much smaller than the number of potential antigens
in the world, so is there some other source of variation used by the immune
system that we have not yet considered? In a sense, yes, but this doesn't
come into play until later. What you must remember is that, in order for
an antibody to 'recognize' an antigen, it does not need to provide an exact
fit to the antigen. The key-lock analogy should be softened a little, since
we are not dealing with rigid metallic keys and locks, we are dealing with
interactions between molecules which have some degree of flexibility. Thus
each species of antibody is capable of recognizing a range of antigens, with
a higher affinity for some antigens than others. There will also be more
than one antibody that is capable of responding to one antigen, though
some antibodies will respond more strongly than others, since they have a
higher affinity (a better fit, in terms of keys and locks) than others. An
arsenal of 10^7 antibodies should be enough for some sort of response to be
generated to almost any type of antigen.

Once an antigen is detected, the immune system is capable of 'fine-
tuning' itself to provide a better response. Through a chain of events to be
considered below, a B cell which encounters an antigen to which it has an
affinity (be it high or low) is triggered to proliferate. Those B cells with a
higher affinity have a better chance of being so activated, thus increasing
the number of B cells available to deal with the antigen. However, when
an activated B cell begins to divide, the genes for the antibody variable
region undergo what is known as *hypermutation*, that is, an enhanced mu-

tation rate. This greatly increases the chance that one of the offspring of the originally activated B cell will produce an antibody that has an even higher affinity for the antigen, which in turn means that that cell will proliferate faster, and so on. The whole process of triggering, proliferation, and hypermutation is known as the *maturation* of the immune response.

This idea, originally proposed by Burnet (1959), is known as the *clonal selection* theory, and is really a version of evolution by mutation and natural selection in miniature. The initial B cell lineage, or clone, is selected by showing an affinity to the antigen, thus allowing it to have more offspring than other B cells which show lower or no affinity. Mutation in successive generations of the B cell clone so chosen produce offspring with even higher affinities for the antigen, so they are selected in preference to other offspring.

8.4 Recognition and processing of antigen

So far, we have only hinted at how T cells and B cells actually do their job of eliminating antigen from the body. The first question we should consider in more detail is: How does an immune cell know that an object is antigen and not part of its own body? More to the point, we should perhaps ask why our own immune system does not kill us.

We know from above that B cells classify a substrate as antigen if there is some affinity between the substrate and the antibody attached to the B cell, but what does the B cell do after that? We have also hinted that killer T cells have a way of detecting an infected cell and killing it, but we have not described how this recognition occurs. To answer both these questions, we need to consider a group of molecules known as the major histocompatibility complex, or MHC.

The MHC group of molecules are rather like a serial number for an organism in that they serve as tags or labels which identify, more or less uniquely, an organism's cells as its own. Investigations into the genetics of the MHC have shown that it has one of the most polymorphic sets of genes known, that is, that there are an enormous number of different genotypes for the MHC in a population. This is, of course, what you would expect if the MHC is to serve as a unique marker for each organism in a population.

MHC molecules are of three main classes, called, not surprisingly, classes I, II, and III. Only classes I and II play a significant role in immunology. Class I MHC proteins are found in the membranes of all cells in an organism (except those, such as red blood cells, that do not have a nucleus). Class II MHC proteins are found only in the membranes of cells, called antigen processing cells, which encounter antigen and process it for presentation to T cells.

Consider first the case of an ordinary cell (one that has nothing to do with the immune system) which has become infected with a virus, such as the common cold. The virus has taken over the cell's protein synthesizing machinery so that the cell now produces viral proteins instead of its own proteins. Some of these proteins are processed by the cell (by means which are largely unknown) and eventually become embedded in the cell membrane where they become associated with MHC I molecules. If such an infected cell should encounter a killer T cell with a receptor molecule on its surface that recognizes the MHC I-viral protein complex, the killer T cell will secrete proteins that kill the infected cell.[2] A killer T cell will *only* respond to a target cell if (i) the target cell exhibits MHC I molecules of the same type as the host, so that the target cell is a 'self' cell; (ii) the MHC I molecules are associated with an antigen.[3]

Now consider the case of antigen which is not contained inside cells of the host, such as an invading bacterial cell (Fig. 8.3). Because this cell is not a 'self' cell, there is a good chance that a B cell will recognize it as an antigen and bind to it. In most cases, binding an antigen is not a sufficient trigger for a B cell to become activated and enter its proliferation mode.[4] However, the B cell may engulf the antigen and partially digest it. The fragments of the antigen cell become associated with MHC II molecules and emerge into the cell membrane where they are displayed on the surface. If a helper T cell should happen along which recognizes the MHC II-antigen fragment complex, the helper T cell will secrete several substances called *interleukins* which will trigger the B cell to enlarge and proliferate, giving rise to clonal selection as described earlier. The proliferating B cell gives rise to a whole generation of B cells which produce antibody similar to that of the original cell. Involved with this production of antibody there is also a phenomenon known as a *class switch*. Antibody molecules come in a variety of forms, but the most common are immunoglobulin G (IgG) and immunoglobulin M (IgM). IgG is the familiar single Y-shaped molecule with two binding sites. IgM consists of five such single molecules bound together in an aggregate with circular symmetry, rather like a flower with five petals. IgM has, as a result of this aggregation, 10 binding sites, since

---

[2]Killer T cells kill their targets by punching holes in the membrane with a protein called perforin and then secreting various enzymes into the target cell which alter its protein synthesis machinery causing the cell to die. Killer T cells also have a defence mechanism so that they don't kill themselves.

[3]In some cases an uninfected foreign cell will be attacked by a killer T cell. Presumably this is because the foreign MHC I molecules on their own resemble host MHC I plus antigen.

[4]There are a few antigens, called T-independent antigens, which will activate B cells without T cell help. In these cases, a crucial event seems to be *cross-linking* of the surface receptors on the B cell: one antigen must be able to bind to more than one receptor, thus linking the surface receptors together.

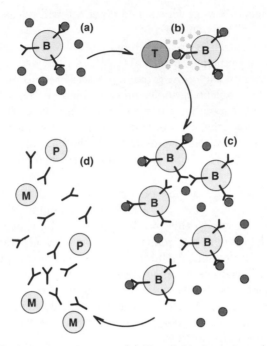

Figure 8.3 The immune response. (a) B cell binds antigen (small circles). (b) Helper T cell secretes interleukins causing (c) B cell to divide. (d) After proliferation, B cells secrete free antibody and differentiate to become memory and plasma cells.

the short arms of each Y-shaped molecule point away from the centre of the circle and are thus freely available to the outside world. IgM is most common at the beginning of an immune response, but after a while, some of the cells switch to the production of IgG.

The proliferation of the B cell population proceeds until the concentration of antigen falls to a certain level, at which point the B cells enter a new phase. They differentiate into either *plasma cells*, which merely secrete antibody as free molecules in the blood, or *memory cell*, which are similar to the original B cells in that they possesses antibody receptors, but remain dormant, awaiting another attack by the same antigen.

There are also numerous other cells which can recognize antigen, although in a non-specific manner. One such cell is the macrophage (literally, 'big eater') which can recognize foreign cells, engulf them and process them in much the same manner as a B cell, displaying the fragments on its surface in association with MHC II molecules. In this case, both a B cell and a helper T cell which recognize the antigen are required to bind to the macrophage, following which the helper cell will release its interleukins and the B cell will become active.

Besides resulting in a greater number of more finely tuned B cells, the trigger provided by helper T cells also causes B cells to secrete their antibody molecules into the body, providing a purely molecular immunological mechanism. Free antibody molecules can bind to the surface of antigen and give rise to the so-called *complement cascade*. Complement is a system of about nine molecular components which act in sequence to destroy the membrane of a target cell, beginning with the binding of the first component of complement to antibody molecules attached to the surface of the cell.

We now have a good idea of how the immune system distinguishes self from non-self cells, but why are there no immune cells that recognize self-cells? The answer to this puzzle appears to be that when T cells are maturing in the thymus, any cells that encounter a substrate that they recognize as antigen die out. Assuming that the only substrates encountered by a maturing T cell belong to the host, this should neatly eliminate all T cells that recognize self-cells while leaving untouched any T cell that does not encounter its antigen while maturing. It is not clear exactly how this procedure is accomplished, nor whether B cells undergo a similar selective procedure in the bone marrow.[5]

8.5   Immune networks

It appears that, with the exception of cells displaying the organism's own brand of MHC molecules, the immune system can recognize virtually any molecule and mount an immune defence against it. This fact prompted Neils Jerne (1974a, 1974b) to suggest that the immune system can recognize itself, in the sense that, for each antibody produced, there is another antibody that will recognize it. If this is true, then the immune system is not merely a collection of isolated cells each producing its own type of antibody. Rather, it is a network of cells and antibodies which, even in the absence of foreign antigens, undergoes an intricate series of interactions within itself. These interactions can determine which part of the complete repertoire is actually expressed at any one time, as well as affecting the response to foreign antigen.

A good review of immune network theory is given by Perelson (1989), including the concept of *shape space*, which we will discuss here. (See also Coutinho (1989) and DeLisi (1983).)

---

[5]A theoretical possibility is that B cells that recognize self *do* exist, but they are suppressed by the immune network (see Section 8.5) so they never have a chance to cause any damage. See Chapter 13.

In order to demonstrate that the idea of an immune network is reasonable, let us investigate how thoroughly an average immune system covers the range of possible antigens.

A lymphocyte's specificity is determined by the antibody molecules it displays on its surface or, once it is stimulated by antigen, the antibodies it secretes. In turn, the antibody molecule is marked as unique by the particular amino acid sequence of its variable regions. The amino acid sequence determines the three-dimensional shape of the variable region and this, in turn, determines the set of antigens which the antibody can recognize. If we want to describe an antibody molecule mathematically, we need to define a number of quantities which can be used to characterize a molecule. These quantities may include such things as shape parameters, for example, size of region, positions of bumps and grooves, and so on[6] and charge distributions (locations of positively and negatively charged regions on the surface). A similar set of quantities may also be defined and determined for the antigen. If an antibody and antigen have complementary values for all or most of these quantities (for example, one has a bump where the other has a groove, and one has a positively charged region where the other has a negatively charged one), then the antigen and antibody have a high chance of 'recognizing' each other, that is, of forming a chemical bond. This collection of parameters describing an antigen or antibody is called the *generalized shape* of the molecule.

Depending on the complexity of the model we are building, the generalized shape could consist of as few as one parameter to as many as our data will allow. In order for an antibody to recognize an antigen, the complementary fit need not be perfect, but the closer the two molecules fit each other, the stronger the affinity between them will be. For however many parameters we have decided to build into our generalized shape, we must define an affinity function which maps the parameter values of the two molecules into a value which measures the attraction of the two molecules. To picture the argument from now on, imagine two spaces: one for the antibody and the other for the antigen. Each space is defined by the parameters defining the generalized shape of the molecule. For simplicity, we will consider a two-dimensional space here, but the argument extends easily to any number of dimensions.

Let us plot the generalized shape (which we will just refer to simply as the 'shape' from now on) of an antigen in the first space. Now there will be (at least) one point in the antibody space corresponding to the shape of antibody which produces the highest affinity for this antigen. Assuming that this point is unique, we plot it on the diagram. Now we know that

---

[6]In general we could define a function which gives the surface shape of the molecule, but this would be too complicated in most applications.

a certain threshold affinity is required to trigger a B cell into proliferative mode. If the maximum affinity corresponding to the point in antibody space is greater than this threshold, then there will be a region around this point in which any antibody would have an affinity high enough to trigger its corresponding B cell. The threshold value of affinity will determine a surface around the point in antibody space, within which any antibody will recognize the antigen. We will call the volume enclosed by this surface the *recognition volume* V_r.

By a similar argument, a single antibody can be mapped into antigen space and a surface can be drawn around the antigen which most closely matches the antibody to determine the set of all antigens which that antibody can recognize. The question we would like to answer is: With a typical immune repertoire, how much of antigen space is covered by the antibodies present?

We can get a feel for the answer to this question using a rough argument as follows. Suppose there are N antibodies present, and that they occupy random positions in shape space. Suppose further that the total volume of the antigen space is V_g.[7] Very roughly, if $NV_r \gg V_g$, we would expect that most, if not all, of antigen space will be recognized by at least one antibody. To make this a bit more definite, we observe that the average number of antibodies that will recognize any one antigen is NV_r/V_g. Since this is a constant over all of antigen space, we can use the Poisson distribution (see appendix B) to find the probability $P(n_A)$ that n_A antibodies will recognize any one antigen. If we define $\lambda \equiv NV_r/V_g$, we have:

$$P(n_A) = \frac{\lambda^{n_A}}{n_A!}e^{-\lambda}. \tag{8.1}$$

In particular, the probability that *no* antibody will recognize the antigen $(n_A = 0)$ is

$$P(0) = e^{-\lambda} = e^{-NV_r/V_g}. \tag{8.2}$$

Experimentally, it is known that the probability of a random B cell recognizing any particular antigen is about 10^{-5}. This is a good estimate of V_r/V_g, since it says that each B cell covers about 10^{-5} of the entire shape space. Putting this into eqn (8.2), we can find the probability of an antigen escaping detection for immune systems with varying repertoire sizes. With a repertoire of 10^6 different types of B cells, for example, we find that $P(0) \approx 4.54 \times 10^{-5}$, so that there is only about one chance in 22,000 that a random antigen will escape detection. With repertoires much smaller than

---

[7] The volume of the antigen space is, in principle, infinite. However, there must be limits to all of the shape and charge parameters due to restrictions on the sizes and charges of the antibody molecules. For example, antibody molecules that recognize a double-decker bus do not exist.

this, there is a significant chance that a few antigens will slip through. It is known that the smallest naturally occurring immune repertoire contains between 10^5 and 10^6 species of antibody, so it would appear that natural selection has found this limit on its own. This should not be surprising, since an immune system that is full of holes in shape space will not be of much use in protecting the animal from infection and will soon lose a contest of fitness and die out.

Most mature animals have immune repertoires larger than 10^6, with a correspondingly smaller probability of there being any holes in its coverage of antigen space. It therefore seems inevitable that antibodies will be recognized as antigens by other antibodies. Jerne's model proposes that each antibody has a *paratope* and an *idiotope*. The paratope is that part of the antibody that recognizes an antigen and binds to it. The idiotope is that part of an antibody which is recognized by another antibody—it is that part which acts as an antigen. Since each antibody is assumed to form a separate species with regard to both the paratope and the idiotope, both these sites must be located in the variable region of the antibody molecule. It is conceivable that the paratope and idiotope overlap, or even that they are identical. In the latter case, two antibodies with complementary binding regions would both recognize and be recognized by their counterpart in the network.

8.5.1 Immune memory

The mechanism of memory in the immune system is still largely unknown, although there are two main theories. The first theory asserts that, after stimulation by an antigen, the B cell enters a proliferative stage that ultimately results in it differentiating into either a plasma cell that does nothing more than secrete antibody, or a long-lived, dormant memory cell. The memory cell is presumed to remain in the immune system, waiting for another encounter with the same antigen that gave it life in the first place. If this should ever happen, the memory cells would spring into life, giving rise to a new and larger generation of proliferating B cells than was present for the first exposure. The problem with this hypothesis is that these memory cells would have to live much longer than the few days or weeks that ordinary immune cells survive, since in many cases, exposure to an antigen results in lifetime immunity to it.

The second hypothesis relies on the dynamics of the immune system. The immune system is presumed to have several stable states, some of which correspond to elevated levels of certain species of B cells. A virgin immune system contains low levels of a large number of B cell types. Triggering one of these species shifts the system into a new stable state in which larger numbers of that species are continually produced by cell division, thus maintaining the immunity to the antigen.

We have seen earlier that the process of maturation of the immune response is similar to a miniature evolving ecosystem where a variety of cell types is produced by mutation and only those with a high fitness, as measured by their affinity to antigen, survive to proliferate further. The network theory gives rise to another, quite different type of analogy.

We will see in the final section of this book that the brain consists of networks of interconnected cells (the neurons) which store information (memories) in the strengths of connections between them. Neurons can send each other excitatory (stimulating) or inhibitory (depressing) signals, which give rise to many different activity patterns in the neural network.

The immune system also consists of a network of cells (B and T cells) which have varying strengths of interaction between them, as measured by the affinities of the various types of cells for each other. Cells can send excitatory signals to each other, as helper T cells do when they cause B cells to proliferate and release free antibody, or they can inhibit each other, as illustrated by the actions of suppressor T cells or antibody–antibody interactions in the network theory. It has been suggested that the immune system functions as a kind of 'second brain' because it can store memories of past experiences in the strengths of the interactions of its constituent cells, and it can generate responses to new and novel events (new antigens). In short, it can both learn and remember.

8.6   Models in immunology

There are many areas where theoretical models can be useful in immunology, but many of these areas are rather specialized. We will concentrate on just two areas: maturation of the immune response and the network theory of regulation.

We will examine several models of the immune network in the chapters that follow. It would be useful to survey these approaches here.

The modelling of a network of, potentially, several million interacting components poses, as you might expect, a non-trivial problem. Clearly, stating and solving several million simultaneous non-linear differential equations is out of the question, even with the power of computers available at present. Simpler approaches are needed.

One of the simplest quantitative approaches to network theory is the plus–minus theory of Hoffmann (Hoffmann, 1975b; Gunther and Hoffmann, 1982). The plus-minus theory reduces the entire network to two components. One component consists of antibodies (the 'plus' antibodies) which recognize the idiotopes on the minus antibodies. The minus antibodies, in turn, recognize the idiotopes on the plus antibodies. The theory is symmetric with respect to the two components.

As simple as this theory may seem, it successfully predicts the existence of four stable states in the network, which correspond to four states observed in real immune systems. The *virgin state* corresponds to an immune system which has never been activated. In the virgin state, the levels of all antibodies are low, although the two species in the model are still interacting.

Two symmetric stable states are also predicted by the model: the *immune state* and the *anti-immune state*. These two states correspond to a high level of one of the two antibody types and a reduced level for the other. This corresponds to a system in which one of the species has been triggered by the other and has mounted an immune response. As a result of this exposure the immune system has moved permanently from the virgin state to an immunized or vaccinated state in which the population of the triggered antibody remains at a high level.

The final state, called the *suppressed state*, consists of elevated levels of both antibody types. This state corresponds to a phenomenon observed in real immune systems which have been overloaded with antigen. In such a case, the system often shows a tolerance for the antigen, so that no immune response is mounted towards it. The immune system thus exhibits both a *low-zone tolerance* (no response if there is insufficient antigen present to trigger any B cells) and *high-zone tolerance* (too much antigen present).

Why an overdose of antigen should cause the immune system to become tolerant is still something of a mystery. Originally, it was thought that an overloaded B cell (one in which almost all of its receptors had become cross-linked with antigen) simply died, but recent experimental evidence seems to suggest that excessive antigen switches the cell off rather than killing it.

Other approaches attempt to confront the complexity of the system more directly. In such models, an attempt is made to represent the paratope and idiotope mathematically and populations consisting of a selection of such discrete molecules are allowed to form and evolve in computer simulations. Although these models offer more biological realism, they are often more difficult to interpret than a simpler, more elegant model such as the plus–minus theory. We will consider several examples of these computer simulation models in later chapters.

The immune system can be viewed as a classic system of coupled components with birth, death, and interaction components. As such, it seems custom-made for a differential equation model, and many such models have been constructed. However, the same caution must be applied when using such continuous models here as in other areas of biology. It must not be forgotten that the immune system is composed of discrete cells and antibody molecules. Even though the total number of immune cells and molecules in an animal may be large, it must be remembered that there are also a great many different species of such cells and molecules, so that the actual number of any one species may not be so great.

Differential equation models are more common than discrete computer simulations of the immune system, possibly because they are easier to construct and, given the availability of computer packages for numerical solution of large systems of equations, easy to solve. A purely discrete, stochastic computer simulation requires a great deal of programming skill to write, and much greater computer resources to run, than a typical continuous simulation. However, with the increasing availability of more powerful computers and more computer-literate immunologists, hopefully this situation will change.

9

Bell's model

9.1 Introduction

One of the first theoretical models of the immune system was that proposed by George Bell in 1970-71 (Bell, 1970, 1971a, 1971b). The model is based entirely on differential equations and therefore cannot realistically simulate an immune system consisting of small numbers of many different kinds of cells, but nevertheless does predict many of the observed properties of a real system.

We will consider the mathematical details of the model in the next section, but a preliminary survey of the model may help readers find their way through a bewildering array of symbols and equations. The system considered by Bell's model begins with a population of B cells, assumed to be present as a result of production from the stem cells in the bone marrow. Each so-called *target cell* is capable of synthesizing one type of antibody molecule. A number of different types of B cells (and therefore different types of antibodies) are allowed, but since each type of B cell introduces 5 differential equations into the model (as we shall see below), the total number of cell types is fairly limited. In Bell's original paper, up to 41 varieties of B cells are simulated.

A single species of antigen is introduced into the system. To give a broad spectrum of antibody responses, the logarithms of the affinities of the B cells for this antigen are chosen to be equally spaced over a biologically realistic range. Logarithms of affinities are used instead of the affinity values themselves in order that the lower range of affinities is represented properly. The antigen and various species of B cells are allowed to interact, with their populations governed by differential equations derived from the principles of chemical reactions. Cells that bind antigen enter a proliferating stage, during which they divide and also produce free antibody of the same species that they exhibit on their surfaces. Eventually, if the concentration of antigen falls to a certain level, these proliferating cells become either plasma cells that do nothing but secrete antibody (they do not divide further), or memory cells, which exhibit antibody on their surfaces and allow a much faster secondary response should the same antigen be encountered again.

The reader may think at this point that it is fairly obvious what will happen: those species of B cells with the highest affinity for the antigen will dominate and all other species will simply not respond. This would be the case except that Bell also attempts to simulate the phenomenon of *high zone tolerance* or *immunologic paralysis*, to which we referred in Chapter 8. Recall that tolerance to an antigen can be induced in an animal in several ways, one of which was the injection of a very large dose of antigen. Bell attempts to model this phenomenon by assuming that any B cell which binds antigen to a large fraction of its surface antibodies will die, thus effectively eliminating the high affinity immune response to that particular antigen. At the time of Bell's paper, the mechanism of tolerance was a mystery. As we discussed in Chapter 8, it is now believed that tolerance is due to certain classes of cells being inactivated rather than killed, although the actual mechanism of this inactivation is not known. However, as the inactivation of a cell effectively removes it from participation in the immune response, for the purposes of a model we might just as well assume the cell has been killed. The introduction of tolerance into the model removes the advantage that would ordinarily be enjoyed by those B cells with high affinity for the antigen.

The model assumes that all antibody molecules have two binding sites, equivalent to the two variable regions at the ends of the arms of the Y-shaped antibody molecule (see Chapter 8). The antigen molecule used in the original model, however, is assumed to be small enough so that it will only bind to one such site on an antibody—such antigens would have to be fairly small molecules. A large antigen, such as a foreign cell, would have many binding sites which could contact many different antibody molecules. In the second version of the model (Bell, 1971a), Bell relaxes this restriction and allows large antigens with many binding sites.

The goal of the model, then, is to see what properties of a real immune system will arise from a purely deterministic model based on these assumptions. We now turn to the construction of the equations.

9.2   Equations of the model

For each species $j \in \{1, \ldots, J\}$ of B cell (J being the number of species), there are five quantities that we wish to keep track of, each as a function of time t. Each of these quantities may be thought of as a chemical concentration using appropriate units (for example, Molar, or moles per litre).

1. The number $N_{1j}(t)$ of target cells, that is, cells that have not changed their state from when they were synthesized in the bone marrow.

2. The number $N_{2j}(t)$ of proliferating cells. These are cells that have been transformed from the target cell state by encountering a sufficient quantity of antigen.

3. The number $N_{3j}(t)$ of plasma cells. These are cells that arise as a terminal phase of proliferating cells, when the antigen concentration has dropped to a low value.

4. The number $N_{4j}(t)$ of memory cells. Memory cells are structurally identical to target cells in this model. They are given their own function so that a record can be kept of their production.

5. The concentration $N_{5j}(t)$ of antibody molecules, including both free antibodies and those bound to antigen. These molecules are produced by proliferating cells and plasma cells. The index j not only labels the species of these cells from which the antibodies arise, but also identifies the species of antibody, since these secreted antibodies are of the same species as the surface receptors in the cells from which they arose.

In addition, we also must keep track of the number $N_6(t)$ of antigen molecules present. If there are a total of J types of B cells, we therefore have a system of $5J + 1$ functions to obtain from the model.

Allowance is also made for external sources of target cells (for example, from the bone marrow), free antibodies (for example, from an external injection) and antigen (which can be present as an initial condition or as a continually injected source, as from constant exposure to a source of infection). These sources are represented by externally specified functions $s_{1j}(t)$, $s_{5j}(t)$, $s_6(t)$ for target cells, antibody, and antigen respectively.

Bell's model contains a distressingly large number of parameters that must be specified before the simulation can begin. We will introduce these as the various equations for the functions above are derived. It should be borne in mind, however, that the presence of such a large number of external parameters indicates that the model has not really come to grips with the fundamentals of the system which it is trying to simulate. A 'deeper' model should be able to predict the values of many of the parameters that must be given as input here.

To get started, we need to specify the set of affinities that each antibody species has for the antigen. Since the affinities of free antibody and cell-surface antibody may not be the same, we need two parameters for each species. We define k_j to be the affinity of free antibody of species j for antigen, and k'_j to be the affinity of the same antibody species for antigen when it is bound to a B cell as a surface receptor.

It is now assumed that both free and receptor antibody are in chemical equilibrium with antigen. This is a reasonable assumption if the reaction rates are much faster than typical cell division times and antibody secretion rates, since it is these effects which determine the dynamics of the model. From what is known experimentally of these rates, the assumption is a good approximation.

This assumption of equilibrium allows us to derive an expression relating the concentration of antigen $N_6(t)$ to the concentration of antibody molecules $N_5(t)$. According to the law of mass action, we must have

$$k_j = \frac{[S_j L]}{S_j L} \tag{9.1}$$

where S_j is the concentration of unoccupied binding sites on free antibodies of type j, L is the concentration of free antigen, and $[S_j L]$ is the concentration of antibody–antigen complex.

Similarly, for the reaction between antigen and cell-surface receptors, we must have

$$k'_j = \frac{[S'_j L]}{S'_j L} \tag{9.2}$$

where S'_j is the concentration of unoccupied binding sites on antibody receptors attached to B cells, and $[S'_j L]$ is the concentration of receptor–antigen complex.

Now, the total number of binding sites on all non-receptor antibodies (free and bound to antigen) is $2N_{5j}(t)$ (since each antibody molecule has two receptor sites), or

$$2N_{5j}(t) = S_j + [S_j L]. \tag{9.3}$$

The total number of receptor sites R_j (= twice the number of antibody receptors embedded in B cells) is

$$R_j = S'_j + [S'_j L]. \tag{9.4}$$

R_j may also be expressed in terms of the concentrations N_{1j} and N_{2j} of target and proliferating cells, respectively.[1] We may write

$$R_j(t) = m(N_{1j}(t) + N_{2j}(t)) \tag{9.5}$$

where m is the number of receptor *sites* (twice the number of receptors!) per cell (assumed to be the same for all types of cell).

---

[1] Depending on the implementation of the model, the number of memory cells, N_{4j}, may also be included.

The total concentration of antigen $N_6(t)$ is the sum of free antigen and antigen bound to free antibody and to receptors:

$$N_6(t) = L + \sum_{j=1}^{J} [S_j L] + \sum_{j=1}^{J} [S'_j L]. \tag{9.6}$$

These equations may be solved algebraically to eliminate explicit dependence on S_j and S'_j to obtain

$$N_6(t) = L \left[1 + 2 \sum_{j=1}^{J} \frac{k_j N_{5j}(t)}{1 + k_j L} + m \sum_{j=1}^{J} \frac{k'_j (N_{1j}(t) + N_{2j}(t))}{1 + k'_j L} \right]. \tag{9.7}$$

Of the quantities in eqn (9.7), the constants m, k_j and k'_j are specified as parameters in the model, but L, the concentration of free antigen, will be a function of time. We will find that we need to know L in order to proceed with the model. Suppose we have obtained values[2] for the various populations N_{ij} ($i = 1, \ldots, 6$) at some time t_1 and we wish to find $L(t_1)$. By examining eqn (9.7) we observe that L is the only quantity we do not know, so we should be able to solve the equation for L. The equation is non-linear, so how can we be sure that a root exists, or of how many there are? If we think of the right-hand side of eqn (9.7) as a function $f(L)$ of L alone (all other quantities are assumed to be known for some time t), we see that it is a sum of a linear term (the first term, L) and $2J$ functions of the form $AL/(1 + BL)$, where A and B are non-negative constants. Now since L is the concentration of free antigen, it must lie in the interval $L \in [0, N_6(t_1)]$. In this interval, any function of form $AL/(1+BL)$ is monotonically increasing (a quick calculation involving the derivative of the function should convince the sceptical) and the sum of several monotonically increasing functions is also monotonically increasing. Now the left-hand side of eqn (9.7), considered as a function $g(L)$ of L, is just a constant $g(L) = N_6(t_1)$, since at some fixed time t_1, $N_6(t_1)$ will be known and constant. Graphically, then, eqn (9.7) is the intersection of a monotonically increasing curve $f(L)$ with a horizontal line $g(L) = N_6(t_1)$, which can give at most one solution.

How do we know that there are *any* solutions? From eqn (9.7), we can find the values of the function $f(L)$, defined over the interval $[0, N_6(t_1)]$, at its end-points. When $L = 0$, $f(0) = 0$. For $L = N_6(t_1)$, $f(N_6(t_1)) \geq N_6(t_1)$, so the range of the function must include the point $f(L) = N_6(t_1)$. Hence, eqn (9.7) always has exactly one solution for L. In practice, the

---

[2]This will be done by solving a system of differential equations.

equation converts into a polynomial in L which can be solved numerically using, for example, the Newton–Raphson iterative method.[3]

Once we have determined L, we can find two more quantities which will be useful in what follows: r_j, the fraction of antibody sites occupied by antigen, and r'_j, the fraction of receptor sites occupied. We need the latter quantity to determine the response of a target cell when it has bound a certain amount of antigen.

The fraction of free antibody binding sites that are occupied is

$$r_j = \frac{[S_j L]}{S_j + [S_j L]}.$$ (9.8)

Using eqn (9.1) we have

$$r_j = \frac{k_j L}{1 + k_j L}.$$ (9.9)

Similarly, for the receptor sites, we have, using eqn (9.2):

$$r'_j = \frac{[S'_j L]}{S'_j + [S'_j L]} = \frac{k'_j L}{1 + k'_j L}$$ (9.10)

from which we have the average number of occupied receptor sites (*not* the number of receptors, since each receptor has two sites!):

$$R'_j = m r'_j.$$ (9.11)

We are now ready to begin constructing the differential equations satisfied by the population functions $N_{ij}(t)$. Consider first the populations of target cells $N_{1j}(t)$. Target cells are synthesized in the bone marrow at a rate given by the source term $s_{1j}(t)$. Target cells are removed when they are transformed into proliferating cells or when they die. Death can result from the model's assumption of high-zone tolerance: if a cell has all or most of its sites occupied, it will die. At intermediate fractions of occupation, the cells will be transformed into proliferating cells, or die at a reduced rate of 'natural' causes. When no sites are occupied, no target cells will be transformed. We would therefore like a function $F(R'_j)$ giving the fraction of cells transforming or dying as a function of the number R'_j of occupied receptor sites. Since $F(R'_j)$ is a proportion of sites, it must satisfy the condition $0 \leq F(R'_j) \leq 1$. This function should be zero when $R'_j = 0$ and asymptotically approach 1 when R'_j gets large. Many such functions exist; Bell chooses the sigmoid form

---

[3]Even in the simplest case where $J = 1$ (there is only one species of antibody), the polynomial is a cubic which is best tackled numerically.

$$F(R'_j) = \frac{R'_j}{1 + R'_j}. \tag{9.12}$$

Note that the actual number R'_j of occupied sites on each cell is used in this formula rather than the fraction r'_j. This is because we could not talk about asymptotic behaviour if we used r'_j, since its maximum value is 1. We would like a function F which always admits some possibility, even if very small, that the cell will not transform into a proliferating cell or die, even when all its sites are occupied.

Loss of target cells due to transformations or death will occur at some characteristic rate. We can represent this by introducing a time parameter T_1 which is a measure of the length of time required for a triggered cell to transform or die.

Finally, a target cell has a finite lifetime even if no antigen is present, and will eventually die of old age (or boredom) with some characteristic time T'_1.[4]

Combining everything, we obtain

$$\frac{dN_{1j}(t)}{dt} = -\frac{F(R'_j(t))N_{1j}(t)}{T_1} + s_{1j}(t) - \frac{N_{1j}(t)}{T'_1}. \tag{9.13}$$

We have written out the time dependence explicitly to illustrate all the terms that are not constant. In practice, this notation will be too cumbersome, so we will abbreviate this equation, and the others that follow, by omitting the explicit time dependence. In this form, this equation becomes

$$\frac{dN_{1j}}{dt} = -\frac{F_j N_{1j}}{T_1} + s_{1j} - \frac{N_{1j}}{T'_1} \tag{9.14}$$

where $F_j \equiv F(R'_j) = R'_j/(1 + R'_j)$.

Note that the time constants T_1 and T'_1 are assumed to be constants independent of the species j of antibody (as are all time constants in the model). This may not be a realistic assumption, but there is little data available to provide a verdict on this point.

Now consider the proliferating cells N_{2j}. They arise initially from transforming target cells, but once some proliferating cells have been formed, they, as their name implies, begin to divide, producing more proliferating cells. Some proliferating cells will, however, differentiate to become plasma or memory cells.

Not all transformed target cells become proliferating cells, since some target cells with most or all of their receptor sites bound to antigen will die, due to the assumption about high zone tolerance. We therefore need

---

[4]This term is not included in Bell's model, but should be present for consistency.

to reduce the term $F_j N_{1j}/T_1$ in eqn (9.14) by some factor depending on r'_j, the fraction of receptor sites occupied by antigen. Again, many possibilities exist, but the simplest, chosen by Bell, is to multiply this term by the factor $(1 - r'_j)$ to give the rate at which target cells are transformed into proliferating cells. This factor has the desired effect: when $r'_j \approx 1$, virtually no cells are transformed since most of them will die. When $r'_j \approx 0$, almost all the triggered target cells become proliferating cells, although when r'_j is small, very few target cells will trigger in the first place, due to the function F_j. We therefore wish to include a term of the form

$$\frac{(1 - r'_j)F_j N_{1j}}{T_1} \tag{9.15}$$

in the equation for dN_{2j}/dt.

Of those proliferating cells already present, some will produce more proliferating cells while others will become plasma and memory cells. According to the assumptions in the model, plasma and memory cells should be produced mainly when the antigen level has dropped to fairly low levels. While there is still enough antigen present to warrant a vigorous response from the immune system, the main effort of the proliferating cells should be towards producing more such cells.

When a proliferating cell divides it will, of course, produce two daughter cells. Let us define a function $H_j \equiv H(R'_j)$ so that, on average, after a proliferating cell divides, there are $1 + H_j$ proliferating cells and $1 - H_j$ other (plasma or memory) cells. We would like a form for H_j such that, if R'_j is large, as will be the case when antigen is still plentiful, $H_j \approx 1$, so that most cell divisions will produce two proliferating cells. If R'_j is small, $H_j \approx -1$, so that very few proliferating cells are produced, and most cell divisions give rise to memory or plasma cells. Thus H_j gives the expected gain or loss (depending on whether H_j is positive or negative) in the number of proliferating cells per cell division. A convenient choice is

$$H_j \equiv \frac{R'_j - 1}{R'_j + 1}. \tag{9.16}$$

This equation introduces the assumption that when only one receptor site is occupied ($R'_j = 1$), there is an equal chance that a daughter cell will be another proliferating cell or a plasma/memory cell. There is no particular reason for this; we could equally well have chosen $H_j = (R'_j - 2)/(R'_j + 2)$ for example. In fact, the choice of the number of receptor sites bound when $H_j = 0$ is another implicit parameter in the model which must be decided before the simulation is run.

Finally, proliferating cells have a finite lifetime with a characteristic time of T'_2.

The equation for the proliferating cells is then

$$\frac{dN_{2j}}{dt} = \frac{(1 - r'_j)F_j N_{1j}}{T_1} + \frac{H_j N_{2j}}{T_2} - \frac{N_{2j}}{T'_2}. \tag{9.17}$$

To construct the equations for the memory and plasma cell populations, we must decide the proportions in which a differentiating proliferating cell will produce each cell type. Again, the simplest choice is that memory and plasma cells are produced with equal probability, although it must be remembered that this is yet another assumption implicit in the model. With this assumption, we obtain

$$\frac{dN_{3j}}{dt} = \frac{(1 - H_j)N_{2j}}{2T_2} - \frac{N_{3j}}{T_3} \tag{9.18}$$

for the plasma cells, where T_3 is the characteristic time for death of a plasma cell, and

$$\frac{dN_{4j}}{dt} = \frac{(1 - H_j)N_{2j}}{2T_2} - \frac{N_{4j}}{T_4} \tag{9.19}$$

for the memory cells. In the simplest form of the model, the memory cells play no further role, since the model has not been used to investigate the secondary response of the system. To do so, one would add the memory cells produced according to eqn (9.19) to the right hand side of eqn (9.14) as a source term for the target cells. Then, the next time antigen is injected into the system, a much increased population of target cells would be waiting for it.

These four equations determine the dynamics of the various types of cells present in the population. We must now examine the equations for free antibody and antigen.

Free antibody molecules are produced, potentially, from three sources: proliferating cells, plasma cells and external injections. Antibodies are eliminated either by combining with antigen (after which they are assumed to be removed from the system by means outside the scope of the model, such as macrophages) or by natural decay.

The rates of antibody production from proliferating and plasma cells are two more parameters that must be specified in the model. Let us define them to be c_2 and c_3 respectively. The external injection source term has been defined above as $s_{5j}(t)$.

To determine the fraction of free antibody that has combined with antigen, we may make use of the quantity r_j, the fraction of free antibody *sites* that are occupied by antigen. Since each antibody molecule has two binding sites, r_j is not the fraction we seek, but we may interpret it as the probability that a single site on an antibody molecule is occupied. Then the probability that both sites are occupied, assuming independence of the two sites, is r_j^2, and the probability that exactly one site is occupied is $2r_j(1 - r_j)$, so the total probability that an antibody has any antigen bound to it is $r_j^2 + 2r_j(1 - r_j) = 2r_j - r_j^2$. If antibody–antigen complexes are removed from the system with characteristic time T_5, and free antibody molecules decay with characteristic time T_5', we have

$$\frac{dN_{5j}}{dt} = c_2 N_{2j} + c_3 N_{3j} + s_{5j} - \frac{(2r_j - r_j^2)N_{5j}}{T_5} - \frac{N_{5j}}{T_5'}. \tag{9.20}$$

Finally, the equation governing the dynamics of antigen will have only one source term (external injection $s_6(t)$), since we are assuming the antigen is inert, so that it does not multiply on its own. Antigen molecules are assumed to have a natural characteristic lifetime T_6. They will also be eliminated by binding to free antibody. In this model, an antigen is not removed by binding to a receptor on a B cell. The amount of antigen bound to free antibody is (total antigen present N_6) − (free antigen L) − (antigen bound to receptors). The last term is given by (number of receptor sites per cell m) × (fraction of receptor sites occupied r_j') × (number of cells present $N_{1j} + N_{2j}$) summed over all species of antibody, that is, over j. Putting this together, we get

$$\frac{dN_6}{dt} = s_6 - \frac{N_6}{T_6} - \frac{1}{T_5}\left[N_6 - L - m\sum_{j=1}^{J} r_j'(N_{1j} + N_{2j})\right]. \tag{9.21}$$

Having constructed all the differential equations needed for the model, a simulation would consist of the following steps.

1. Specify values for the parameters and initial conditions.

2. Determine the value of L, the amount of free antigen, by numerically solving eqn (9.7).

3. Numerically solve the differential equations for the next time step.

4. Repeat steps 2 and 3 until the desired time is reached.

9.3   Results

The model can be used to investigate responses of the immune system to various conditions. We will briefly describe some of the experiments done by Bell. Readers interested in the quantitative details should consult the original papers by Bell (1970,1971a,1971b).

In the following series of experiments, the following parameter values were used.

- $c_2 = c_3 = 7 \times 10^6 \text{ hr}^{-1}$.

- $m = 10^3$.

- $T_1 = T_2 = 10$. (As mentioned above, in Bell's model the term containing T_1' did not appear. In practice, a large value such as $T_1' \approx 10^6$ hours may be used.)

- $T_3 = 50$, $T_4 = 10^6$, $T_5 = 10$, $T_6 = 100$, $T_2' = 10^6$, $T_5' = 200$.

All these values are based on experimental evidence, references for which may be found in Bell (1970).

A perpetual problem in using differential equations to model discrete objects (such as cells) is what to do when the equations predict the presence of less than one cell at some time. It may be argued that the solutions of a system of differential equations are predictions of the *average* behaviour of the system, so that a prediction of, say 0.75 cells could mean that in 75 per cent of real systems, one cell is present and that in the remaining 25 per cent, no cells are present.

Another possible way of handling fractional cells is to impose the condition that whenever the number of cells present is predicted to be less than one, the number of cells is set to zero. This is in fact what is done in Bell's model. Since the cell populations are represented not by absolute numbers, but by concentrations, this condition must be imposed as follows. The concentration of one species of target cell is given by N_{1j} which has units of moles/litre. If only one cell is present in a system with a volume of V litres, then the concentration is $N_{min} \equiv (6.02 \times 10^{23} V)^{-1}$ moles/litre, since the number of cells in one mole is Avogadro's number, or 6.02×10^{23}. The convention used in dealing with small values of N_{1j} is that if $N_{1j} < N_{min}$ at some time, then N_{1j} is set to zero at that time step.

This artifice can have potentially drastic effects on the system, since it means that it is possible for cell populations to die out entirely, rather than simply be reduced to very low, but non-zero, levels. For a model such as this in which only a single species of antigen is being considered, this may not make much difference, but if another species of antigen is introduced later for which the now extinct species of antibody had a high affinity, the ability of the system to respond to the new antigen has been drastically reduced.

If the antigen is delivered to the system all at once, for example, by injection at time $t = 0$, then the source function $s_6(t) \equiv 0$ for $t > 0$. We can investigate the effect of varying the initial dose of antigen.

A typical experiment is monitored by observing several key quantities. One such quantity is the mean affinity $\bar{K}$, defined as follows. We first calculate the weighted average of the logarithm of the antibody affinities:

$$\overline{\log k} \equiv \frac{\sum_{j=1}^{J} N_{5j} \log k_j}{\sum_{j=1}^{J} N_{5j}} \tag{9.22}$$

Then we define $\bar{K}$ as

$$\bar{K} \equiv e^{\overline{\log k}} \tag{9.23}$$

This quantity gives a good measure of the overall affinity of the antibody population.

The initial population of target cells contain receptors with values of k_j' ranging over values from 10^4 to 10^8, with initial concentrations in the region of 10^{-20} moles/litre.

The results are much what would be expected in that for very large doses of antigen, the cells with the highest affinities are killed off due to the high zone tolerance assumption. As a result, the response of the system is slower for high initial doses of antigen, and the resulting population of memory cells has a much lower average affinity $\bar{K}$ than in systems exposed to a lower antigen dose, although the population of memory cells is much greater for higher doses.

Rather than introduce all the antigen into the system at the start, antigen can be continuously fed into the system over a prolonged period (up to 1000 hours). This can be accomplished by setting the source function $s_6(t)$ to some non-zero value (either a constant, if the antigen is to be introduced steadily, or some other form if desired). In this way, overloading B cells with too much antigen at a time can be avoided, thus preventing them from dying. As expected, the response of the system is better in this case, with a much higher value of $\bar{K}$ for the resulting memory cell population and fewer species of target cells being killed.

Secondary immune responses can be simulated by allowing the effect of the first injection or exposure to antigen to pass through the system and then injecting a second dose of the same antigen into the trained system. The memory cells produced by the first exposure will have increased the ability of the system to respond to the antigen, since many more target cells of the correct affinity will be present at the second injection. The response of the model reflects this: a faster and more intense response occurs for the second injection.

By appropriate choices of parameter values and initial conditions, many of the observed features of real immune systems can be simulated using Bell's model. However, the model does not allow for any new species of antibodies to arise during the maturation process, nor for class switching, both of which are now known to be important processes. Indeed, it would be difficult to incorporate such effects into a differential equation model, since it would require introducing new equations into the model as a simulation was in progress. A more realistic approach to a system which can generate variety as it progresses is to use a fully stochastic simulation. We will examine such a model in subsequent chapters.

Bell's model is a valuable illustration of the construction of a differential equation model of a complex biological system, however. The biological goals are always kept firmly in view, and the parameters used are, as far as possible, taken from experimental data.

Several deficiencies in the model are corrected in Bell's second paper. One of the main restrictions of the model presented here is that an antigen molecule has only a single binding site. Another is that no limit is placed on the proliferation of triggered target cells, with the result that in extreme cases, the immune system can become larger than the entire animal. Both of these problems are tackled in the revised paper, but these modifications are beyond the scope of this book.

10

Adaptive walks

10.1 Introduction

We have seen in Chapter 8 that the process of maturation of the immune response is equivalent to evolution on a cellular scale. Once a B cell is triggered by encountering enough antigen, it enters a phase of rapid proliferation, during which the genes coding for the variable region on the antibodies produced by the B cell mutate at an enhanced rate, thus increasing the chances that an antibody with even higher affinity for the antigen will be produced. One theoretical framework which has proven useful in analysing evolving systems is that of the *adaptive walk*.

The concept of an adaptive walk on a fitness landscape was designed originally to provide a framework in which quantitative models of evolution could be constructed. The idea is not new, as it dates back at least as far as the 1930s in biology, and considerably further than that in physics. However, like so many theoretical techniques, its full potential can only be realized when it is incorporated into computer simulations.

We shall describe some of the properties of adaptive walks in general before proceeding to consider its application to a model of the maturation of the immune response. The work we will review here is primarily that of Stuart Kauffman and his collaborators (see Kauffman and Levin (1987), Kauffman and Weinberger (1989) and Kauffman *et al.* (1988)).

To keep things fairly general as well as simple, let us consider an abstract organism for which we can define a quantity called its *fitness*. We won't worry too much about precisely what we mean by fitness at this point, except to note that the higher an organism's fitness, the better off it will be. The fitness of an organism is determined by two factors: the internal state of the organism, and the environment in which it lives.

We will represent the internal state of an organism by means of a binary string (a sequence of zeroes and ones). This, in principle, places no limitations on our description of the organism, since any information can be represented as a binary string (all information stored on a computer is represented this way). However, for our purposes, it will be easier if we provide some definite interpretation for each bit in the string. We may think of the binary string as the base sequence of a DNA molecule in which only two bases are used (as we did in the spin glass model of the origin of life in Chapter 4), or as the amino acid sequence of a protein in which only two amino acids are used. We may even expand our horizons a bit and think of the binary string as an entire genome, with each bit representing a single gene coding for some trait of the organism such as eye colour, height, and so on Each gene has two different types, or *alleles* (represented by 0 or 1) so there are two possibilities for each trait, such as blue or brown eyes, tall or short growth patterns, and so on. The precise interpretation of the string of bits does not matter in this general version of the theory, except that each bit must code for something which can affect the fitness of the organism.

Before we introduce the environmental contribution to fitness, let us consider the concept of a *landscape*. Having defined the internal traits of the organisms, we can represent each distinct organism type as a point in some space. For ease of visualization, we will use a two-dimensional space and plot our organisms so that each type is assigned a grid point in this space. The method by which we distribute the organisms over this space may be based on some rule, or we may choose to scatter the organisms randomly. For example, suppose we have organisms represented by strings of, say, 4 bits, such as 0000, 1011, and so on. We may decide to plot them so that the first two bits provide the x coordinate and the last two the y coordinate (in binary). Then the binary string 0000 would be placed at the origin, 1011 at the point (2,3) (since 10 is binary for the integer 2, and 11 for 3) and so on. Another possibility is to arrange the organisms so that bit strings differing by single bits are adjacent (or as close to each other as possible), while those with a larger difference in their bit strings are further apart. Plotted in this way, the distance between two organisms could be used as a measure of their relatedness.

Now that we have the organisms spread over the space, we can introduce the environment and, with it, the concept of fitness. One of the central ideas of the theory of evolution is that the fitness of an organism can only be measured relative to its environment. Fish are well adapted for life in water, but are not found in the middle of a desert. If you move a fish from the sea into a desert, you have not changed the fish, only the environment, but the fitness of the fish has dropped considerably. We can, in a sense, define the environment by specifying a fitness for each organism that could be placed in it. An environment in which the fitnesses of animals with thick fur, birds with insulating down, and plants with tough ground-hugging branches are high and that of palm trees, monkeys and iguanas are low would be found in a place such as the arctic. Another environment in which the fitnesses are reversed for the same organisms would be found in a sub-tropical location.

We can introduce fitnesses and the environment they define into the model by simply specifying a fitness for each type of organism. Since we have represented the organisms by binary strings plotted on a two-dimensional surface, we can introduce fitnesses by turning the surface from a plane into a more rugged landscape, with the peaks corresponding to high fitnesses and the valleys to low fitnesses. The shape of the landscape will depend on how we have plotted the points corresponding to the binary strings and on how we have defined the environment.

We can model the evolution of a population on a fitness landscape as follows. If we consider an idealized population in which all members are genetically identical, then the entire population will occupy a single point on the landscape. If we are using two traits to specify the genotype of the population, we may think of placing the population at one point on a plane, rather like placing a piece on a chessboard, except that the squares can be at different heights. The fitness of the population would be indicated by the height of the point at which it was placed.

To be a bit more realistic, we must recognize that populations consist of individuals with a variety of genotypes, each with its own fitness. If the population contains only genotypes that are fairly similar, we may picture its members as occupying a region centred at a point in the landscape, rather than a geometric point corresponding to complete genetic uniformity.

The genotype of an individual is determined at its conception, and cannot be changed over the course of its life. This is true of both entire organisms and individual B cells. Therefore the only way the population can change its location on the landscape is to have offspring with different genotypes to their parents. The rules of the adaptive walk, however, state that a population cannot take a step on the landscape unless that step is uphill, in the direction of higher fitness. Downward steps are not allowed because they produce organisms that are less well adapted to their environment, and therefore stand less of a chance of survival. Such a journey on the fitness landscape is called an *adaptive walk*.

This condition is rigorously observed in the model that follows, but its application to real systems is still somewhat uncertain. The idea of life constantly striving towards loftier peaks on the fitness landscape has led to the view of man as the ultimate peak of evolutionary perfection. It also seems to indicate that evolution has some ultimate goal, or that the processes of mutation and natural selection are directed in some way. This is not the case. Mutation seems to be totally blind, and the process of selection is determined by the interaction of organisms with their environment. We must leave the question of whether there really is any ultimate goal or direction to evolution to the philosophers, as it is much too large a topic for this book. However, the basic theory of evolution itself makes no provision for any such goal.

The adaptive walk is often used in the purely mathematical problem of maximizing a function of several variables. A starting point is chosen and the direction of maximum gradient of the function is calculated. A step in this direction is taken to arrive at a new point on the surface, at which the direction of maximum gradient is calculated again, and so on.

Both the biological and mathematical applications of this hill-climbing technique for maximizing functions suffer from the drawback of local maxima. Once you have reached a hilltop in your walk, the method will not allow you to take any more steps, even if you know that there is a higher peak somewhere else. In the mathematical application, this can be a serious problem if the function is known to have many local maxima and the global maximum (the largest value assumed by the function in its entire range) is required. Various methods have been devised to circumvent this problem, including using several starting points, trying longer step lengths to 'step over' small hilltops, and so on.

From the biological point of view, however, the problem is not so serious, since we want to simulate what real populations actually do, which is not necessarily the best that they can do. Real organisms face the same problem of local maxima as the theoretical model, so if we simply build a model that uses adaptive walks to find local maxima, we should have a reasonable model of what biologically evolving systems do.

10.2   Uncorrelated landscapes

To get a feel for how adaptive walks work we will begin with the easiest case to analyse: that of the uncorrelated landscape. In such a landscape, each bit string is assigned a fitness at random, so that two strings which differ by only a single bit may have vastly different fitnesses. This is not a particularly realistic situation from a biological point of view, since two organisms whose genes are identical except for a very few point mutations are likely to be very similar to each other. However, the uncorrelated case allows us to develop a good picture of some of the properties of fitness landscapes using some very simple statistical arguments.

We will consider a population in which each organism is characterized by a gene (bit string) containing N bits, each of which can have the value 0 or 1. There are therefore 2^N possible types of organisms. Since the adaptive walk algorithm deals only with relative fitnesses (a step is taken on the landscape if a point with a higher fitness is found—how much higher is not considered), we do not need to assign absolute fitness values to each string. We can therefore rank the strings in order of increasing fitness, with a rank order of 1 indicating the lowest fitness, and 2^N the highest. To maintain the uncorrelated nature of the landscape, we will list the strings in random order, and assign rank order fitnesses in the order the strings are listed.

At each stage in the adaptive walk, the parent organism generates a sequence of offspring by mutating one (or more) of its bits (if the bit is a zero, it mutates to a 1 and vice versa). In the simplest case, only one bit at a time may be mutated. In systems where larger single steps across the landscape are allowed, more than one mutation may be allowed per generation. In the single-mutation case, the N bits are mutated one at a time, in random order, until a fitter mutant has been found or until all N bits have been mutated and no fitter mutant is found. In the latter case, the current organism is the fittest in its local area, and we have arrived at a local maximum in the fitness landscape. When this happens, the process terminates.

We can now investigate a few basic properties of such landscapes using the simplest of probabilistic arguments.

How many local maxima are there?

The number of local maxima depends on how large each step is allowed to be. To see this, suppose you have arrived a point in the landscape where the fitness is greater than at all points which can be reached by single mutations from your current location. If we are restricting ourselves to single mutations then we are at a local optimum. However, if a point that can be reached after two mutations has a higher fitness, and we allow two mutations per generation, then that point can be reached from our current location in a single step, and the current location no longer qualifies as a local maximum.

The notion of a local maximum as used here is different from that commonly used in the calculus of continuous functions. There, a point is either a local maximum or it isn't: there is no dependence on step size. The definition of a maximum here is a functional one—it is a point from which an organism cannot move without either breaking the rules of the simulation (by taking a larger step than is allowed) or reducing its fitness.

To estimate the number of local maxima, let us consider the one-mutation case. Here, each bit string has N other strings which are accessible by a single mutation or step on the landscape. Since all the strings are assigned unique rank order fitnesses, the chance that any one string has a higher fitness than any of its N nearest neighbours is

$$P_1 = \frac{1}{N+1}. \tag{10.1}$$

The average number of local maxima in a population is then

$$M_1 = \frac{2^N}{N+1}. \tag{10.2}$$

If $N = 4$, giving 16 string types, $M_1 = 16/5 \approx 3$, so we would expect about 3 local maxima in a population consisting of genes containing 4 bits. Note that this is only an average value, since the actual number of local maxima depends on the arrangement of the genes in rank fitness order. If we arrange things so that a path exists from the lowest fitness to the highest through intermediate strings, each separated from the next by a single mutation, there will be only one maximum, while if we arrange the strings so that fitnesses occur in alternating peaks and troughs, there could be as many as 8 local maxima.

If we allow more than one mutation per generation, the chance of any one string having a locally optimum fitness decreases. The number of 2-mutant neighbours of a single string is the number of ways of choosing two bits from N, which is just the binomial coefficient $\binom{N}{2} = N(N-1)/2$. The total number of 1-mutant and 2-mutant neighbours of any string is then $N + N(N-1)/2$. The chance that a string has a higher fitness than any of its neighbours now becomes

$$P_2 = \frac{1}{1 + N + N(N-1)/2} \tag{10.3}$$

so the average number of local optima becomes

$$M_2 = \frac{2^N}{1 + N + N(N-1)/2}. \tag{10.4}$$

If we allow each step to contain up to k mutations, the corresponding terms become

$$P_k = \frac{1}{\sum_{r=0}^{k} \binom{N}{r}} \tag{10.5}$$

and

$$M_k = \frac{2^N}{\sum_{r=0}^{k} \binom{N}{r}}. \tag{10.6}$$

In the extreme case where we allow all of the bits to mutate at once, we may use the fact that $\sum_{r=0}^{N} \binom{N}{r} = 2^N$ to show that

$$P_N = \frac{1}{2^N} \tag{10.7}$$

$$M_N = 1. \tag{10.8}$$

The latter condition arises from the fact that if all strings are accessible at each generation, there can be only one maximum.

For smaller values of k, however, there are many local maxima. For the single mutation model ($k = 1$) for example, if $N = 10$ there will be about 100 local maxima. This means that any system restricted to steps of a certain length will have many possible states in which it will stop evolving, all but one of which will be less fit than the best it could be.

In the more general case where the string representing the organism's type consists of units, each of which can be of B types (rather than the 2 types we have considered in the binary strings so far), the above equations can be generalized. If only single mutations are allowed, then each string of length N has $(B - 1)N$ single-mutant neighbours. We define D_1 to be the number of single mutant neighbours, so that

$$D_1 \equiv (B - 1)N. \tag{10.9}$$

The probability that a randomly chosen string will be the fittest in its one-mutant neighbourhood is

$$P_1 = \frac{1}{D_1 + 1}. \tag{10.10}$$

The total number of strings of length N is then B^N, so the average number of local optima is

$$M_1 = \frac{B^N}{D_1 + 1}. \tag{10.11}$$

In the completely general case where up to k mutations are allowed per generation, the number of neighbours accessible by a single step D_k may be calculated as follows. The number of ways of choosing k sites from N as the ones to be mutated is, as before, the binomial coefficient $\binom{N}{k}$. Each of these k sites can mutate to $B - 1$ possible values, so each choice of k sites results in $(B - 1)^k$ possible mutations. Thus the total number of neighbours is

$$D_k = \sum_{r=0}^{k} (B - 1)^r \binom{N}{r} \tag{10.12}$$

and the average number of local optima is

$$M_k = \frac{B^N}{D_k + 1} \tag{10.13}$$

How likely is it that a particular organism of fitness rank X will be a local maximum?

In the one-mutant neighbour case, any string has $D = (B-1)N$ neighbours. In order that a string of rank X is a local maximum, all of these neighbours must have a lower rank. The number of ways of choosing D strings from the $X - 1$ available strings of rank lower than X is $\binom{X-1}{D}$. The total number of possible choices of D strings from the $T - 1$ strings remaining (where $T = B^N$ is the total number of string types) is $\binom{T-1}{D}$, so the probability that X is a local maximum must be the ratio of these two coefficients:

$$P_m = \frac{\binom{X-1}{D}}{\binom{T-1}{D}} = \frac{(X-1)!(T-D-1)!}{(T-1)!(X-D-1)!}. \tag{10.14}$$

Using Stirling's approximation for $n!$

$$n! \approx \sqrt{2\pi n}\, n^n e^{-n} \tag{10.15}$$

we can derive an approximation to this equation if we assume that both X and T are much larger than D, so that $X - 1 \approx X - D - 1 \approx X$ and $T - 1 \approx T - D - 1 \approx T$. In this case

$$P_m \approx \frac{\sqrt{(X-1)(T-D-1)}(X-1)^{X-1}(T-D-1)^{T-D-1}}{\sqrt{(T-1)(X-D-1)}(T-1)^{T-1}(X-D-1)^{X-D-1}} \approx \left(\frac{X}{T}\right)^D. \tag{10.16}$$

The last form was obtained by applying the approximations assumed above to all factors except the exponents in the first expression.

The probability that an organism is a local optimum is, as we should expect, low if its rank fitness is low and rapidly approaches 1.0 as its rank X approaches the largest possible rank T.

How long is the walk before a local optimum is reached?
To get an upper bound, let us assume that we begin with the least fit string. Then any mutation will improve its fitness, and on average will result in a string with fitness $T/2$. If this is not a local maximum, then if we choose one of the fitter mutants available to this organism it, on average, will be half again as fit, so that its fitness will be $3T/4$. After k steps, the average fitness will be, assuming that a local optimum has not been found along the way,

$$F_k = T(1 - (1/2)^k). \tag{10.17}$$

At each step, the fitness of the string improves, but what is the probability that we have arrived at a local maximum after k steps? After the first step we will have a string with an average fitness of rank $T/2$. In order for this to be a local optimum, it must be fitter than all its D neighbours. We know for certain that it is fitter than at least one of its neighbours, since it just mutated from a less fit string, and this string is one that could be reached from the new string by a single mutation. Therefore all we need to worry about are the remaining $D-1$ neighbours. Using the approximate form (10.16) for the probability that a given string is a local optimum (replacing D by $D-1$ for the reason just given), we obtain the probability that we have arrived at a local maximum after one mutation (using $X = T/2$):

$$P_1 = \frac{1}{2^{D-1}}. \tag{10.18}$$

In order for the walk to continue beyond any step, the current point must not be a local optimum. The probability W_1 that the walk continues past the first step is then

$$W_1 = 1 - P_1 = 1 - \frac{1}{2^{D-1}}. \tag{10.19}$$

We can iterate this argument to obtain the general expression. The average fitness of the string after k steps, assuming we have not attained a local maximum in that time, is $F_k = T(1 - 1/2^k)$. The probability that this string will be a local optimum is

$$P_k = \left(1 - \frac{1}{2^k}\right)^{D-1}. \tag{10.20}$$

The probability that the walk will continue past step k, given that it has reached step k in the first place, is

$$W_k = 1 - P_k = 1 - \left(1 - \frac{1}{2^k}\right)^{D-1}. \tag{10.21}$$

The probability that the walk starting with the least fit string will continue past step k is then the product of the k terms W_r, $r = 1, \ldots, k$ since the walk must make it through each step independently. We have therefore the probability L_k that the walk will last through the kth step:

$$L_k = \prod_{r=1}^{k} \left[1 - \left(1 - \frac{1}{2^r}\right)^{D-1}\right]. \tag{10.22}$$

Most walks will proceed until the probability of their continuation is less than 0.5. For some value of D, let us see if we can find the value of k where this happens. If we suppose for now that $D-1$ is a power of 2, then there will be a term in eqn (10.22) where $r = R \equiv \log_2(D - 1)$ is an integer, where $\log_2$ indicates a base-two logarithm, defined so that

$$2^{\log_2 x} \equiv x. \tag{10.23}$$

Using this fact, that term will have the form

$$1 - \left(1 - \frac{1}{D - 1}\right)^{D-1}. \tag{10.24}$$

Now, one way of defining the the exponential function e^x is as a limit:

$$e^x = \lim_{n \to \infty} \left(1 + \frac{x}{n}\right)^n. \tag{10.25}$$

If $D - 1$ is large enough, the last term in eqn (10.24) is well approximated by $e^{-1} = 1/e$, and we have

$$1 - \left(1 - \frac{1}{D - 1}\right)^{D-1} \approx 1 - e^{-1} = 0.632 \tag{10.26}$$

to 3 decimal places. Now the term in eqn (10.22) with $r = R - 1$ will have one less factor of two in the denominator and may be written:

$$1 - \left(1 - \frac{2}{D - 1}\right)^{D-1} \approx 1 - e^{-2} = 0.865. \tag{10.27}$$

Backing up up two more terms, we get reasonable approximations from the expressions $1 - e^{-4} = 0.982$ and $1 - e^{-8} = 0.9997$. Terms before this may be taken to be 1.0 without much loss of accuracy. Similarly, terms following $R = \log_2(D - 1)$ may be approximated by $1 - e^{-0.5} = 0.393$, $1 - e^{-0.25} = 0.221$, and so on.

Putting all these approximations together gives us the following behaviour for L_k around $R = \log_2(D - 1)$.

k	L_k
$R - 2$	0.982
$R - 1$	0.849
$R = \log_2(D - 1)$	0.537
$R + 1$	0.211
$R + 2$	0.047

This table is a surprisingly accurate description of the behaviour of systems with fairly small values of R. For $R = 4$ ($D = 17$), the values are already accurate to within 5 per cent, while for $R = 10$ ($D = 1025$), they are almost exact.

This result indicates that most walks will stop within a step or two of $\log_2(D-1)$, since the cutoff in the value of L_k is quite sharp. It is a good programming exercise to write a small program which generates a population of strings and calculates the mean walk length as a function of D. You should find that the average walk length is near to R.

10.3   Correlated landscapes—*NK* models

The uncorrelated landscapes treated in the previous section are a useful introduction to adaptive walks, since they allow us to get a feel for the concepts involved by means of simple statistical arguments. However, real evolving systems will have some degree of correlation present. A step in a landscape is taken whenever an organism's genome sustains a mutation of some sort. Mutations come in various forms, each of which can cause different types of steps to be taken. Point mutations, involving changes in single bases in the DNA sequence, usually give rise to changes that are either neutral (have no effect on the organism) or of minor importance (a slight change in hair colour, for example). In this case, the two DNA sequences are separated by only a single mutation, and have fitness values that are the same or very similar.

Other types of mutations can have more serious effects. A *frameshift mutation*, in which a single DNA base has been deleted or inserted causing all the remaining bases to be shifted one frame from their original position, can change the amino acid sequence of a large section of a protein. Such a mutation usually drastically reduces the fitness of the organism, since it is highly unlikely that the resulting protein will have a function remotely similar to the original form, or indeed that it will have any function at all. In such a case, a single mutation results in an enormous drop in fitness, so that the two strings are not closely correlated in the landscape.

We will consider only point mutations in what follows. To introduce correlations into the landscape, we will assume that each site in the string (a 'site' corresponds to a base in a DNA sequence, an amino acid in a protein, and so on.) has an individual fitness associated with it, and that the fitness of the entire string is obtained by calculating the arithmetic average of the fitnesses of each individual site. The fitness of a site will depend on the identity of the bit at that site (we are reverting to the use of binary strings to represent sequences) and on the identities of K other sites, where K is a parameter that can vary from $K=0$ (where all sites are independent) to $K=N-1$, where the fitness of each site depends on all other sites in the string. Models of this sort are called *NK* models.

Another characteristic of the model is the manner in which the K sites are chosen. They may be chosen to be sites that are physically closest to the current site (for example, $K/2$ bases on either side of a base in a DNA sequence), or they may be chosen randomly from the entire sequence. There is some rationale for choosing sites from disparate locations in a sequence, since distant sites in a protein can approach each other when the amino acid string folds up so that the protein assumes its three-dimensional shape. The fitness of one site will be altered if the amino acid present at the distant location to which the first site binds is changed by a mutation, although mutations in adjacent sites may not affect the fitness of the site at all.

Having chosen the value of K and the manner in which the K sites are to be chosen, the fitness of each site must be calculated. Then the fitness of the entire string is taken to be the average of the fitnesses of all the sites. Since the fitness of each site depends on $K + 1$ bits (the site itself and the other K sites on which it depends), each of which can take on 2 different values, there are 2^{K+1} different fitnesses possible for each site. Ideally, to study such a system, we would create a catalogue of all possible fitnesses at each site and use this list to calculate the fitness of the string at each stage in the simulation. If we wish to write a computer simulation to study the behaviour of a system with a large value of K (around 50 or more), we cannot store a catalogue of all the different fitnesses, since there are far too many ($2^{50} \approx 10^{15}$). However, in any simulation only a small fraction of all possible sequences will arise, and the fitness of each sequence can be calculated and stored as it is needed.

In the absence of any experimental data on the fitnesses of distinct configurations the best we can do is assign a random fitness to each configuration for each site in the string. For convenience, this random fitness may be chosen from the flat distribution over the unit interval $[0, 1)$, since most random number generators produce numbers this way. This may seem contrary to our intention of introducing correlations into the landscape: after all, if altering a site (or any of the K other sites on which it depends) causes its fitness to change at random, then it may seem that two sequences that are similar in structure may have widely different fitnesses, just as in the uncorrelated case. However, the point to notice is that the fitness of the whole string is the *average* of the fitnesses of all the individual sites. Changing the fitness of a single site, even by a large amount, will not greatly affect the fitness of the entire string if there are many sites present.

We may now see how the value of K bears on the degree of correlation present in the model. If $K = N - 1$, then every site affects every other site, and a single mutation will change the fitness of every site in the string. In this case, the fitness of the entire string is the average of N random numbers, all of which change every time there is a mutation. This produces a system which is similar to the uncorrelated system considered in the previous section. It is not precisely the same, since there is no guarantee here that all strings will have different fitnesses, so it may not be possible to produce a rank ordering of fitnesses with each string allotted a unique position. However, most of the conclusions of the previous section should apply to $K = N - 1$ strings, since we would not expect many strings to have the same fitness.

Since we are now assigning actual values to the fitness, rather than just providing a rank order, we can investigate the behaviour of these values in the $K = N - 1$ model. Since the fitness of each site is a random number chosen from the unit interval, the fitness of the entire string will be the average of N such random numbers. Now the mean of the unit distribution is $1/2$ and the variance is $1/12$ so, by the central limit theorem[1] the average of N numbers drawn from such a distribution becomes a normal variable with mean 0.5 and variance $1/12N$ as N becomes large. Therefore, the fitness of any string will approach 0.5 as its length increases. There will always be a slight bias towards fitnesses greater than 0.5, since the evolution algorithm requires us to take a step only if that step will result in an increase in fitness, but as N increases, the probability that such a step will be found decreases. In fact, we can do a simple calculation to determine the probability that we will be allowed to take a step from our current position.

If we are dealing with a single-mutation model, then for a string of length N, there are N possible mutations from any given starting string. If we are not at a local optimum, at least one of these mutations must produce a string with a greater fitness. If the fitness of the starting string is f_0, we therefore want the probability that we will find at least one string with a fitness $f > f_0$ in N mutations. Let p_f be the probability that a single mutation produces a fitness $f > f_0$. Then the probability that a mutation does not produce a greater fitness is $1 - p_f$. The probability that none of the mutations produces a fitness $f > f_0$ is therefore $(1 - p_f)^N$. The probability that a step is taken is therefore

$$Prob(step) = 1 - (1 - p_f)^N. \qquad (10.28)$$

Since the probability p_f of the fitness of a mutant being greater than f_0 is obtained from the normal distribution[2], it is easily found from tables or a calculator with statistical functions. As an example, suppose we have a string with $N = 100$ and would like to know the probability that a fitness greater than $2/3$ (which turns out to be the average fitness in a $K = 0$ model—see below) is obtained in a single mutation. In this case we need $p_f = Prob(f > 2/3)$ from a normal distribution with mean 0.5 and variance $1/12N = 1/1200$. (The fact that the variance is so small should tell you that p_f is going to be vanishingly small,

---

[1]See Appendix B if you are unfamiliar with means, variances, and the central limit theorem.

[2]See Appendix B.

but we will continue with the calculation anyway.) This is equivalent to $Prob(z > (2/3 - 0.5)\sqrt{1200}) = Prob(z > 5.77)$ where z is a normal variable with mean 0 and variance 1 (the standard mean and variance listed in most tables of the normal distribution). From tables, we find that $p_f \approx 4 \times 10^{-9}$. For such a small value of p_f, the probability of a step given by eqn (10.28) is well approximated by $Np_f = 4 \times 10^{-7}$.

In fact, for a string of length $N = 100$, the probability p_f has dropped to around 0.1 when $f_0 = 0.53$, so strings of this length will virtually never achieve fitnesses significantly greater than the average of 0.5. Kauffman refers to this phenomenon as a 'complexity catastrophe'. As we will see, the less correlated a landscape is, the more local optima it has, so we can say that uncorrelated landscapes are, in the sense of optima available to the system, more complex than highly correlated landscapes which have few optima. This added richness in variety comes at the cost of most of these optima being of only mediocre fitness.

At the other extreme, the case $K = 0$ corresponds to a highly correlated system. In this case, all sites are independent, so that any mutation at a site affects the fitness of that site only. This produces a highly correlated system, since changing a single site only changes one of the N fitness values that go into the fitness of the whole string. We would expect similar strings to have similar fitness values.

A single mutation will produce a fitter string if it increases the fitness of the site at which the mutation occurs. Since we are considering sites with only two possible occupants (0 or 1), there are only two possible fitness values for each site, both of which are random numbers chosen from the uniform unit interval [0,1). The average maximum fitness for a single site is then the average value of the larger of a pair of random numbers. Although the mean value of random numbers chosen from the unit interval is 0.5, we would expect the average of the larger of two numbers to be greater than 0.5. We can work out this value using the following argument.

The probability density function (pdf) for the unit interval is $f(x) = 1$ if $0 < x < 1$ and zero otherwise. The probability that the larger of a pair of random numbers lies in the interval $[x, x + dx]$ is twice the probability that the first number lies in that interval, which is $f(x)dx$, times the probability that the other number is less than x, which is just x, since x is the fraction of the unit interval in the region $[0, x]$. The probability is *twice* this quantity because either the first or the second number in the pair could be the maximum. Thus the overall probability that the larger of a pair of random numbers lies in the interval $[x, x + dx]$ is $2xf(x)dx = 2xdx$, since $f(x) = 1$ in the interval. The mean of this quantity is then

$$2 \int_0^1 x^2 dx = \frac{2}{3}. \tag{10.29}$$

We would therefore expect the mean fitness of any site that has mutated to be 2/3. The mean fitness of the entire string is therefore also 2/3, since it is just the average of N random variables, each of which has mean 2/3. A similar calculation shows that the variance of optimal fitness of each site is 1/18, so by the central limit theorem, the variance of the optimal fitness of the entire string will tend to $1/18N$ as N gets large. Long strings are virtually guaranteed to have fitnesses of 2/3 if they are allowed to evolve long enough.

This is an obvious improvement over the $K = N - 1$ uncorrelated landscape, but it comes at the cost of having only a single optimal state in the landscape. This must occur because, for any string that is not in its optimal state, there must be at least one single mutation that will improve its fitness, so there is an unbroken path from any suboptimal string to the optimal string. The fitness landscape must resemble a cone (or to be more picturesque, Mount Fuji).

We have already derived an estimate for the walk length on an uncorrelated landscape and found that most walks will end after about $\log_2 N$ steps (since $D = (B - 1)N = N$ if $B = 2$). Let us consider walk lengths on the correlated landscape where $K = 0$. Since each site has two possible values (0 and 1) and one of these has a higher fitness than the other, we may take the higher fitness to be the 'correct' fitness and the lower to be the 'incorrect' fitness. If a string has c correct sites, it requires $N - c$ mutations to attain the optimal fitness. If mutations occur at random sites in the string, we would expect only a fraction $p_m \equiv (N - c)/N$ of these mutations to occur at incorrect sites, that is, at sites where a mutation will improve the fitness. Mutations at correct sites will be ignored, since they would cause a decrease in fitness. However, we are interested in the total time required for the optimal fitness to be reached, so we will have to count mutations that result in lower fitness even though the string remains unchanged (that is, the mutated string is thrown away in favour of keeping the original string).

The probability of finding the first mutation that improves the fitness on the nth try is the probability that the first $n - 1$ mutations decrease the fitness and the nth improves it. This is $(1 - p_m)^{n-1} p_m$. The mean number of steps until the first improvement is then

$$\bar{n} = \sum_{k=1}^{\infty} k p_m (1 - p_m)^{k-1}. \tag{10.30}$$

This sum can be evaluated by observing that it is equivalent to

$$\bar{n} = \frac{p_m}{1 - p_m} \frac{d}{ds} \sum_{k=1}^{\infty} [(1 - p_m)s]^k \bigg|_{s=1} \tag{10.31}$$

where s is just a parameter introduced for convenience.[3] The sum is now an infinite geometric series, which we may sum to get

$$\bar{n} = \frac{p_m}{1 - p_m} \frac{d}{ds} \frac{1}{1 - (1 - p_m)s}\bigg|_{s=1} = \frac{1}{p_m}. \tag{10.32}$$

On average, we require $1/p_m = N/(N - c)$ mutations to take a single step upwards on the landscape. Using a similar calculation, we may find that the variance is

$$\sigma_n^2 = \frac{1 - p_m}{p_m^2} = \frac{Nc}{(N - c)^2}. \tag{10.33}$$

How many mutations will we need to reach the optimal fitness? In the worst case, we would start with a string in which none of the sites is correct, so that $c = 0$. Since the average time to take a step is given by eqn (10.32), the total time to go from $c = 0$ to $c = N$ is

$$T_N = \sum_{c=0}^{N-1} \frac{N}{N - c} = \sum_{c=0}^{N-1} \frac{1}{1 - c/N}. \tag{10.34}$$

If N is large, we may approximate this by an integral:

$$T_N \approx \int_0^{N-1} \frac{dx}{1 - x/N} = N \ln N. \tag{10.35}$$

The variance may be evaluated in a similar manner to give

$$\sigma_N^2 = \sum_{c=0}^{N-1} \frac{Nc}{(N - c)^2} \approx \int_0^{N-1} \frac{Nx\,dx}{(N - x)^2} = N^2 - N - N \ln N. \tag{10.36}$$

The walk lengths are therefore much longer on a correlated landscape ($N \ln N$) than on an uncorrelated one ($\ln N$), although these longer walks lead to much higher peaks than the gentle hilltops in an uncorrelated landscape.

It is not easy to analyse those values of K between 0 and $N - 1$ in the same fashion as for the extreme cases considered above. The easiest way to get a feel for the results is to do some numerical simulations, such as those reported by Kauffman *et al.* (1988).[4] The most significant finding,

---

[3]This 'trick' is a simple application of a more general statistical technique called a *generating function*, which can be used to generate means, variances, and higher moments of some distributions.

[4]You will find that computer simulations involving random numbers are referred to by Kauffman and some other authors as *Monte Carlo* simulations. The term presumably arises from the famous casino in Monte Carlo in which the fates of some people's lives are determined by random number generation.

apart from the fact that the theoretical results presented in this chapter are confirmed by numerical simulation, is that as K is increased from 0, the fitness values of the local optima increase slightly from the value of $2/3$ when $K = 0$ to values around 0.70 before declining to values just above 0.5 as K approaches $N - 1$ and the complexity catastrophe rears its ugly head. The number of local optima steadily increases as K increases, and the average walk length to a local optimum steadily decreases. All this would indicate that there is some optimal value of K at which a reasonable amount of variety can be generated in the form of several local optima, while at the same time allowing these optima to possess respectable fitness values, rather than the sea of mediocrity present for an uncorrelated landscape. The question arises: Is evolution able to find these values of K which allow a richness in the population, while still allowing the organisms present to be fit enough to survive?

There is another form of complexity catastrophe which has already been mentioned in Chapter 2, when we discussed Eigen and Schuster's model of the origin of life. In the $K = 0$ case, we argued that the landscape was highly correlated because the fitness of an individual site had a relatively small effect on the total fitness of the string. This was due to the fact that the string's fitness is the average of N random variables, so changing one variable will not affect the average if N is fairly large, and the larger N is, the smaller the effect of each site. Now suppose we have a string that has evolved until it is at or very near the maximum in the fitness space (recall that the $K = 0$ model has only a single maximum). The probability of any given site mutating remains the same for a highly fit string as for any other string, so this optimal string will constantly be producing slightly inferior copies of itself in addition to those copies that are accurate reproductions and hence still optimally fit. In order that the fittest strings retain their position as the majority of the population, the difference in fitness between them and their slightly inferior offspring must be enough that the optimal strings can outlive and outperform their children. If this is not the case, there will be a steady increase of these inferior copies at the expense of the fitter parents.

The larger the value of N, the smaller is the individual contribution of each site to the total fitness. This means that for very long strings, the difference between the optimal string and a mutant with a single incorrect site will be very small, so small that there will be no difference in the success of the two string types in the population. In other words, there will be a critical value of N at which the selection pressure which pushes strings towards higher and higher fitness peaks is not discerning enough to distinguish between the numerous slightly inferior offspring and the optimal parent, so that increasing numbers of suboptimal strings are tolerated in the population. Thus for correlated landscapes, there would appear to be a limit to the size of string which can be maintained in the population, just as Eigen and Schuster found when discussing the origin of life. It is not known whether this catastrophe occurs in less correlated landscapes, but it should be a field open to numerical investigation.

10.4 Adaptive walks in maturation of the immune response

10.4.1 The model

After this lengthy description of adaptive walks on fitness landscapes, it is finally time to see how they apply to the immune system (Kauffman and Weinberger, 1989).

As we mentioned at the beginning of this chapter, the main application of adaptive walk theory to immunology is as a model of the maturation process, especially the hypermutations that occur as the stimulated B cell proliferates. We wish to follow the descendents of a B cell after it has been triggered by antigen in an attempt to learn something about its journey through the adaptive landscape.

We may picture the adaptive landscape for the immune system as a space in which a species of antibody (and the B cells that secrete them) occupies a point determined by the structure of the molecule. The *structure*, in this model, will be represented by the amino acid sequence of the variable region of the antibody. Thus N, the number of individual sites, each of which contributes towards the fitness of the molecule as a whole, is the number of amino acids in the molecule. It is known from the DNA sequences of the genes coding for the variable region that there are between 110 and 120 such sites.

Each of these sites can have one of 20 identities, since there are 20 different amino acids from which to choose. Ideally, at this point we should choose the correlation parameter K, which determines how many other sites a particular amino acid will affect. However, we have no data on which to base such a choice. In fact, the determination of K and, therefore, the degree of correlation of the walk on the landscape, is one of the goals of the model. We will therefore run the model with several different values of K in an attempt to find the range of values which give the most realistic behaviour.

The fitness of each antibody is determined according to the prescription given in the previous section. The fitness of each site is chosen as a random number from the uniform distribution over the unit interval [0,1). The fitness of the entire molecule is the average of the fitnesses at each site. The value of K determines at how many sites fitnesses will change when a single amino acid is altered. The higher the value of K, the less correlated is the landscape.

In order to begin a simulation run, some initial conditions need to be set. In particular, we need to specify the population of B cells which have been stimulated to begin proliferation. It is known from experimental studies that for any given antigen, only about one in 10^5 B cells has an affinity high enough to be triggered. Since the fitness of an antibody is the average of between 110 and 120 (in practice, Kauffman and Weinberger used $N = 112$) random numbers chosen from the unit interval, by the central limit theorem[5] this fitness will have a normal distribution with a mean of 0.5 and a variance of $1/12N$. From tables of the normal distribution, we find that, if $N = 112$, a fitness greater than about 0.617 occurs with probability of 10^{-5}, so this is the minimum required fitness for an initial antibody.

Having chosen our initial population, we begin the proliferation process by allowing a single mutation in the antibody string. If we define a mutation to be a single amino acid substitution, there are $19N$ nearest neighbours to any given antibody. However, if we are representing the antibody not by an amino acid string, but by a DNA sequence, it must be realized that not all amino acid substitutions are possible from a single mutation in the DNA sequence. If we choose to use DNA as our string rather than amino acids, we must restrict the number of possible mutations accordingly.[6]

We now must make a choice for K. It is believed from experimental data that between six and eight mutations occur in the average antibody as it goes through the maturation process. Although this is only a rough guide, it would make sense to experiment with values of K until a walk length of this size was found.

We also need to specify how the K sites are to be distributed over the string. Again, Kauffman and Weinberger tried several possibilities (nearest neighbours, random placement, and so on.), but found that this did not affect the results significantly.

10.4.2 Results

For a string with $N = 112$, it was found that a value of K near 40 produced walk lengths in the required range. If K is reduced to near 30, the walk lengths become too long (> 10) and if K is increased to around 50, the walk lengths drop to values below 5.

This value of K would indicate that each amino acid interacts with about 40 others in the antibody. There is very little experimental data with which to compare most of the results in this model, but an experiment on the protein cytochrome C (which is, admittedly, not an antibody, although it has a length of 106 amino acids so it is similar in size) suggests that one

---

[5]See Appendix B.

[6]This restriction reduces the number of single-step mutations to about a third of the possible single amino acid substitutions. It turns out that the model is relatively insensitive to which method is used.

site can affect around 30 other sites in the same molecule. The value of $K = 40$ is therefore in a realistic region.

The model also predicts a realistic value for the fraction of single-mutant variants which will be fitter than the starting antibody. We typically find around 1 per cent of the mutants are fitter in the first generation. As the local optimum is approached, however, the number of fitter variants declines towards zero. Again, indirect experiments on other proteins indicate that this is a reasonable value.

Computer experiments have been performed to determine the number of accessible local optima from a single starting point. Usually, several hundred such peaks are found. There are essentially no data on this point, however, so the significance of this finding is unknown.

Probably the most interesting prediction to come out of the NK model of the immune system concerns the existence of *conserved sites* in the antibody molecule. One method that biologists have used to trace evolutionary lineages among organisms is to compare the DNA and amino acid sequences for a single protein from various organisms. One of the most heavily studied is the protein cytochrome C, but the same technique can be applied to any protein. When the sequences from several different organisms are compared, it is often found that certain sites in the protein never change, while other sites tend to be occupied by different amino acids in different animals. The constant sites are called conserved sites, because the identities of the amino acids at these places seems to be very important. The most obvious interpretation of this phenomenon is that conserved sites represent locations that determine the function or activity of the protein, while the other sites (where the identity of the amino acids isn't so vital) are merely filler sites which are there merely to ensure that the conserved sites are at the correct locations in the molecule.

Since the NK model of the immune system constructs antibodies without any explicit mention of their three-dimensional structure, it may come as something of a surprise to find that the model predicts the existence of several conserved sites in the antibody as it walks towards a local maximum in the adaptive landscape. Not only that, but the actual proportion of the total molecule that these sites represent (about 1-2 per cent) agrees roughly with experimental data on other similar proteins.

The model allows conserved sites because, with $K = 40$, considerably below the uncorrelated value of $N - 1 = 111$, it is possible for no more than one or two sites in the molecule to be connected to other sites whose fitness values drop drastically when the original sites mutate, thus effectively eliminating the affinity of the molecule. If the value of K were to increase to 50, however, we find that almost any amino acid substitution will have this effect because the range of influence of each site has grown too large for the effects of a mutation to be damped out by the rest of the molecule.

On the other hand, if K falls to 30, most amino acid substitutions have very little effect. When $K = 40$, however, we have a variety of different sites. Some can tolerate almost any substitution, others must be strictly conserved, while still others are tolerant of a mutation to some amino acids but not to others.

Thus, the value of $K = 40$, which was chosen solely on the basis that it provided the correct number of steps in the adaptive walk, seems also to be the level at which the maximum variety of amino acid site type (conserved or variable) occurs.

The adaptive walk model of the immune system is capable of making some powerful and general predictions. However, there is, as yet, very little data against which to test these results. One of the marks of a successful theory is that it points the direction in which future experiments should go.

11

Maturation of the immune response

11.1 Introduction

The models of the immune system we have considered so far have treated the various components (B cells, antibodies, antigens, and so on.) as abstract objects which may be characterized by a few numerical parameters. While this sort of model is useful for getting a feel for how a complex system operates, we would like a model which allows us to include a bit more of the experimentally determined features of the cells and molecules of the immune system. We will examine such a model, proposed by Weinand (1990), in this chapter. Weinand's model deals with the specific problem of initial stimulation of the immune system with an antigen, and the subsequent maturation of the response through proliferation and hypermutation of the B cells.

11.2 Representation of components of the immune system

Rather than view the components of the immune system as abstract objects described by a few numerical parameters, Weinand represents them as molecules with a specified three-dimensional geometry. The parameters determining the type and magnitude of interactions between antigen and antibody then arise naturally as a consequence of the structures of the molecules.

The most critical parameter in determining the strength of the interaction between an antigen and an antibody (whether or not the antibody is attached to a B cell) is the affinity between the two molecules. On the atomic level, this affinity is determined by various types of chemical bonds which are formed (or not) according to the shapes of the antibody and antigen, and their positions relative to each other when they meet. If the two molecules have even a mild affinity for each other, they will tend to adjust their relative positions to find the best fit. If this best fit produces a strong enough bond, the antigen and antibody will have a high probability of remaining attached to each other long enough for the chain of events leading to proliferation of the B cell to begin.

One simple way of modelling such a system would be to consider a single antigen and then define a population of antibodies with a certain distribution of affinities for that antigen, much as Bell (1970) did in his model (see Chapter 9). Although such a model is relatively easy to implement, it is not very satisfying because it gives no insight into how the affinity arises, nor does it allow a natural treatment of the mutation that occurs in the variable region of the antibody when the B cells proliferate.

The solution adopted by Weinand is to represent each type of antibody by the stretch of DNA that codes for the variable region of antibody molecule. If we have a way of mapping the DNA sequence onto the three-dimensional structure of the resulting molecule, and of using this structure to determine the affinity of the antibody for a given antigen, it is then easy and natural to examine the effect of a mutation in the DNA sequence when the B cell proliferates.

As usual with any computer model of a biological system, limitations on memory and time drastically restrict the degree of realism that can be simulated. A typical antibody molecule contains more than one hundred amino acids in its variable region, and there can be several million different types of antibody present in a normal immune system. Storing such a large amount of data would be beyond the capacity of most university computing systems, and, even if enough space were available, attempting to run a simulation using such a vast amount of space and time is not a good way to make friends with the other members of your department.

For these reasons, the model actually implemented by Weinand is a scaled-down version of a real immune system. Each antibody molecule has a variable region that consists of only four amino acids. Each amino acid can be one of 16 possible types (rather than the 20 found in nature), so there is a total possible repertoire of $16^4 = 65\ 536$ possible antibody types. An antibody can then be represented in the computer by the sequence of 12 DNA bases required to code for the four amino acids in the variable region. Even with such a reduced system, several megabytes of disk space are necessary to store the characteristics of the full repertoire, including their base sequences, affinities for various antigens, and so on.

The paratope (antibody–antigen combining site) is represented by a square region divided into an 8 by 8 grid, rather like a chessboard. There are two amino acids on the top and bottom of this square, with side chains that project towards the horizontal midline of the region (see Fig. 11.1). Each of the 16 amino acid types is assigned a shape, consisting of a backbone of four units and a side chain of between zero and three units projecting from each of the four backbone units (Fig. 11.2). These shapes are based, very roughly, on the actual shapes of the amino acid molecules used in building proteins.

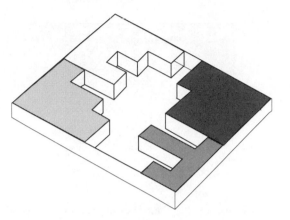

Figure 11.1 A binding site on an antibody molecule. Four amino acids enclose an area into which an antigen may bind.

It can be seen that each choice of four amino acids determines a different shape for the paratope region in the square. An antigen is assumed to consist of a pattern of blocks which can slot into the space formed by the amino acid side chains, like a piece in a jigsaw puzzle. Antigens need not consist of totally connected patterns of blocks, since a large antigen, such as a foreign cell, may have several projections which slot into separate parts of the paratope.

In order for an antigen to have a chance of binding to the antibody, it must be able to fit entirely into the binding site formed by the four amino acids. Only those surfaces of the antigen which lie next to surfaces in the antibody can contribute to the binding strength or affinity. The antigen can be translated and/or rotated through multiples of 90 degrees to obtain the best fit (highest affinity).

The calculation of the affinity may be done by various means. Probably the simplest is just to count up the number of antigen surfaces that lie next to antibody surfaces. Included in the count are those surfaces that lie on the floor of the paratope region as well as those that lie adjacent to a block in one of the side chains of an amino acid.

For added realism, Weinand introduces several different 'classes' of surface on the antibody and antigen molecules, reflecting the fact that different sorts of molecular subunits have different affinities for each other. Some surfaces, for example, may be charged and therefore have a high affinity for other surfaces with an opposite charge. Other surfaces may have a shape that fits more closely on the atomic scale with certain types of subunit than with others. Each unit surface area on an amino acid side chain is assigned

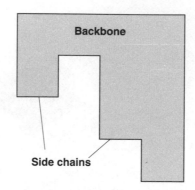

Figure 11.2   Model of an amino acid.

one functional type or class, which may be related to the actual properties of that amino acid, or may be chosen arbitrarily. Similarly, each unit area on the antigen is also assigned a class. Since antigens can be virtually any substance, these classes would be chosen at random. When two unit surfaces come into contact in the binding site, a contribution to the total binding force is obtained by pairing off the adjacent faces on the antigen and antibody, and consulting a table of binding forces. Weinand used five functional types, and proposed the following table of binding forces:

Type	1	2	3	4	5
1	1.0	1.0	1.0	1.0	1.0
2	1.0	-4.0	6.0	1.0	1.0
3	1.0	6.0	-4.0	1.0	1.0
4	1.0	1.0	1.0	4.0	1.0
5	1.0	1.0	1.0	1.0	11.0

Since the interactions are symmetric, it does not matter whether the rows are assumed to represent the antigen and the columns the antibody or vice versa. For example, if a unit area of type 2 on the antibody contacted an area of type 3 on the antigen the contribution to the binding force is 6.0.

The units of force used in this method are more or less arbitrary, and in practice, the binding force would be transformed to give biologically realistic values. One such transformation is

$$K_{ij} = c_1 c_2^{B_{ij}} \qquad (11.1)$$

where B_{ij} is the binding force calculated using the table above and c_1 and c_2 are constants. The quantity K_{ij} is then the equilibrium constant for the reaction between antibody i and antigen j. In terms of the concentrations $[Ag]$, $[Ab]$, and $[AgAb]$ of antigen, antibody, and antigen–antibody complex, respectively, K_{ij} would be written

$$K_{ij} = \frac{[AgAb]}{[Ag][Ab]}. \tag{11.2}$$

The values of c_1 and c_2 used in the model are $c_1 = 5 \times 10^{-11}$ and $c_2 = 1.72$. These parameter values yield affinity strengths in line with those observed experimentally. The exponential transformation has the effect of greatly enhancing the affinity of those antibodies that bind strongly to an antigen.

As described in Chapter 8, a B cell must be triggered by binding sufficient antigen before it will begin to proliferate and differentiate to produce more copies of itself, some of which will ultimately release free antibody. In the model, a B cell cannot be triggered unless the binding force between antibody and antigen exceeds a threshold value, and the B cell binds at least a critical number of antigen molecules. These two quantities become parameters in the model.

11.3 Steps in the simulation

A repertoire of antibodies is determined by deciding on the side chain shapes of the individual amino acids and the form of the binding force and then generating a table giving the 65 536 possible antibody structures. Even with the ability of the antibody genes to generate diversity by permuting their components, a real system is not capable of storing enough genetic information to produce every possible antibody structure. Similarly, in the model, only a fraction of the complete repertoire can be generated directly from the genes present in the organism. In practice, only about 6000 of the 65 536 possible antibodies may be produced by direct translation of the DNA code. It is hoped that many of the remaining antibodies will be produced by hypermutated offspring of these genetically produced cells.

The model considers the response of the immune system to a single antigen. To start the cycle, several genes, chosen at random, are activated so that a starting set of about 120 B cell types are produced, with about 50 copies of each type. During each cycle of the model, another batch of 120 B cell types, with 50 copies of each, are introduced into the system. The average lifetime of a B cell is seven cycles, giving an observed average of around 1800 species of B cells present in the system, after enough cycles have elapsed to bring things into equilibrium.

After the introduction of B cells, the antigen is introduced and allowed to interact with the B cells that are present. Any B cells that display antibody on their surfaces that has a high enough affinity for the antigen will eventually bind enough antigen to be triggered. At this stage, enough antigen is present to saturate the system. The interaction between antigen and antibody is done according to the methods given above: the shapes of the antigen and antibody are matched to obtain the highest bonding force, and if this force exceeds the threshold for activation of the B cell, the bond triggers the cell.

A triggered B cell will begin to multiply. At this stage, the mutation rate must be determined. Experiments with different mutation rates may be performed to see how quickly the immune response can 'fine-tune' itself to the antigen, that is, produce an antibody with the maximum affinity. In the simulation reported by Weinand, several runs were done with between 0 per cent and 50 per cent of the daughter cells being mutants. It is believed that many real immune systems show mutation rates approaching 50 per cent.[1]

The mutation is implemented by randomly changing one of the bases out of the 12 that are being used to represent a particular antibody. Due to the degeneracy of the genetic code, this may not actually change the amino acid for which the mutated codon codes. If no change in the amino acid composition occurs, the mutation is called *silent* and no change will be observed in the affinity for the antigen. However, silent mutations can have an effect if the cell should divide again, since a further mutation will now cause the new cell to be two steps removed from the original cell. This two-step change may give rise to a new amino acid which could not be reached in a single step from original cell, but only by using the silent mutation as an intermediary.

The most common type of mutation will be one which does change the amino acid at one of the sites, however. Of these mutations, most will decrease the affinity of the antibody, usually by an amount that will reduce the binding force below the threshold required to trigger the B cell. Such offspring will be of no use in the fight against the antigen, and will die without producing any further offspring, since they cannot be triggered.

Several of the offspring, however, will produce antibodies with an increased affinity for the antigen. These cells will be triggered in the next generation, going on to proliferate further and, possibly, enhance the affinity even more.

During the proliferation phase, some of the B cells will differentiate to become *antibody-forming cells*. These cells are no longer capable of going

---

[1] A mutation rate of 50 per cent means here that half the daughter cells contain at least one mutation, *not* that half the sites on the DNA have mutated! In this case, a 50 per cent mutation rate means that about one DNA base in 24 will have changed. This is still much larger than a real mutation rate, but the main purpose of this aspect of the model is to simulate the number of actual cells that are mutants, and not the molecular mutation rate.

through the proliferation cycle. Their only job is to produce antibodies which they release into the bloodstream. The antibodies then deal with antigen by purely molecular means such as the complement cascade described in Chapter 8. This process is important for the model because it affects the concentration of antigen in the system, so the model takes account of antibody production by keeping track of antibodies produced and removing antigen which they encounter.

In summary, one cycle of the model involves the following steps:

1. Synthesize some B cells directly from the genetic repertoire.

2. Allow B cells and antigen to interact.

3. Determine which B cells have been triggered by the interaction.

4. Create copies of the B cells, applying a mutation procedure to the offspring.

5. Create antibody-forming cells.

6. Determine how much antigen is removed by free antibody.

11.4 Results of the model

In a typical test of the model, one antigen species is selected and presented to the immune system. The effects of varying the mutation rates, bonding strengths, and so on can be studied by running the simulation with different parameter sets. In addition, for each parameter set, the stability of the model can be tested by running it with various random number seeds, which results in different initial sets of synthesized B cells. This latter test is important because we wish to see how much of the complete B cell repertoire is eventually expressed through mutation after some of the initial B cells are triggered by the antigen. As we mentioned above, only a fraction of the total possible number of antibodies is assumed to be coded in the genes (in Weinand's model, about 6000 antibodies could be generated directly from genes). If the system ultimately reaches the same repertoire from several initial populations of B cells, it is stable.

One way of measuring the effectiveness of an immune system against a particular antigen is by the average value of the affinities of the cells for the antigen. We can therefore examine the ability of mutation to increase the affinity of the system for an antigen.

In most runs of the model, only a few of the species of B cells that can be synthesized directly from genes have an affinity high enough to be triggered by an encounter with antigen. In most cases, not all of these will be present when the antigen is first introduced, so the first defence against an antigen will be mounted by only one or two species of B cells. Once these cells have been triggered, the process of affinity maturation can begin.

If we initially examine what happens if no mutation is allowed on proliferation, we find, not surprisingly, that the average affinity of the immune system increases only slightly as the response progresses. The increase is due to the increased number of cells with an affinity for the antigen due to their proliferation after the initial contact, and to the introduction of the remaining species of B cell which have an affinity for the antigen during later cycles of cell synthesis. However, unless one of these other species of B cells happens, by chance, to have a very high affinity for the antigen, the system is limited in its response by those few species available.

If we now switch on the mutation, we can examine its effect by varying the mutation rate. The average affinity after 100 cell cycles increases dramatically (by more than a factor of 10) as the mutation rate increases from zero to around 20 per cent (one in every 5 cells mutates), then declines as the mutation rate is increased further. When the mutation rate approaches 50 per cent, the affinity actually dips below the rate when there is no mutation at all.

There should be nothing particularly surprising about any of these results, since we would expect that too high a mutation rate would lead to the system losing any new, high-affinity species just as fast (or faster) than it gained them.

The most important observation from these experiments is not that the average affinity increases, up to a point, with increased mutation rate, but that the manner in which the affinity increases is *not* random, despite the random nature of the mutation process. In the set of antibodies that are directly encoded in the genes, we have noted that there are only a few (typically 10 or so) that express a triggerable affinity for any given antigen. There are considerably more antibodies in the complete repertoire of 65 536 possible antibodies which have high affinities for the same antigen, but these antibodies are not directly encoded in the genes and can only be reached, if at all, by mutation. However, in the experimental runs, it was found that if one starts with the same initially generated B cells but uses different random number sequences for the succeeding mutations, only a limited subset of these extra high-affinity antibodies is generated, no matter how often the simulation is run.

To understand why this is the case, remember that a single mutation is really a change of one base in the DNA sequence encoding one of the four amino acids that make up the antibody's binding site. In most cases, a single mutation will result in a new antibody which has a sub-threshold affinity for the antigen and will, therefore, never be triggered. Any such mutation will thus lead to a dead end as far as attempting to adapt to the antigen is concerned. Now, many of the high-affinity antibodies not encoded in the genes cannot be obtained from those that are encoded by a single mutation. If any of the intermediate mutations required to generate a new high-affinity antibody from one that has just been triggered result in an antibody with low affinity for the antigen, then that path cannot be used to generate the high-affinity antigen. Therefore, if *all* the paths leading to this high-affinity antibody pass through low-affinity intermediaries, there is no way this new antibody can be generated. Given a fixed set of initial high-affinity B cells, only a limited number of other cells not encoded in the genes can ever be generated.

This restriction leads to the concept of a *mutation set*. If we start with one of the high-affinity antibodies encoded in the genes and present when the antigen is introduced, we can draw a graph (in the graph-theoretic sense) indicating all other high-affinity antibodies which can be reached by single-step mutations from the starting antibody. If we extend the graph by adding all high-affinity antibodies that can be reached by single mutations from these new antibodies and continue in this fashion until no more antibodies can be added, we will have derived the complete set of antibodies that can arise by mutation from the single starting antibody. Such a set is called the mutation set of the initial antibody. We can do this for all high-affinity antibodies present in the immune system when the antigen is introduced and hence discover the complete set of antibodies that may appear in the system for the given set of initial conditions. From the way these sets are constructed, they must be disjoint (have no elements in common), although we may find that two or more of the initial antibodies end up in the same mutation set.

The concept of mutation sets may help explain why the immune system does not attack the cells of its own body. Although the main reason, as we have seen, why there are no antibodies that recognize 'self' cells is believed to be that the T cells that do recognize self molecules are destroyed in the thymus while they are maturing, this does not explain why cells that recognize self do not appear by mutation during a B cell's proliferative phase. The answer may be that antibodies against self lie in a separate mutation set, so they cannot be produced by mutations from other B cells. This is unlikely to be the whole answer, however. The partition of the antibodies in an organism into mutation sets will be different for every antigen, since it is determined by the threshold affinity for the antigen. It is unlikely that no mutation set for any antigen will contain any antibodies against self, so there must be some other regulatory process which prevents auto-immune cells from running wild. One of the defects that does occur in the immune system is *auto-immune disease*, in which the body attacks itself with its own immune system.

11.5 Other approaches

Another approach to affinity maturation is that of Weinand and Conrad
(1988). This model uses a more traditional approach, reminiscent of Bell
(1970). Differential equations are used to model the population sizes of a
set of 'specialist' B cell species which cover a broad range of affinities for
the antigen. The specialist cells behave in the normal manner, requiring a
certain threshold level of antigen to trigger them into proliferating. However, the existence of another set of *generalist* cells is proposed to overcome
Bell's difficulties in predicting high- and low-zone tolerance to antigen.
These generalist cells have very low thresholds and, instead of entering a
proliferative mode, move immediately to the plasma cell state and secrete
antibodies.

The Weinand–Conrad model does not consider mutation of proliferating
specialist cells. Rather, they claim that when the system is fighting inert
antigen (antigen that does not reproduce on its own), this combination of
generalist and specialist cells is sufficient to cleanse the system of antigen
without the need for fine tuning through hypermutation. In addition, their
model successfully explains low- and high-zone tolerance. They suggest
that hypermutation is only needed if the antigen is capable of proliferating
itself (as with bacteria or viruses) so that a prolonged immune response is
required.

Although Weinand's hypermutation model presented in this chapter
treats some aspects of the immune system with attention to biological
detail, it consciously neglects many other features, such as the roles of the
various forms of T cells, the network theory, and so on. The immune system
is sufficiently complex that no one has yet produced a comprehensive theory
covering all its major features. However, Perelson (1988) has sketched an
outline of what such a theory should include.

Perelson's scenario includes some interesting suggestions, some of which
have been implemented by various authors in different guises. Being a pro-
ponent of the shape space approach (see Chapter 8) he naturally supports
the concept as a foundation of a general theory. The representation of
an antibody as a bit string (compare with Kauffman's approach in Chapter 10) is suggested as a way of modelling the idiotope and paratope sites.
However, besides providing a description of an antibody which may be used
to define its fitness in an adaptive walk model, the bit string may also be
thought of as a description of the actual shape of the binding site. Thus
an antigen, also represented by a bit string, would match the antibody if
enough of its bits were complementary to those on the paratope.

Immune networks can be constructed by collecting together sets of antibodies which are complementary to each other (this idea is developed more
fully in Chapter 13).

Superimposed on these representations of antibodies and networks is a system of differential equations to model the dynamics of B cells, antibodies and (possibly live) antigen.

Such a grand overall model does not appear to have yet been constructed. However, in the next two chapters, we shall consider models of another aspect of the immune system that has not yet played a role in our discussions: the network.

12

The symmetric immune network model

12.1   Introduction

One of the first models based on Jerne's network theory was proposed by Hoffmann in 1975, with several modifications and extensions since then. The model avoids the problems of the huge number of variables in a full immune network by grouping all the cells and antibodies into two classes: plus cells (and related antibodies) and minus cells and antibodies.

The model is designed to simulate a network of lymphocytes without any external antigen being injected into the system. Many of the features of real immune systems are incorporated into the model, although since only two variables are treated, the amount of detail is minimal.

We will examine in detail some of the more recent versions of the model. In particular, we will study a model by Gunther and Hoffmann (1982) in which the switch from production of immunoglobulin M (IgM) type antibodies to IgG antibodies is modelled, and an extension of the model by Hoffmann *et al.* (1988) to handle more than just two types of cells. Besides being useful models of the immune network, these papers illustrate graphical methods of exploring the parameter space in differential equation models.

12.2   The plus–minus model: two species

In the simplest version of the model, there are two species of cells, each with receptors that recognize idiotopes on the other species. The species are called plus and minus, respectively, and have B and T cells of types B_+, T_+, B_-, T_-.

As mentioned in Chapter 8, one way of triggering a lymphocyte is to cross-link its surface receptors with antigen. Large antigens, such as entire cells, are very good at cross-linking receptors since they can cover large areas on the surface of the recipient cell. Individual antibodies are also fairly proficient at cross-linking, since even the smallest version of antibody, IgG, has two binding sites which can each bind to a separate surface receptor. The larger IgM, with 10 binding sites, is even more efficient at cross-linking.

As mentioned in Chapter 8, helper T cells become activated when they bind to a B cell displaying antigen and self-MHC molecules. Activated T cells produce various molecular factors with diverse effects on B cells, one of which is helping them proliferate. It is also believed, however, that some of these factors released by T cells can inhibit other T cells and B cells from binding further antigen. The T cell factors may do this because they have only a single binding site, rather than the multiple binding sites of antigen and the various types of antibodies. If a T cell factor binds to a single surface receptor, that receptor cannot be cross-linked, so the potential for the cell to trigger is reduced, since there are fewer receptors available for binding antigen.

Once free antibody of either the plus or minus variety is produced, it will kill cells of the opposite species by initiating the complement cascade, as described in Chapter 8. Other methods of cell death (besides natural death through age), such as killer T cells, are also treated in this model.

We must now construct a mathematical model incorporating these features. We define x_+ and x_- to be the population of plus and minus cells respectively. No distinction is made between the various members of each population: B cells, T cells, and free antibody are all included in the one variable. This assumption obviously detracts from the realism of the model, especially as it has been shown in other models (see Chapter 13) that by ignoring the time lag between the stimulation of B cells and the production of antibody, some important dynamical features are being missed. However, our goal at this stage is a simple model with minimal complications.

A general form for the differential equations satisfied by x_+ and x_- is

$$\dot{x}_+ = x_+[R(x_-, x_+) - D(x_-, x_+) - k_4] + S \qquad (12.1)$$
$$\dot{x}_- = x_-[R(x_+, x_-) - D(x_+, x_-) - k_4] + S. \qquad (12.2)$$

The term S represents a constant rate of synthesis of cells due to production of B and T cells from the bone marrow and background cell division, unrelated to any stimulation by the opposite species. This term is assumed to be the same for both the plus and minus types.

The constant background death rate is given the by parameter k_4. Note that this is a death rate *per cell* (since it multiplies the population variable x in each case), rather than a constant death rate. Again, this is assumed to be the same for the two species.

The function R represents the the stimulation of a species by interactions with the opposite species. Since the plus–minus model is symmetric, the minus species is assumed to have the same effect on the plus species as the plus species on the minus species. This is reflected in the fact that the same function R is used in the two equations, except the order of the independent variables is reversed.

The function D represents the killing of one species by antibody produced by the other. Again, to preserve the symmetry of the model, the same function is used in both equations with arguments reversed.

The form assumed for the stimulation function R is

$$R(x,y) = k_1 x e_1(x,y) \tag{12.3}$$

where

$$e_1(x,y) = \frac{1}{1 + [xy/c_1^2]^{n_1}}. \tag{12.4}$$

$R(x,y)$ has a factor directly proportional to its first argument x which corresponds to a linear dependence on the antigen population. The function e_1 determines the probability that an encounter between a plus cell and a minus cell will result in triggering a cell to proliferate. We wish to include the effect of tolerance, that is, the fact that, for very high or very low concentrations of antigen, the immune system produces very little response. The form of e_1 is such that if either x or y is large, the probability of an effective interaction is reduced.[1] The parameters c_1 and n_1 determine respectively, the point at which $e_1 = 0.5$ and the sharpness of the transition from small values of e_1 (near zero) to large values (near 1). They are constants for any particular instance of the model.

The function D includes terms describing the death of antigen from cellular interactions (for example, killer T cells) and antibody interactions (for example, the complement cascade). We would like to model antibody interactions arising from both IgG and IgM reactions. Killer T cells kill target cells on their own—all that is needed for the T cell to recognize its target is that the target cell is displaying antigen and the correct MHC molecule on its surface. Similarly, IgM (the complex of 5 antibody molecules) can attach to a target cell singly and initiate a complement attack which destroys the cell. Since both these methods of cell death involve objects (cells or molecules) acting on their own, they can be modelled by a linear term in the function D.

The interaction involving IgG (the single antibody molecule) is more complex. We know that IgG must cross-link some of the receptors on the target cell in order to begin a complement cascade. Although a single IgG molecule can cross-link two receptors, it is believed that at least two IgG molecules must attach to receptors in order that complement can begin its work. Other mechanisms involving IgG are also known to lead to cell death,

---

[1]If one of the variables is *very* small, of course, e_1 will still be close to 1, but if the population of one of the species is close to zero, the overall response to an interaction is very small due to the other terms in the differential equation.

but all of these require at least two IgG molecules to be present. Using standard mass-action theory from chemistry we know that in a reaction involving two reactants, the rate of change of the product of the reaction depends on the product of the concentrations of the reactants, so to model the effects of IgG, must include a term proportional to the square of the antibody concentration.

A suitable form for D is then

$$D(x,y) = k_2 x e_2(x,y) + k_3 x^2 e_3(x,y) \tag{12.5}$$

where the functions e_2 and e_3 have the same form as e_1:

$$e_i(x,y) = \frac{1}{1 + [xy/c_i^2]^{n_i}} \tag{12.6}$$

for $i = 1, 2, 3$. The parameters c_i and n_i have the same interpretation as before, and are constants.

The final form of the equations in the two-species model are then:

$$\dot{x}_+ = x_+[k_1 x_- e_1 - k_2 x_- e_2 - k_3 x_-^2 e_3 - k_4] + S \tag{12.7}$$
$$\dot{x}_- = x_-[k_1 x_+ e_1 - k_2 x_+ e_2 - k_3 x_+^2 e_3 - k_4] + S \tag{12.8}$$

where the explicit dependence of the functions e_i on x_- and x_+ is omitted for simplicity.[2]

Before we consider ways of examining the behaviour of these equations, we can have a look at some trajectories for a particular choice of parameters. There are 11 parameters in the model (4 k_is, 3 c_is, 3 n_is, and S) so we cannot use trial and error to explore the entire 11-dimensional parameter space, but it is often a good idea to try a few numerical solutions of the equations to get an idea of how they behave before doing a more general analysis.

Using any standard numerical integration package (or writing your own using a simple integration method such as Euler's rule) it is fairly easy to write a simple program to numerically integrate the two equations. Since the populations x_i can vary over a large range of values (several orders of magnitude), it is easier to view the results if we plot trajectories on a graph of $\log x_-$ versus $\log x_+$. By choosing a selection of initial conditions and numerically integrating the equations until the trajectories either converge to a stable point or leave the graph, we can construct a map of the behaviour of the solutions (Fig. 12.1) Such a map is often called a phase-plane diagram.[3]

---

[2]Note that the functions $e_i(x,y)$ are symmetric in x and y: $e_i(x,y) \equiv e_i(y,x)$, so there is no confusion arising from omitting the functional dependence.

[3]Phase-plane diagrams such as the one shown in Fig. 12.1 are obtained by numerical integration of the eqns (12.7) using methods similar to those described in Appendix

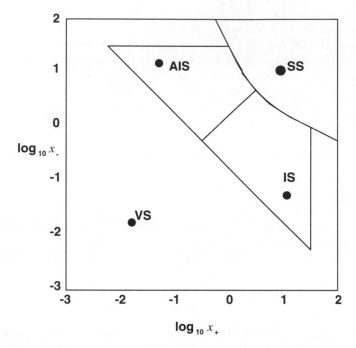

Figure 12.1   Phase-plane map of solutions to the plus–minus system. The stable attractors are shown as black dots. The region around each attractor is its basin of attraction. If the initial conditions lie within one of the regions, the solution will converge onto the attractor within that region.

It shows the solutions not as functions of time but as curves in the space of variables x_+ and x_-. We have already seen some phase-plane diagrams in the solution of the hypercycle equations in Chapter 6.

We can see from Fig. 12.1 that one possible solution of the equations contains four stable points and, at least in the area shown by the graph, no other fixed points. We discussed the nature of these points briefly in Chapter 8, but we will summarize their interpretations again here.

The virgin state (VS in the figure) corresponds to the state before any stimulation of the immune system has occurred. In this state, both species have low populations. The anti-immune state (AIS) and immune state (IS)

A. These equations appear to be very sensitive to the method of numerical solution, the step size used, and so on. The author attempted to reproduce Fig. 2 in Gunther and Hoffmann (1982), but despite finding the points VS and SS, could not find any trajectories which converged on the points AIS and IS. The figure shown here uses the same parameter values as Hoffman *et al.* (1988).

correspond to two symmetric states in which one of the two species has been triggered to respond to the other species. In the AIS state, for example, there is a reduced population of plus cells and an increased population of minus cells, indicating that the minus cells have mounted an immune reaction against the plus cells and drastically reduced their number. Finally, the suppressed state (SS) corresponds to a situation where both populations are large, but no immune response takes place. This corresponds to the naturally observed phenomenon of high-zone tolerance, in which a large dose of antigen results in indifference from the immune system, with no reaction taking place.

The key point about these four states is that they are stable and, as we can see from the figure, all four states have fairly large *basins of attraction*, or areas on the graph where trajectories flow into that state. If these equations described a real immune system, all four states could easily be realized at some time in the life of the organism. In particular, if the system started out in the virgin state and received enough of a jolt to enter the immune state (IS), it would remain in that state unless another large shock was administered to the system. This is a reasonable simulation of memory in the immune system; a memory resulting from a fixed point in the dynamics of a continually evolving system rather than from the creation of long-lived memory cells. Remember that all cells and antibodies have the same natural death rate given by the parameter k_4, so no provision is made for some special memory cell that lives much longer than the other cells.

12.3 Exploring the parameter space

We now examine some techniques for exploring a large parameter space, such as the 11-dimensional space of the plus–minus model.

In a differential equation model, such as the plus–minus theory, it is often possible to learn a lot about the system without explicitly solving the equations, either analytically or numerically. Such is the case here.

In attempting to study the behaviour of the equations in the plus–minus theory, it is a good idea to express them in a form which emphasizes any symmetries or regularities they may have. Examining the equations we see that the combination x_+x_- occurs frequently, so we can try introducing a new variable $p \equiv x_+x_-$. Rewriting the equations in this form we have

$$\dot{x}_+ = k_1e_1p - k_2e_2p - k_3e_3px_- - k_4x_+ + S \qquad (12.9)$$
$$\dot{x}_- = k_1e_1p - k_2e_2p - k_3e_3px_+ - k_4x_- + S. \qquad (12.10)$$

Note also that $e_i = 1/[1 + (p/c_i^2)^{n_i}]$ is a function of p only.

The first two terms and the last term in eqns (12.7) are identical, so we can group them together with the definition

$$C \equiv k_1 e_1 p - k_2 e_2 p + S. \tag{12.11}$$

With the additional definitions

$$A \equiv k_3 p e_3; \qquad B \equiv k_4 \tag{12.12}$$

we have

$$\dot{x}_+ = C - Ax_- - Bx_+ \tag{12.13}$$
$$\dot{x}_- = C - Ax_+ - Bx_- \tag{12.14}$$

where A and C are functions of p only and B is a constant.

One of the things we would like to know about these equations is the location of their stable points, that is, places where $\dot{x}_+ = \dot{x}_- = 0$. Now for a particular value of p, eqns (12.13)–(12.14) are linear in x_- and x_+. On a graph of x_+ vs x_-, we can draw these lines (Fig 12.1). The point where they intersect is a possible fixed point, but only if this point also satisfies the condition $x_- x_+ = p$ which, for fixed p, defines a rectangular hyperbola. Therefore, the condition for a fixed point is that the two lines $\dot{x}_- = 0$, $\dot{x}_+ = 0$, and the hyperbola $x_- x_+ = p$ all intersect at a common point.

In general, if we choose some value of p and draw the three curves (the two lines and the hyperbola), they will not intersect in a common point, but we can still use this graph to tell us something about the dynamics of the system. For values of x_- above the line $\dot{x}_- = 0$, we see from eqn (12.13)–(12.14) that $\dot{x}_- < 0$. Similarly, to the right of the line $\dot{x}_+ = 0$, we see that $\dot{x}_+ < 0$. In the region of the graph that is above and to the right of both lines, both x_- and x_+ are decreasing.

Now let us return to the condition for a fixed point. Due to the symmetry of the equations for the two lines, they always intersect along the line $x_- = x_+$ unless the two lines are identical, in which case, of course, all values of x_- and x_+ will satisfy them. Thus, any fixed point must either satisfy the condition

$$x_- = x_+ \tag{12.15}$$

(recall the two points VS and SS in Fig. 12.1) or else the two lines are identical. In this case, there are three possibilities.

1. The single line representing the two equations $\dot{x}_- = \dot{x}_+ = 0$ intersects the hyperbola twice, giving rise to two more fixed points symmetrically placed on either side of the line $x_- = x_+$ (recall the points AIS and IS in Fig. 12.1).

2. The single line is tangential to the hyperbola giving one fixed point. This case can be effectively discounted, since it occurs for only one precise set of parameter values which would not occur in nature.

3. The single line lies entirely below the hyperbola and does not intersect it at all. No fixed points exist.

However, any of these conditions could hold as we vary p, so how do we find the value(s) of p for which fixed points actually exist? Consider first the fixed points in the case where the lines $\dot{x}_+ = 0$ and $\dot{x}_- = 0$ intersect at only one point. This will give us the symmetric fixed points VS and SS in Fig. 12.1. In this case, the fixed point must occur for those value(s) of p such that the intersection point of the two lines occurs on the hyperbola. We already know that the intersection of the lines occurs only when $x_- = x_+ \equiv x_0$. In this case the two eqns (12.13)–(12.14) become identical, so we can substitute $x_0 = \sqrt{p}$ into one of them and set it equal to zero to get the condition

$$C(p) - [A(p) + B]\sqrt{p} = 0. \tag{12.16}$$

For convenience, let us define the left-hand side of this equation to be a function $G(p)$:

$$G(p) \equiv C(p) - [A(p) + B]\sqrt{p}. \tag{12.17}$$

From the definitions of $C(p)$ and $A(p)$, solving the equation $G(p) = 0$ is equivalent to finding the roots of a polynomial in p (assuming the numbers n_i, $i = 1, 2, 3$ are all integers). In general this polynomial could have a fairly large degree (certainly larger than 2, so that the quadratic formula cannot be used), so the solution of this algebraic equation will have to be done numerically. Various numbers of solutions will be found, depending on the degree of the polynomial and the values of the other parameters. Each value of $p \geq 0$ will give rise to a fixed point with population values $x_- = x_+ = \sqrt{p}$.

Now consider the case where the straight lines $\dot{x}_+ = 0$ and $\dot{x}_- = 0$ are identical. In this case, we have, by subtracting eqn (12.13) from eqn (12.14),

$$B = A(p) \tag{12.18}$$

or, using the definitions of B and $A(p)$:

$$k_4 - k_3 \frac{p}{1 + (p/c_3^2)^{n_3}} = 0 \tag{12.19}$$

If $n_3 > 1$, plotting several graphs of this function shows that it can have 0, 1, or 2 solutions. For each solution p of this equation (which again will have to be found numerically if $n_3 > 2$), we have a possible pair of asymmetric solutions (like AIS and IS in Fig. 12.1). Once these values of p (if any) have been found, we must satisfy the two conditions

$$x_- x_+ = p \tag{12.20}$$

and

$$C(p) - B(x_- + x_+) = 0. \tag{12.21}$$

These equations can be solved directly to yield a quadratic equation in one of x_- or x_+:

$$Bx_+^2 - C(p)x_+ + Bp = 0. \tag{12.22}$$

If this equation has real roots, the corresponding values of x_- and x_+ are the coordinates of the fixed point.

Once the fixed points are found, we would like to determine their nature, that is, are they stable, unstable, saddle points,[4] etc.? It is possible to apply a more advanced method to determine this analytically, but this is beyond the scope of this book. Interested readers may consult Gunther and Hoffmann (1982). More pedestrian readers may be satisfied with finding the fixed points and testing their stability via numerical simulation, which may be done by starting the system off near each fixed point and observing its behaviour.

However it is done, the analysis of the stability of the fixed points shows that a great many types of dynamics are possible. Various numbers and combinations of stable, unstable, and saddle points can exist for appropriate parameter values. We are seeking those ranges of the parameters that provide us with phase-plane portrait similar to that shown in Fig. 12.1, where we have four stable points corresponding to the immune and anti-immune states (IS and AIS), and the suppressed (SS) and virgin (VS) states. The complete analysis is shown in Gunther and Hoffmann (1982), with the result that if the set of parameters satisfies either of the conditions

$$\frac{k_4}{k_3} < c_3^2 < \frac{S}{k_2} < c_2^2 < \frac{S^2}{k_4^2} \tag{12.23}$$

or

$$\frac{S}{k_2} < c_2^2 < \frac{k_4}{k_3} < c_3^2 < \frac{S^2}{k_4^2} \tag{12.24}$$

the required dynamics are obtained.

Comparison of these conditions with experimental data shows that these restrictions are reasonable. It is possible to investigate the feasibility of an immune system consisting of only one type of immunoglobulin (IgG or

---

[4]In Gunther and Hoffmann (1982), a saddle point is given the rather unconventional name of *col*, which is a mountaineering term meaning a pass through a mountain range.

IgM). If we set $k_3 = 0$, we eliminate the term corresponding to IgG (the form of antibody with two receptors). Doing so requires a new analysis of the equations, but it turns out that no immune or anti-immune states can exist without the presence of IgG.

Setting $k_2 = 0$ to simulate the effect of eliminating IgM from the model does produce the required dynamics for certain conditions on the remaining parameters. However, the resulting immune state (IS) contains just as much of the plus species as the virgin state, although the population of the minus species has been greatly reduced, contrary to what is observed. In an immunized system, the antibody population should be considerably larger than in the virgin state, since this is what allows the larger and faster response on second exposure to antigen.

12.4 Extension to many species

One obvious problem with the plus–minus theory is that it considers only two species. An extension of the model to cope with, in principle, any number of species was proposed by Hoffmann *et al.* (1988).

The extension is straightforward enough. Instead of the plus and minus species, we now have N species whose populations are represented by the variables x_i, $i = 1, \ldots, N$. Then the system's dynamics are given by solutions of the set of differential equations:

$$\frac{dx_i}{dt} = S - k_2 x_i Y_i e_{2i} - k_3 x_i Y_i^2 e_{3i} - k_4 x_i. \tag{12.25}$$

Here S, k_2, k_3, and k_4 have the same meanings as in the two-species model. The variable Y_i is given by

$$Y_i \equiv \sum_{j=1}^{N} K_{ij} x_j. \tag{12.26}$$

It represents the total interaction between species i and all other species j, with the interaction strengths given by the $N \times N$ matrix K. In keeping with the symmetry of the earlier model, K is assumed to be a symmetric matrix: $K_{ij} = K_{ji}$.

The functions e_{qi}, $q = 2, 3$; $i = 1, \ldots, N$, have similar definitions to before:

$$e_{qi} = \frac{1}{1 + (x_i Y_i / C_q)^{n_q}} \tag{12.27}$$

where the parameter C_q has replaced the c_q^2 in the earlier model.

The behaviour of any one species of antibody embedded in the network can be observed by plotting phase-plane diagrams similar to the plus–minus theory, except that the ordinate is now occupied by Y_i, which represents the behaviour of the network as a whole, while the abscissa is given to the single species x_i. On such simple plots, similar behaviour to the two-species model is observed: four stable states for certain values of the parameters.

12.5   Summary

The plus–minus theory models a simple two-species network, incorporating effects due to B cells, T cells, free antibody of both IgG and IgM types, and natural birth and death terms. Although the model is simple in construction, it has the advantage that it incorporates many of the observed phenomena in the immune response in a formulation that is relatively easy to study. The locations and stability properties of the fixed points can all be found analytically, and conditions can be derived which the parameters must satisfy in order that the model predicts the four stable fixed points required. It is also straightforward enough to generalize the model to a system of N species, although the analysis of the fixed points is no longer so easy.

Although it is capable of predicting the states of an immune system after exposure to antigen, the model does not correctly describe the dynamics of the immune response as it occurs. For example, an immune response should be triggered by an increase in the population of the antigen species, which in turn should lead to proliferation of the antibody species. From the dynamical portrait in Fig. 12.1, let us begin at the virgin state VS, and try to stimulate the system so that it migrates to the immune state IS. At IS, the plus species is the antibody and the minus species is the antigen, so we should expect that if we increase the value of x_-, the system should respond by stimulating the growth of the plus species which will cause the population of minus cells will drop and the system to converge on IS. However, if we examine the diagram we see that if we increase x_- (starting from VS), we will never reach IS, since all trajectories in the region above VS lead to other stable points. In other words, the model accurately predicts the existence of the four stable points, but tells us little about how a real immune system arrives at them.

The model also predicts that the immune system will only possess such states if the parameters satisfy certain conditions (eqns (12.23) and (12.24)). Outside these areas in parameter space, the system will have other behaviour, but does this behaviour accurately reflect the behaviour of a real immune system with similar parameter values? We do not know.

Although the distinction between the two forms of antibody, IgG and IgM, is built into the model in the form of two distinct terms in eqn (12.7), the model does not predict which of the two forms is used, nor when (or even if) the experimentally observed switch from IgM to IgG occurs. As observed in the last section, the model predicts that the required behaviour cannot be obtained if IgG is absent, and although it can be obtained if IgM is absent, the resulting dynamics are not realistic. However, since no distinction between free antibody types, or even between antibodies and cells, is made in the model, we cannot tell what is happening to the individual components.

The lack of biological detail in the symmetric network model clearly detracts from the accuracy of its predictions. As our final example of a model of the immune system we shall consider a network model which attempts to include a more detailed representation of the components of the immune system. The model is more realistic than the plus–minus theory, but this realism is obtained by sacrificing the clear analysis that was possible in the simpler model.

13

A shape space network model

13.1   Introduction

While the plus–minus model of Hoffmann, considered in the last chapter, succeeds in predicting several observed states of real immune systems from a minimum of assumptions, it would be interesting to examine a model which incorporates more of the features of a functioning immune network. This can only be done, as you might expect, by a considerable increase in the complexity of the model. We will study one such model, that of De Boer and Perelson (1991), in this chapter. The paper which forms the main source for this chapter is one of a large collection of models by a group of researchers which has been working on models of the immune system for many years.

The model combines stochastic and deterministic simulation methods to produce a system in which many species of lymphocytes and antibodies may appear and interact. The type of antibody produced by a lymphocyte is determined randomly, just as it is believed to occur in natural immune systems. Once formed, a new lymphocyte species interacts with those species already present, and may become stimulated to proliferate as a result. The dynamics of the system are determined by a set of differential equations. This model goes some way towards implementing the suggestions of Perelson (1988).

13.2   Representation of antibodies

We will consider first the stochastic part of the model. The structure of an antibody molecule is represented by a bit string—a sequence of zeroes and ones. The bit string is an abstraction of the variable region on the two arms of the Y-shaped molecule. The sequence of bits is an indication of the 'generalized shape' of the region, which is a combination of the physical shape, the charge distribution and any other properties which help determine the antibody's affinity for other molecules.

The total number of possible antibodies which can be represented in the model depends on the length of the bit string, since in an n-bit string, there are 2^n possible bit sequences. This *total repertoire* is a reservoir from which those antibodies actually present in the system may be drawn at random, in much the same way as a new B or T cell being synthesized in the bone marrow is drawn from the total repertoire of such cells by choosing one gene fragment from each region in the DNA. In a real immune system, only a small fraction of the total repertoire is expressed in the body at any given time. Similarly, in this model, only a few of the 2^n possible antibodies are present at a time.

Each cell generated by the bone marrow produces antibody of only one type. Once such a cell (or group of identical cells) is produced, it will interact with other cells already present.[1] The strength of interaction between two antibodies is modelled by matching up the bit strings of two molecules. A 'match' occurs between two opposing bits (one from each antibody) if the bits are different (a zero in one string lies next to a one in the other). Such differing bits are said to be *complementary* to each other. The affinity J_{ij} of antibody i for antibody j is then defined as a function of the number of matches obtained between the two bit strings.

There are several ways in which this affinity could be calculated. We could simply sum up the number of complementary bits without regard to their relative positions and define the affinity as an increasing function of this number. In De Boer and Perelson's model, a threshold number T of *consecutive* complementary bits must be found on the two molecules in order for any affinity between them to exist. Pairs of antibodies which match in exactly T consecutive locations are assigned a low affinity value: $J_{ij} = 0.1$. If they match in more than T locations, a high affinity of $J_{ij} = 1.0$ is assigned. If this seems too artificial, it would be easy enough to define some other function in which the affinity J_{ij} is a steadily increasing function of the number of complementary bits. Since the affinity depends only on the number of complementary bits in two strings, it must be symmetric: $J_{ij} = J_{ji}$. The model also imposes the restriction that a species cannot recognize itself, so that $J_{ii} = 0$.

The probability of two antibodies having a non-zero affinity may be estimated from probability theory. The problem is an example of a general problem in probability theory: the *success run*. Simply stated, we wish to find the probability of finding a specific pattern of length T bits somewhere in a sequence of total length n bits, given that the probability of a single bit being zero is p and of a single bit being one is $q \equiv 1 - p$. The problem turns out to be surprisingly non-trivial, but an approximate formula for $P(T, n)$, the probability of a success run of length T in a string of total

---

[1] To start things off, the animal is assumed to inherit some antibodies (but not lymphocytes) from its mother at birth.

length n, is:

$$P(T,n) \approx 1 - \frac{1 - px}{(T + 1 - Tx)qx^{n+1}} \qquad (13.1)$$

where x is the largest root of the polynomial equation in variable s:

$$s = 1 + qp^T s^{T+1}. \qquad (13.2)$$

The value of x may be found using a numerical polynomial solver, or the approximation formula

$$x \approx 1 + qp^T + (T + 1)(qp^T)^2 \qquad (13.3)$$

may be used.

Equation (13.1) is accurate to within 1 per cent for $n > 3$, which is certainly good enough for our purposes.

The set of all 2^n possible antibodies defines a *shape space* in which each antibody occupies a single point, defined by its particular bit string. We have already discussed the concept of shape space in Chapter 8, where we observed that each point in the space is surrounded by a region within which any other antibody (or any molecule for that matter) will be 'recognized', in the sense that a non-zero affinity will exist between that molecule and the original antibody. In our original discussion of shape space, however, we assumed that the antibodies that were present were scattered randomly over the space, so that we could use the Poisson distribution to estimate their coverage of the space. In the present model, we are still assuming that antibodies (or at least the B cells that secrete them) are generated randomly in the bone marrow, but after their creation, these cells and antibodies interact with other molecules already present. Because of these interactions, we can no longer be certain that those antibodies present are still randomly distributed over the shape space. The interactions may favour some areas of the space or eliminate antibodies in another area.

A measure of the influence of a particular species of antibody is provided by the *field* associated with it. The field $\bar{A}_i$ of species i is defined as

$$\bar{A}_i \equiv \sum_{j=1}^{n} J_{ij} A_j \qquad (13.4)$$

where A_j is the population of species j. Thus the field of species i is a weighted sum of the affinities that this species has for the other species present. Species that interact with many other species, especially populous ones, have a large field, while species that can find few other species with which they have a non-zero affinity have small fields.

The field of an antibody species gives a measure of how likely that species is to encounter another antibody with which it can interact. As we saw in Chapter 8, a cell which becomes saturated with antigen often produces no response to it (the phenomenon of high-zone tolerance), so we would expect that species with very high fields would suffer from this effect. Similarly, species require a minimal level of interaction before they can be triggered to proliferate. Thus molecules with low fields will also be unresponsive. We can therefore map the fields onto an *activation function* $f(\bar{A}_i)$ which has these properties. Again, various possibilities exist, but the one chosen by De Boer and Perelson is

$$f(\bar{A}_i) = \frac{\bar{A}_i{}^{\eta}}{\theta_1^{\eta} + \bar{A}_i{}^{\eta}} \frac{\theta_2^{\eta}}{\theta_2^{\eta} + \bar{A}_i{}^{\eta}}. \tag{13.5}$$

This function is the product of two sigmoid functions. The first factor starts at zero when the field is zero, and rises to one as the field becomes large. The second factor inverts the behaviour, starting at one and falling to zero as the field becomes large. The three parameters η, θ_1, and θ_2 define the shape of the function. The steepness of the transition is governed by η: the larger its value, the closer to a step function each sigmoid becomes. The parameters θ_1 and θ_2 determine the values of the field at which the steps in the two sigmoids occur. If we choose $\theta_2 \gg \theta_1$, the two steps will be well separated, so that the function will start at zero, rise to nearly 1.0 and remain on a plateau in the interval (θ_1, θ_2) before falling through the downward step to return to zero. The region of this plateau gives the range of field values for which a B cell will be triggered.

A little calculus shows that the maximum value of $f(\bar{A}_i)$ occurs at the geometric mean of θ_1 and θ_2, that is, at $\bar{A}_i = \sqrt{\theta_1\theta_2}$. This value of the field may be considered the dividing line between stimulative and suppressive behaviour, although if $\theta_2 \gg \theta_1$, the maximum value occurs in the middle of a long, flat plateau, so that little change in the behaviour of an antibody will be noticed unless its field value is near either end of the plateau. For convenience, we shall refer to the activation function for species i as f_i from now on:

$$f_i \equiv f(\bar{A}_i) \tag{13.6}$$

13.3 Dynamics

Having defined the representation to be used for antibody molecules and their interactions, we must now build the dynamics of the system. The dynamics of the B cells follow the usual pattern of birth, proliferation, and death. The cells are produced at a constant rate m, proliferate at a rate p per cell, weighted by the activation function f in eqn (13.5), and die at a rate d_B per cell. The resulting differential equation is

$$\frac{dB_i}{dt} = m + B_i[pf_i - d_B]. \tag{13.7}$$

From the form of this equation, it cannot produce negative values of B_i provided that the initial condition is a positive number of cells, but it can predict values of B_i less than one. We will see how to patch up this inconsistency later on.

One of the advantages of the shape space model over simpler models such as the plus–minus model is that it treats antibodies and B cells separately. Many models assume that, since antibodies are produced by B cells, their populations should always be proportional to one another. However, due to the time required for the immune response to mature (see chapter 8) there is always a time lag between the appearance of a new B cell and its secretion of antibody, so it is not correct to assume that the population of antibody species i will suddenly increase as soon as a new B cell of type i is produced.

To account for this delay, a 'gearing-up' function $G_i(t)$ is introduced. The gearing-up function just specifies the fraction of B cells of type i that are producing antibody at time t, so $G_i(t)$ is restricted to the interval [0,1]. De Boer and Perelson define G_i as the solution of the differential equation

$$\frac{dG_i}{dt} = k[f_i - G_i] \tag{13.8}$$

where k is another parameter.

This equation states that the rate of change of the gearing-up function is proportional to the difference between the current activation function f_i for species i and the current value of G_i. The activation function f_i is a property of the environment in which the B cell finds itself, and not of the state of development of the cell itself. In a sense, it represents the state of activity which the cell would 'like' to have, if it were fully mature, while G_i represents the actual state of activity, taking into account the cell's state of development. The parameter k determines the rate at which the cells respond to their environment: a low value of k, for example, means that a cell's response will be sluggish and it may not manage to adjust to its environment significantly before the environment changes again.

The changing environment is an important feature of eqn (13.8). Since new species are constantly being introduced and old ones proliferating or dying off, the field felt by a B cell is constantly changing, so that its activation function f_i is also changing. Thus eqn (13.8) represents a constant race for the cell to keep up with the latest developments in its field.[2]

As mentioned by De Boer and Perelson, other models have explicitly incorporated the time delay by making the antibody production depend on the B cell population at some time $t - \tau$ in the past. They criticize this approach because the antibody production at time t depends on the

---

[2]Pun intended.

B cells that are present at time t. While this is certainly true, it is not clear that eqn (13.8) provides a truly realistic solution to the problem. For example, assuming that there are no B cells present at time $t = 0$, there must be a finite time lag before *any* antibody can be produced, since those B cells that are created at $t = 0$ take a finite time to mature, proliferate and finally secrete antibody. However, since some antibodies and B cells will be present in the system from $t = 0$, the field f_i of any new cells will be non-zero at $t = 0$. Thus, even if $G_i(0) = 0$ (as it is assumed to be in the model), $G_i(t)$ will be non-zero for $t > 0$, which indicates that some antibody will be produced immediately after the system is started, which is impossible. A model in which antibody production at time t depends on the B cell population at time $t - \tau$ will not suffer from this problem. Since $B_i(t) = 0$ for all $t \le 0$, no antibody will be produced until at least time $t = \tau$.

Once a form for dealing with antibody secretion has been decided, the differential equation describing the antibody population can be written. Antibodies are produced only from activated B cells. We assume that all cells have the same maximum rate s of antibody production. Free antibody may form complexes with other free antibody molecules, or it may bind to B cells to begin the activation process. Both of these processes will remove free antibody from solution. In addition, free antibody will decay naturally. An equation incorporating all these effects is

$$\frac{dA_i}{dt} = sB_iG_i - A_i(d_C\bar{A}_i + d_A). \tag{13.9}$$

Here, the first term accounts for antibody production, taking into account the gearing-up function G_i. The second term describes the two methods of removing antibody from solution. The constant d_C gives the rate at which antibody combines with other antibodies and B cells. The overall rate at which antibodies of species i react will depend on the number A_i of species i molecules present and on the field $\bar{A}_i$ felt by each of them. Finally, the constant d_A gives the decay rate, per molecule, of free antibody.

The model therefore consists of the stochastic simulation resulting in the production of the B cells with their associated antibodies, and the differential equations (13.7), (13.8), and (13.9). Since new species are being introduced and old ones die off, the number and types of species present will be constantly changing, so that the number of differential equations will not be constant throughout a simulation. This should not pose any problems, since the equations will be solved numerically.

13.4 Simulation results

The above model may be simulated in a two-species system similar to that considered in the plus–minus model in the previous chapter. For most realistic values of the parameters, some form of oscillatory behaviour occurs. For some regions of parameter space, chaotic behaviour occurs, so that the populations of the two species of antibody fluctuate in a seemingly random manner.

The main value of the shape space model, however, is in its ability to study networks with a large and changing antibody population. We shall therefore examine a typical simulation and discuss the results and their implications for real immune systems.

First, the size and matching requirement for the antibodies must be decided. De Boer and Perelson have chosen the length L of the bit string to be 32 bits, and have experimented with various values of T, the number of consecutive complementary bits that must match before an affinity can develop between two antibody species. Using eqn (13.1), we find that for $T > 6$, $P(T, 32) < 0.1$.

Next, we must seed the system by introducing some 'maternal' antibodies (molecules that would be inherited from the animal's mother). We would like these initial antibodies to give a fairly complete covering of shape space. The average proportion of shape space accessible to an antibody is just $P(T, 32)$, the probability that it will match another random molecule. We will call this probability p for the moment, just to keep the notation simple. We would like to derive an estimate of how many random strings we need to cover a certain fraction of shape space. Since p is the probability that an antibody will match another antibody, $1 - p$ is the probability that it will *not* match. The probability that an antibody at one point in shape space will not match any of the n antibodies present is, therefore, $(1 - p)^n$. Therefore the fraction S of shape space covered by n random antibodies is

$$S = 1 - (1 - p)^n. \tag{13.10}$$

Solving for n we obtain

$$n = \frac{\ln(1 - S)}{\ln(1 - p)}. \tag{13.11}$$

Let us find the number n_{99} of strings we need to cover 99 per cent of shape space ($S = 0.99$). For values of $p < 0.1$, as is the case if we require a match in more than 6 bits in a string of length 32, $\ln(1 - p)$ is well approximated by $-p$. With $S = 0.99$, $\ln 0.01 \approx -4.6$ so

$$n_{99} \approx \frac{4.6}{p}. \tag{13.12}$$

We may therefore seed the system with approximately $4.6/P(T, 32)$ different species. If $T = 7$, $P(7, 32) \approx 0.1$, so we could use 50 species.

Once we have the initial conditions set up, we begin the simulation. Each cycle begins with the introduction of some novel species of B cells into the system. The model requires that all new cell species added to the system satisfy three conditions:

- The species is not currently part of the network.

- The species must match (have an affinity for) at least one species already present.

- The interaction between the new species and the network must result in the new species growing (that is, $dB_i/dt > 0$), at least at first.

These assumptions are partly for convenience, but they have far-reaching consequences for the meaning of the immune network. Some researchers believe that the network encompasses only about one-fifth of the total number of cell species present in the immune system. The cells that are outside the network are those which do most of the work in actually attacking antigen. The network itself does possess some ability to respond to antigen, but its main function is to stabilize the system, and to determine the overall immune repertoire by accepting into or rejecting from the network new species of B cells produced in the bone marrow. Thus the requirement that new species must be able to recognize part of the network and that they initially thrive within the network environment are instrumental in determining which species will become part of the regulatory network and which will be relegated to defence of the organism. Notice that those species not accepted into the network do not necessarily die out—they are simply not considered further in this model. The network model considered here makes no attempt to include the response to antigen, so these other cells may be present in the system. They do not, however, have any further influence on the dynamics of the network.

At this stage, those species already in the network are checked to see if any of them have died out. The criteria for death of a species are: (i) $B_i < 1$ (less than a single cell is present); (ii) $A_i < \theta_1/10$, so that the antibody population is less than a tenth the level required for stimulation. Any such species are eliminated from further consideration.

The differential equations are then solved numerically for one day of system time. Following this, the cycle begins again with the introduction of new species.

The model shows a remarkable behaviour to stabilize itself. During the first 30 days or so, the number of species tends to peak (the more new species introduced each day, the higher the peak), but then falls back to a stable level of around 200 species which remains essentially unchanged (except for statistical fluctuations) for several hundred days. Similarly, the average number of connections per species (the number of other species each antibody recognizes) peaks during the first 30 days, but then falls back to a constant, low level (around 6 to 9 connections per species).

By varying the required number of matching bits (T), we can plot a graph of the number of species present (after stabilization) versus $P(T, 32)$. This graph has a similar shape to that for $n_{99} = 4.6/P(T, 32)$, except that a few more species are present. This would seem to indicate that the system is attempting to cover shape space as much as possible. What appears to be happening is that the system evolves towards a stable state in which the network covers most of the shape space, but with antibodies that are fairly selective in their affinities.

The antibodies evolve to become selective because of the activation function f_i. Initially, when the number of species and connections per species peak, there are species present with very large field values, since they can recognize many species. Species with field values larger than θ_2 will die out, since they are suppressed by the network. The tendency, then, is for those antibodies which recognize fewer species, and hence have field values in the acceptable region between θ_1 and θ_2, to survive.

One question may have occurred to the observant reader at this point. We have stated that the network evolves towards a state in which it covers all of shape space, and yet a great many new species are not accepted into the network. If the network can recognize every molecule, why does it reject so many?

The answer appears to be that the rejected species *are* in fact recognized by the network, but their field values cause them to fall into the heavily suppressed region of the activation function, so they cannot proliferate. One of the conditions for acceptance into the network was that the species must be able to grow on its first day. These rejected species cannot do this. However, it has been postulated that it is just these rejected antibodies that form the core of the body's defense system. In fact, the argument has been reversed to propose that the network may offer a solution to the problem of discriminating self from non-self antigens. Although the network covers all of shape space, it may be concentrated very heavily in that area of the space where self molecules reside (remember that each animal has its own 'serial number' in the form of unique MHC molecules). If any randomly produced B cell produces antibody that would recognize self, it is immediately incorporated into the network where it is suppressed by interaction with other antibodies.

There are many things this model does not include. The equations do not allow for the existence of foreign antigen, they make no mention of T cells (either helper or killer), they assume that the immune system is a 'well-stirred' system (ignoring the fact that it is compartmentalized in various parts of the body), and so on. Immunological modelling is still in its infancy, although the models we have seen (and many more that we have not had the space to include) have all shed rays of light from different angles on a complex topic. We can only look forward to further developments when the cooperation of theory and experiment may provide a more complete explanation on the functioning of the immune system.

Some further studies that have been done on some of the aspects covered in this chapter may be found in the following papers.

Perelson and Weisbuch (1992) discuss a model in which the compartmentalization of the immune system is taken into account. The immune system contains several organs, such as the thymus, bone marrow, and spleen, in addition to the lymphatic system, all of which can affect its maturation and functioning.

The problem of memory in an immune network is studied by Weisbuch *et al.* (1990). T cells are explicitly included in a network model by De Boer and Hogeweg (1989). Automata and their application to the immune system are discussed by Neumann and Weisbuch (1992) and Atlan (1989).

14

AIDS

14.1   The biology of AIDS

Acquired Immune Deficiency Syndrome, or AIDS, has been claiming head-lines for several years as a new and potentially devastating disease. Since it is a disease of the immune system, and several theoretical models have been proposed to simulate its behaviour, it seems appropriate to include a chapter on AIDS in this section of the book.

There are several forms of AIDS, but the one of most concern to the medical profession is, of course, the strain that attacks humans, known as the Human Immunodeficiency Virus, or HIV.

To understand how HIV works, we need to know a bit about viruses in general. A virus consists essentially of a strand of RNA or DNA (and possibly a few other proteins) enclosed in a protein sheath. Since the virus contains little else, it is not a free-living cell and cannot reproduce without a host cell in which to do it. Indeed, there is an ongoing debate as to whether viruses are really a form of life or constitute some form of matter intermediate between an inanimate object and a truly living organism.

The virus is able to reproduce by invading a host cell and causing the host's reproductive machinery to produce copies of the components re-quired for assembling more virus particles rather than the components it needs for its own reproduction. The strand of nucleic acid in the virus contains only a few genes, but these genes contain the information for con-structing the viral coat protein, as well as code which allows the viral DNA or RNA to direct the reproductive machinery of the host cell to produce viral proteins and copies of the viral genome. As the host cell starts to produce these components, they self-assemble and produce more viral par-ticles which, when released from the host cell, are free to infect other hosts and perpetuate the process.

Whether viruses are considered as a form of life or not, they are highly successful at achieving their ends. Every form of life is vulnerable to some form of viral attack. Humans, of course, are susceptible to a huge variety of viral infections, from the common cold and influenza to more serious diseases such as HIV. Plants have their own viruses to contend with. One of the most intensely studied viruses is the tobacco mosaic virus, which infects the leaves of tobacco plants, causing a mottled pattern to form on them (hence the name 'mosaic').[1] Even bacteria suffer from viral invasions. A special class of viruses known as bacteriophages (literally, 'eaters of bacteria') can infect and kill bacterial cells.

To the human immune system, most viruses are recognized as foreign objects and cause an immune response to be mounted which, in most cases, is eventually successful in eliminating the viruses. HIV, however, has found a way to avoid attack by the immune system. In its protein coat, an HIV particle contains a protein known as gp120, which has a shape complementary to the surface receptor distinguishing a helper T cell. Rather than triggering the T cell into action, however, this particular complementarity allows the HIV particle to merge with the cell membrane of the T cell. After such a merger has taken place, the virus is able to release its genetic material, which in the case of HIV consists of two strands of RNA, along with a few enzyme molecules, into the interior of the T cell.

As described in Chapter 1, in a normal cell, protein synthesis occurs by transcription of the DNA gene into messenger RNA and the subsequent translation of the mRNA into protein via the ribosome. In order for the RNA genome of the virus to be translated into the viral protein, its genes must first be converted into DNA, after which they are transcribed and translated in the usual way. Because the conversion of RNA into DNA is opposite to the normal flow of events in a cell, RNA viruses are called *retroviruses*. The virus produces its own version of DNA polymerase, which is able to synthesize a single (not a double helix) DNA strand from an RNA template. The original RNA is then destroyed by the enzyme ribonuclease. The DNA polymerase is then able to create a complementary strand to the single DNA strand, by using the original strand as a template. The two strands can now join by using the complementary base-pairing rules to form a strand of double-helix DNA. This DNA strand is able to integrate itself into the host cell's DNA in the nucleus of the cell, effectively elongating the host cell's genome. Since the viral genetic message has now been integrated into the host cell's genome, the viral DNA is duplicated along with that of the host every time the host divides.

A helper T cell, however, will not divide until it is triggered by immune response to a foreign invader. As well, a *specific* T cell will not divide until some antigen with a high affinity for the T cell's receptors is encountered. Thus, if only a few T cells in the body are infected with HIV, this may not become known for quite some time if the person concerned is not exposed to the antigen to which the infected T cells are sensitive. Once a T cell does

---

[1] Efficient though viruses are, the tobacco mosaic virus is not nearly effective enough for the author's taste.

divide, the viral DNA directs the host cell to produce RNA transcripts of its own genetic material. Some of this RNA is used as mRNA to produce viral proteins, while other RNA strands become the genomes of new virus particles. The viral proteins and genetic material assemble into new viral particles within the host cell. Depending on the speed with which these events occur, the host cell may release new HIV particles slowly, or may give rise to so many new viruses that it literally explodes. Either way, the cell gives rise to a new generation of viruses that are now free to infect more T cells.

Although T cells are the main targets of HIV, many other cells in the body are also susceptible to infection, although in these cases the results are usually not fatal to the host cell. This is not to say that the infected cells show no ill effects: in many cases the functioning of these cells is impaired or distorted, sometimes leading to cancer. The macrophage (the non-specific lymphocyte) is a common target.

Clinically, the main effect of an HIV infection is the steady decline of the helper T cell population over several years. This deficiency in the immune system, combined with the side-effects of HIV infection in other cell types, can lead to a bewildering array of symptoms. Ultimately, however, the loss of an effective immune response will kill the infected person. The fact that HIV infection is always fatal, combined with the fact that, at present, there is no cure for AIDS, is what makes the disease so frightening.

Theoretical models of AIDS fall into two main categories. The first group of models attempts to predict the pattern of infection in a population. Since this is really a branch of epidemiology (the study of epidemics) and does not concentrate on the cellular action of HIV within the organism, we will not consider such models in this book. The second, and considerably smaller, group of models attempts to simulate the behaviour of a single immune system during the course of an HIV infection.

We will examine in detail one such model: that of R. B. Pandey (1991). The model illustrates an interesting application of cellular automata, which we met in Chapter 7.

14.2   Cellular automata, the immune system, and AIDS

14.2.1   A single cell automaton model of HIV infection

Recall from Chapter 7 that a cellular automaton is a system consisting of a collection of cells, each of which can exist in one of a number of specified states. The automaton evolves through time, with the state of each cell at the next time step being determined by its own state, and those of its neighbours, at the current time step.

In applying cellular automata to a model of HIV infection, Pandey (1991) views an organism (such as a person) as a cellular automaton. Because the word 'cell' has two meanings in this context: one as a biological cell and the other as a cell in the cellular automaton, we shall use the word 'cube' to refer to a cell in the cellular automaton (since Pandey's model is three dimensional) and the word 'cell' in the biological sense.

The individual cubes in the automaton correspond to spatial locations in the body.[2] The state of a cube describes the cellular composition of that location in the body: how many helper T cells, killer T cells, macrophages, and so on, there are at that point. Because the immune system consists of several types of cells, each cube actually has several states or attributes, rather than the single attribute found in many other cellular automata.

As with other aspects of the immune system, the biology of HIV infection is sufficiently complicated that it would unrealistic to attempt to model the system in molecular and cellular detail.[3] The specific aspects of HIV infection that Pandey has chosen to model are as follows.

As mentioned in the previous section, HIV primarily attacks the helper T cells, although it can infect and multiply in other cell types, most notably the macrophages. The chain of events to be considered in the model are:

1. Introduction of HIV into the immune system, causing a non-specific immune response from the macrophages. Macrophages will engulf the HIV particles and attempt to digest them in order to present them to the helper T cells. In the process, however, some macrophages will become infected with HIV, becoming reservoirs for virus growth and a safe haven from attack by other components of the immune system.

2. The macrophages present the partially digested components of the virus to the helper T cells, causing them to release *lymphokines*, proteins which trigger the killer T cells into action.

3. The infection and subsequent destruction of helper T cells by HIV virus, concurrently with other events described here.

4. The proliferation of killer T cells in response to the lymphokines released by the helper T cells.

5. The destruction of infected cells by the killer T cells.

---

[2]The habit of physical scientists of simplifying biological models is nicely summarized in the following story. A dairy farmer, a veterinarian, and a physicist were asked to give their views on how milk production in cows could be improved. The farmer said that it was important to feed the cows on the right sort of grass. The vet said that it was important to make sure that the cow was properly inoculated against disease, and kept in a clean, dry barn. The physicist began his remarks by saying 'Let us approximate the cow by a sphere...'.

[3]Even if you are fortunate enough to have access to a Cray supercomputer, as was used by Pandey for his model.

6. The spread of the virus by both means mentioned in the last section: rapid growth causing rupture of the host cell and slower growth
causing new viruses to be released gradually by budding from the cell
membrane.

This list of events makes no explicit mention of many of the molecular details, but contains an overview of the experimentally determined
sequence of events.

The cell types considered by Pandey are: (i) stimulated macrophages,
that is, macrophages that have encountered HIV; (ii) healthy helper T cells,
referred to in the model as T4 cells, since the surface marker on a helper T
cell is composed of a set of proteins known collectively as CD4 (standing
for *cluster of differentiation, type 4*); (iii) killer T cells, known as T8 cells
(since their surface markers are known as CD8); (iv) cells infected by HIV
or free virus particles, referred to as *virions*.

Rather than dealing with actual cell populations, Pandey's model uses a
binary code to describe the state of a cube. If a cube has a high population
of a particular cell type, say macrophages, the macrophage state is defined
to be 1, while if the population of that cell type is low or absent, the state
is defined to be 0. It is important to note that if the state of a cell type is 0,
this does *not* necessarily mean that there are *no* cells of that type present;
rather, it means that the cell population is low.

The state of each cube in the automaton is specified by four values: the
binary code describing the state of each of the four cell types. Since the cell
types are all functions of time t, the state of a cube is described by the four
functions $M(t)$ for macrophages, $T4(t)$ for helper T cells, $T8(t)$ for killer
T cells, and $V(t)$ for virions. Since there are four binary states, there are
$2^4 = 16$ possible states for a cube. If we order the states as $[M, V, T4, T8]$,
we may represent the state of a cube as a 4-bit binary number, and refer to
the state by its decimal equivalent. For example, if a cube had high levels
of macrophages and virions, and low levels of T4 and T8 cells, its state
could be given by the binary number 1100, which is 12 in decimal.

The dynamics of the automaton come in two varieties: one for each of
the two infection modes (fast replication followed by rupture of the cell,
and slower reproduction). The dynamical rules are given in the form of
logical statements, using the Boolean operators NOT, AND, and OR. The
NOT operator returns the opposite of its operand: NOT (1) = 0 and NOT
(0) = 1. The AND operator links two operands, and returns a 1 if and only
if both its operands are 1: 1 AND 1 = 1, but 0 AND 1 = 1 AND 0 = 0
AND 0 = 0. The OR operator returns a 1 if either or both of its operands
are 1: 1 OR 1 = 0 OR 1 = 1 OR 0 = 1, but 0 OR 0 = 0.

At time $t + 1$, the state of each of the four cell types depends on the states of the cell types at time t. The first set of dynamical rules is as follows:

$$M(t+1) \quad = \quad M(t) \text{ OR } V(t) \tag{14.1}$$
$$V(t+1) \quad = \quad [V(t) \text{ OR } M(t) \text{ OR } T4(t)] \text{ AND } [\text{ NOT } T8(t)] \tag{14.2}$$
$$T4(t+1) \quad = \quad [M(t) \text{ OR } T4(t)] \text{ AND } [\text{ NOT } V(t)] \tag{14.3}$$
$$T8(t+1) \quad = \quad T4(t) \text{ AND } M(t) \text{ AND } V(t). \tag{14.4}$$

Equation (14.1) says that the activated macrophage population will be high in the next time cycle if it is high in the current cycle, or if there are a large number of virions present, or both. In other words, if there are infected cells present, these will be recognized by the macrophages and cause them to become active. Also, if there are a large number of activated macrophages already present, they will multiply and maintain their population number.

Equation (14.2) says that there will be a high population of virions if either (i) there are many virions present now or (ii) there are many activated macrophages (since activated macrophages act as reservoirs for virus) or (iii) there are many helper T cells (since viruses infect helper T cells) AND that the population of killer T cells is low (since they destroy virions).

Equation (14.3) states that helper T cells will proliferate if there are activated macrophages present (since macrophages present digested antigen to helper cells, triggering them to multiply), or there are a lot of helper cells present, but only if there are not very many virions present (since virions attack helper cells).

Finally, eqn (14.4) says that killer T cells will multiply only if helper T cells, macrophages, and virions are present, since the helper T cells are required to produce the lymphokines, and macrophages are required to present the infected cells for killing.

To get a feel for how these rules operate, we can consider the so-called *mean-field approximation*, which means we approximate the automaton by a single cube, and apply the rules above to that single compartment. This is equivalent to regarding the entire organism as a single compartment in which all cells are allowed to interact with each other.

Within this single cube, we can choose one of the 16 possible states as an initial condition. Let us choose state 11, which is 1011 in binary notation, meaning that $M(t)$, $T4(t)$, and $T8(t)$ are high (1) and $V(t)$ is low (0). Applying the rules above, we find that $M(t+1) = 1 \text{ OR } 0 = 1$; $V(t+1) = 0$ because of the NOT $T8$ term in equation 14.2; $T4(t+1) =$

[1 OR 1] AND [NOT 0] = 1 and $T8(t+1) = 0$ since $V(t) = 0$. We have therefore arrived in state 1010, or decimal number 10.

We can completely map out the trajectories followed by this system by starting at each of the 16 possible combinations of cell states and applying the rules until we hit a fixed point or a stable cycle of states. We find that there are two fixed points in the dynamics and a stable cycle of three states.

The fixed points are the states 0000, which means that none of the cell types is active, so that the person is healthy; and 1100, corresponding to high populations of macrophages and virions, but low counts of both types of T cells, indicating loss of immune function. A person in the latter state would be seriously ill.

The cycle consists of the three states 1110, 1101, and 1000 endlessly repeated in that order. The first state is an infected state (low T8, but high for the other 3 cell types), but because the healthy helper T cell population is high, the killer T cells are triggered in the next cycle. However, the presence of virions means that the helper T cells are killed off in this second stage, resulting in a serious infection. The killer T cells come to the rescue by the third stage however, having killed off the virion population. However, a reserve of virus particles is contained in the macrophage population, which remains high, so the infection cycle begins again.

The cycle could be interpreted as the rapid mode of virus reproduction. The infection in state 1110 causes the T4 cells to rupture and spread the infection by the second stage. The killer T cells are able to restore the balance temporarily, until the next round of infection begins.

The second set of dynamical rules is as follows:

$$M(t+1) \;=\; M(t) \text{ OR } V(t) \tag{14.5}$$

$$V(t+1) \;=\; [V(t) \text{ OR } T4(t)] \text{ AND } \{ \text{ NOT } [T4(t) \text{ AND } T8(t)]\} \tag{14.6}$$

$$T4(t+1) \;=\; \{T4(t) \text{ OR } [M(t) \text{ AND } V(t)]\} \text{ AND } [\text{ NOT } V(t)] \tag{14.7}$$

$$T8(t+1) \;=\; T8(t) \text{ OR } [T4(t) \text{ AND } M(t) \text{ AND } V(t)] \tag{14.8}$$

Equation (14.5) is the same as eqn (14.1). Equation (14.6) states that the virion population will be high if there is either a high virion population or a high T4 population, and not both of the T4 and T8 cell levels are high. Previously (eqn (14.2)) we only required the absence of T8 cells, and allowed virion proliferation if activated macrophages were present. This rule simulates the condition where viruses inside macrophages are dormant, which is one mode of behaviour observed in actual AIDS cases.

Equation (14.7) is an attempt to allow T4 proliferation when macrophage and virion are present, since macrophages process virions and present them to T4 cells, causing them to proliferate. However, Pandey's equation as it is written here does not allow this condition. The final NOT $V(t)$ term means that virion concentration must be low in order for $T4(t+1)$ to be high, which means that the term $[M(t) \text{ AND } V(t)]$ in the first part of the equation is always 0 and can therefore be omitted. The effective form of this equation is then

$$T4(t+1) = T4(t) \text{ AND } [\text{ NOT } V(t)] \qquad (14.9)$$

which does not have the desired effect. Equation (14.3) from the first set of rules would appear to be sufficient for our purposes here, and perhaps could be tried in a modified version of the model. However, since the model requires a significant amount of time on a supercomputer, it is not a change that can be easily tested.

The final equation (14.8) allows killer T cells to proliferate either from their own population or from the presence of the other three cell types as in eqn (14.4).

This set of rules has seven fixed points and no cycles. The two fixed points 0000 and 1100 are still present. Of the five remaining fixed points, four (0011, 1001, 1000, and 1011) have low virion population levels, so do not correspond to infected cases. The final fixed point, 1101, is the badly infected state that was present as part of the cycle of three states in the first set of rules.

In this model, state 1110 (all cells present except T8) leads to state 1101 (all cells present except T4), just as in the first model, but unlike that model, state 1101 is now a fixed point. Since both virions and killer T cells are present in this state, this would imply that the virus and killer T cells are in equilibrium. This model therefore corresponds to a slower and steadier interaction than the cycle in the first model, where the virus would expand rapidly, followed by equally rapid killing by T8 cells, followed by another viral expansion, and so on.

14.2.2 A three-dimensional model of HIV infection

The mean field model of the previous section crudely reproduces some of the symptoms seen in a real AIDS patient. However, to increase the realism of the model, we need to introduce some spatial dependence. We can do this by considering a three-dimensional model in which the organism is represented by a lattice composed of individual cubes, within each of which cellular interactions of the sort considered in the last section are going on.

In a real system, of course, the various locations in the body interact through processes such as blood flow and diffusion. We can model this in our lattice model by allowing each cube to interact with its six nearest neighbours.

We consider a system to consist of a cubic lattice of size $L \times L \times L$. Within each cube in this lattice, we have the same four cell types as in the last section. If a particular cell type is in the high population state, cells of that type will tend to spread to neighbouring cubes. To model this, we shall impose the following inter-cube interaction rule for each cell type, which is to be performed at each time step, before the cell interaction rules of the last section. For a given cube and a given cell type, if the concentration of that cell type is high either within the cube or within any of its six nearest neighbours, then the concentration of that cell type will be high at the beginning of the next time step. In other words, if a cube contains a lot of a given cell type it will keep those cells at least until the cell interaction rules are applied, or if any of its neighbours has a high concentration of that cell type, some of those cells will diffuse or flow into the cube before the cell interaction rules for the next time step can be applied. Each time step now consists of two steps: (i) apply the rules for cell transport between cubes; (ii) apply the rules for cell interaction within cubes.

Pandey performed several experiments on such a system, using lattice sizes of $L = 64$ and $L = 192$. We shall consider a few of his results here.

In the first experiment, a certain fraction p_i of cubes are seeded with large populations of cell type i, and the first of the two cell interaction rules in the last section is used. It is found that for low values of p_i, where very few cubes have high population values, that the system tends to a steady state in which the virus spreads to all cubes and the T4 cells are killed off everywhere. As the value of p_i is increased for all cell types except virions (the virus is assumed to start in only one cube), the infection spreads to a lesser extent, and more cubes contain healthy populations of helper T cells. At a value of p_i around 0.07, the number of cubes containing healthy T4 cells surpasses the number of infected cells (in the steady state). This trend continues until for values of p_i exceeding 0.15 the infection is virtually eliminated. These are general trends—the oscillation observed in the single-cube model is still present in the larger model, but to a lesser extent. The oscillations have a smaller amplitude, so that both the virion and T4 population values tend to oscillate about fixed values.

For the second cell interaction model, the virus always spreads to all cubes no matter what the initial value of p_i.

However, it was pointed out in the last section that the two sets of rules for cell interaction are characteristic of the same HIV infection at different times and places. It is therefore not quite correct to model an HIV infection using only one behaviour pattern. Pandey has therefore extended his model to account for this.

Two possibilities are catered for: (i) to model the observed habit of HIV to become dormant after an initial infection, the possibility of the effects of the virus 'switching off' every so often is allowed; (ii) the fact that both of the cell interaction models above may occur in the same system at different places is allowed.

To model these possibilities, Pandey introduces a *latency parameter B*. In case (i), where the virus becomes dormant at certain times, B represents the probability that the virus is active in a given cube at a given time cycle. If the virus chooses to fall dormant during a time cycle, then all other cell types in that cube behave as though $V(t) = 0$ in that cube, even if there are a great many virus particles present. Thus the virus has the ability to trick the defence mechanism into believing that it has been eradicated. If the defence system is deactivated because of this false belief, the virus can reactivate later on and take advantage of a defenceless cube. These models are called *dilution models*, because the influence of the virus is diluted over time.

In the second model, the virus never becomes dormant, but cubes switch between the two sets of rules for cell interaction. Here the parameter B is the probability that a cube uses the first set of interaction rules during a particular time cycle, and $1 - B$ is therefore the probability that the other set of rules is used.

Consider first the dilution models. Whichever set of interaction rules is used, we find qualitatively similar behaviour as B increases from 0 to 1. For small values of B, there is very little cell activity. This is what one might expect, since if the virus spends most of its time in the dormant state, it cannot do much damage and host defences will not be stimulated into action very often. As B increases, the population of killer T8 cells steadily increases. The behaviour of the virus and the helper T4 cells, however, is somewhat more complex. At first, the virus population increases steadily but, at around $B = 0.5$, it tends to drop off (or at least slow its rate of increase—the precise effect depends on the starting value of p_i, the initial populations of the various cell types). The T4 population shows a corresponding increase around the point. The viral population reaches a local minimum with respect to B around $B = 0.6$, after which it increases so that, when $B = 1$, it has managed to infect virtually the entire lattice. The helper T4 cells show a local maximum, also around $B = 0.6$. It appears, therefore, that if the virus is active around 60 per cent of the time, it causes the maximum response from the immune system without causing so much damage that it incapacitates it. Admittedly, this is a fairly rough model, but it suggests a possible clinical application: if the virus can be induced into a state of partial dormancy, the body's immune system can provide a peak level of defence against the infection. Supplemented with external treatment, this may help a cure.

In the second model, where the system switches between the two patterns of cellular activity, the parameter B represents the probability that the first set of interaction rules is being used. The general trend here is that the steady state level of virus tends to drop as B increases from 0 to 1, with a corresponding rise in the population of T4 cells. This would seem to indicate that first set of interaction rules, although characterized by cycles of explosive viral growth, also has periods of relative inactivity during which the immune defences can restore some semblance of order. The second set of rules, as observed above, always leads to total infection sooner or later.

Part III

The Brain

15

Neurons and synapses

15.1 Introduction

The human brain is without doubt the most complex object in the known universe. It is a lump of tissue about the size of two clenched fists, yet it contains more than 10^{12} cells and is the seat of essentially everything a human being is. The brain controls and initiates virtually every act a person performs in his life, from relatively simple, but vital, functions such as breathing and heartbeat, to the height of creativity as exemplified by the composition of great symphonies and the formulation of intricate scientific theories.

In attempting to explain the brain, we are attempting to explain ourselves. We may expect such an attempt to be the most challenging project we shall ever undertake. Indeed we may seriously question whether such an explanation is even possible.

As we will see, the gap between the theoretical models of various brain functions and the experimental data in the same areas is immense, so large in some cases that the traditional interplay between theory and experiment has not yet taken place. To some, it may seem premature to include theories of brain function in a book on models in biology. But however large the gulf between theory, experiment, and reality may be, the intellectual rewards to be gained by studying the brain are even greater.

Because the number of functions of the brain is very large, we will consider only one aspect of neural modelling in this book: memory. This choice is made mainly because there are many theoretical models of memory, most of which are amenable to computer simulation. Even within this one area, however, we will find that there are far too many models for a book of this size to consider them all.

The first two chapters in this part of the book will provide some biological background on the nature of neurons (this chapter) and the nature of biological memory (Chapter 16). Readers interested in pursuing a study of the neural system are referred to the excellent (though very heavy) book by Kandel and Schwartz (1985).

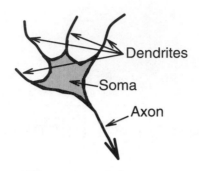

Figure 15.1   A neuron.

15.2 Neurons

The nervous system of any animal is composed of specialized cells called
neurons. Despite their exceptional properties, neurons share many of the
properties of most other cells. They contain nuclei in which the genetic
material of the organism is stored in DNA, and thus possess the ability to
synthesize proteins. The cells are bounded by a cell membrane, which, as
in other cells, is composed of a double layer of lipid (fat) molecules. In
the lipid membrane are embedded many specialized proteins which permit
various ions and molecules to pass through the membrane under certain
conditions.

Neurons differ from other cells in many ways. One of the most striking
differences is their shape: neurons usually possess many tendrils which can
extend out from the main body of the cell for a considerable distance.
Broadly speaking, a neuron can be divided into three parts: the cell body
or *soma*, those tendrils which carry information into a nerve cell, called
dendrites, and the tendril which carries information out of the cell, called
the *axon* (see Fig. 15.1).

Note that a neuron can have many inputs, but in general, only one
output. The axon, however, can branch after it has left the soma and thus
carry information to many different locations. Needless to say, there are
many variants on this basic model, but most neurons follow this pattern.

The nerves are composed of bundles of fibres leading from their points of
origin (sensory receptors such as touch, taste, smell and so on) to neurons in
the spinal cord. These fibres form strands much like the individual strands
in stranded copper wire.

The analogy between nerves and copper wire is deeper than merely
structural. Just as copper wire can conduct electric current, so too can
nerves. This is the main way that neurons communicate with each other,

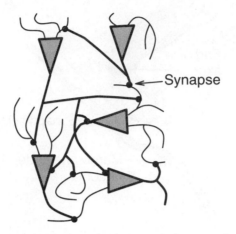

←—Synapse

Figure 15.2 A simple neural network. Axons are drawn as heavy lines; dendrites as light lines. Black dots are synapses. Note that axons may make synapses on the dendrites, soma, or even the axon of another neuron.

both in transmission of messages from the extremities of the body to the brain, and intercellular communication between various parts of the brain. However, whereas a copper wire requires a voltage along its length in order for a current to flow, electrical conduction in a nerve is a bit more complex. In neurons, electrical signals can be transmitted in two ways. The first, *passive transmission*, occurs in all neural tissue: dendrites, soma, and axon. Passive transmission can only transmit electrical signals over relatively short distances (around 1 mm or less). The second, the *action potential*, occurs only in axons and can transmit impulses over any distance. The action potential is therefore the means of communication between the brain and the rest of the body. Signals from sensory receptors are encoded into action potentials which are transmitted along nerves to the central nervous system (the brain and spinal cord). The brain interprets these incoming, or *afferent* signals, decides on an appropriate response, and sends messages back to the correct parts of the body (usually a signal to the muscles) by means of more action potentials. For a given nerve, an action potential consists of a single sharp electrical pulse which travels down the nerve in much the same way as a single pulse can be transmitted down a rope by giving one end a rapid jerk. The intensity of a signal in a nerve is varied by varying the frequency at which the action potentials are generated, not by varying their amplitude. All action potentials in a nerve have the same amplitude.

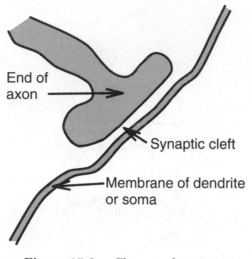

Figure 15.3   Close-up of a synapse.

When an action potential reaches the end of an axon, the information it contains must be transmitted to the neuron to which the axon is joined. The coupling between an axon and another neuron is called a *synapse*. Between the end of the axon and the adjacent cell there is a small gap called the *synaptic cleft* (see Figs 15.2 and 15.3).

In most synapses, the electrical signal from the action potential reaching the end of the axon is transmitted across the synaptic cleft by the diffusion of a chemical substance called a *transmitter* or *neurotransmitter*, rather than by any direct electrical connection. The transmitter is released from the end of the axon, drifts across the synaptic cleft and attaches to receptors on the other neuron. If enough transmitter molecules are received by the target cell, another action potential is generated in that cell which is passed on to other neurons in the network.

Because these methods of neural communication are fundamental to all brain models, we will devote the rest of this chapter to a more detailed examination of them.

15.3   Passive transmission

An electrical impulse can be initiated in a nerve by many mechanisms. If the nerve is a sensory nerve, the impulse can be generated by specialized receptors which respond to various stimuli. The sense of touch, for example, has receptors that are sensitive to such things as pressure, heat, cold, pain, and so on. Each of these receptors can start an electrical impulse which propagates down the nerve.

To understand how the impulse travels, by either passive or active transmission, we must examine the nerve cell membrane. This membrane is a double layer of lipid molecules with various types of proteins embedded in it. This membrane serves as a barrier between two solutions: the cytoplasm, or fluid inside the cell, and the extracellular fluid, which surrounds the nerve cell. The concentrations of various ions, such as potassium (K^+), sodium (Na^+), chloride (Cl^-) and calcium (Ca^{++}) are different on each side of the membrane. Since these ions are charged and not in electrical equilibrium, there is a net voltage across the membrane. The membrane potential V_m, measured in millivolts (mV or thousandths of a volt), is defined to be the potential of the inside of the membrane relative to the outside. In other words, it is the change in electrical potential experienced as you travel from the outside of the membrane to the inside. In most neurons, this potential is in the range -40 to -75 mV. The negative potential indicates that there is an excess of negative ions on the inside of the cell.

The potential V_m results in an electrical force which tends to pull positive ions into the cell and push negative ions out. However, there is also a concentration gradient for each ion species across the membrane. In a resting membrane (one not conducting an action potential), there tends to be an excess of sodium and chloride ions on the outside and an excess of potassium ions on the inside. In an attempt to equalize the concentrations of each ion species, there will be a tendency for sodium and chloride ions to diffuse into the cell and for potassium ions to diffuse outwards.

We therefore have two forces operating on any given ion: an electrical force resulting from the potential difference across the membrane, and a chemical force resulting from the concentration gradient of that ion species. Let us examine the effects of these forces on the potassium ion. The potassium ion is a positive ion, and is observed to have a higher concentration inside the cell. Since there is a negative potential difference across the membrane, the electrical force tends to attract potassium into the cell, but the concentration gradient tends to force potassium out of the cell. The two forces tend to oppose each other. It seems reasonable that there is some particular value of membrane potential at which the electrical and chemical forces would exactly balance each other, so that there would be no net movement of potassium ions across the membrane. This potential, E_K, (the subscript K refers to potassium), can be calculated from the *Nernst formula* which is derived from thermodynamic theory:

$$E_K = \frac{RT}{ZF} \ln \frac{[K^+]_o}{[K^+]_i} \tag{15.1}$$

where $[K^+]_o$ ($[K^+]_i$) is the concentration of potassium ions on the outside (inside) of the membrane, R is the gas constant, T is the absolute temperature (in degrees Kelvin), Z is the valence of the ion (+1, for potassium) and F is the Faraday constant. At a temperature of 25°C (298 Kelvin), $RT/F = 26$ mV.

In one system used in early studies of the membrane potential, the giant axon in the squid (used because its large size made experiments easier), the concentration of potassium in the cytoplasm is 400 mM (millimolar)[1] and the concentration in the extracellular fluid is 20 mM. Substituting these numbers into Nernst's formula gives an equilibrium potential of about −75 mV. In the squid axon, the resting potential is around −60 mV.

Similar calculations for sodium give an equilibrium potential of +55 mV and for chloride of −60 mV. The sodium potential is positive, since the concentration of sodium is greater on the outside of the membrane, so a positive interior voltage is required to maintain this difference.

We see that only the chloride potential is the same as the actual resting potential of the membrane. Since potassium and sodium ions are clearly not in either chemical or electrical equilibrium, how are these ionic populations maintained? The answer lies in the fact that the membrane restricts the movement of the various ions. The proteins embedded in the lipid membrane serve as channels which will only allow specific ions to pass through. Each channel is, in general, permeable to only one species of ion. However, there can be more than one channel for each ion type. Some of these channels are always open, so that an ion of the correct type is free to diffuse through. Other channels are *voltage-gated*, that is, they only open when the voltage across the membrane reaches a certain value. Still others can be mediated by other molecules, such as proteins, whose concentration determines if the channel is open or not. The full range of various channels is probably not yet known. At the time of writing, there are two sodium channels, seven potassium channels, and three calcium channels known (Shepherd, 1990).

For the moment, we will consider only those channels which are always open, since these are responsible for passive transmission. We will assume, for simplicity, that we have only two types of these passive channels: one for sodium and one for potassium.

At rest, the membrane is much more permeable to potassium than sodium, but there is a much stronger electrical force (+55 − (−60) = 115 mV) on the sodium than on the potassium ((−60) − (−75) = 15 mV). The differences are such that the leakage of sodium into the cell is just balanced by the leakage of potassium outwards. Since sodium and potassium

---

[1]A 1 molar solution is one where there is 1 mole of molecules per litre. A mole is given by Avogadro's number, approximately 6.02 $\times 10^{23}$.

ions have the same charge, there is no change in the membrane potential. You may wonder why this leakage does not cause the Nernst potentials of the ions to change, since the diffusion would alter the concentrations of the two ions on either side of the membrane. To prevent this, there is a metabolically driven sodium–potassium 'pump' which restores the sodium and potassium concentrations to their original values. Since the pump is opposing the natural tendency towards equilibrium, it requires energy to run. It is a bit like a continual recharging of the nerve's 'battery' to maintain the correct voltage across the membrane.

Because the Nernst potential for chloride ions is the same as the resting membrane potential, there is no net force on chloride ions in either direction, so we can disregard them.

Let us re-examine the properties of the resting nerve membrane with an eye to simplifying our representation of it. It is a barrier which maintains, via the sodium–potassium pump, non-equilibrium concentrations of sodium and potassium ions on either side. The membrane allows a certain amount of both ion species to flow through selected locations (the ion channels), so it is not a perfect insulator. In addition, the membrane can store charge on its two surfaces at locations where no current is allowed to flow through. These three properties are analogous to components found in simple electric circuits.

The non-equilibrium concentrations of ions are equivalent to voltage sources, that is, batteries. Each battery will have a voltage equal to the Nernst potential of its corresponding ion. These potentials have been given above: $E_K = -75$ mV, $E_{Na} = +55$ mV, and $E_{Cl} = -60$ mV.

The ion channels are equivalent to resistors, since they allow limited flow of current through the membrane. Rather than measure the resistance R of a membrane channel, it is conventional to use the reciprocal quantity, known as the conductance g. The unit of conductance is the siemen, abbreviated S, and defined by 1 S $= 1$ ohm^{-1}. [2] The conductance of a patch of membrane depends on the number of channels per unit area. Conductance values are usually given as siemens per square centimetre, although the area unit is often omitted. Typical values are: $g_K = 10 \times 10^{-6}$S/cm^2; $g_{Na} = 0.5 \times 10^{-6}$S/cm^2. Note that g_K is 20 times that of g_{Na}.

The ability of the membrane to store charge is equivalent to a capacitance. A capacitor is a circuit element which stores an amount of charge Q equal to the product of the voltage V across the capacitor and the capacitance C: $Q = CV$. Capacitance is measured in farads, with one farad being 1 coulomb of charge per volt of potential difference across the capacitor. The farad is an enormous unit: most capacitors in ordinary electric circuits have capacitances measured in microfarads, or 10^{-6} farads. A typ-

---

[2]Engineers tend to use the mho, ohm spelled backwards, as the unit of conductance.

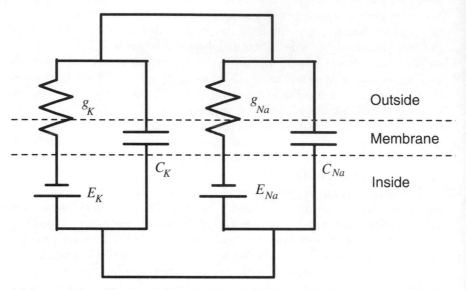

Figure 15.4   The equivalent electric circuit for a patch of nerve membrane. Only one sodium and one potassium channel are shown.

ical membrane capacitance is about 1 microfarad per square centimetre of membrane area.

Considering only the passive potassium and sodium channels, an equivalent circuit for a patch of membrane is as shown in Fig. 15.4.

We can use a bit of elementary circuit theory to work out the resting potential V_R of the membrane from this circuit. Since the membrane is resting, the net current across it must be zero, so that the sum of the sodium current I_{Na} and the potassium current I_K is zero:

$$I_{Na} + I_K = 0. \tag{15.2}$$

As well, in a resting membrane the capacitors would be fully discharged, so we can ignore them for now.

Now according to circuit theory, the total potential difference between two points is the sum of the differences along any path joining those two points. Using Ohm's law (which states that potential difference V is the product of current I and resistance R: $V = IR$, or, in terms of conductance, $V = I/g$), the potential difference across the resistor in the sodium channel is I_{Na}/g_{Na}, so the resting membrane potential V_R calculated along the sodium channel must be

$$V_R = E_{Na} + I_{Na}/g_{Na} \tag{15.3}$$

and similarly for the potassium channel:

$$V_R = E_K + I_K/g_K. \tag{15.4}$$

Rearranging these equations to solve for the currents, we get

$$I_{Na} = g_{Na}(V_R - E_{Na}) \tag{15.5}$$

and

$$I_K = g_K(V_R - E_K). \tag{15.6}$$

Adding these equations, using the current equilibrium condition and solving for V_R gives

$$V_R = \frac{E_{Na}g_{Na} + E_Kg_K}{g_{Na} + g_K}. \tag{15.7}$$

This is a weighted mean of the Nernst potentials, with the weights being the conductances. The channel with the largest conductance has the most influence on the resting potential, which is what you would expect.

For more sophisticated modelling of neurons, we need a more complete mathematical description of a passive neuron. Although this model makes no mention of the voltage-gated channels and therefore does not apply to the action potential, it is a useful description for those parts of a neuron, such as the dendrites, that do not generate action potentials.

Our goal is a model which will allow us to calculate the membrane potential as a function of position x and time t in a non-resting state. Such a state can arise when a dendrite receives input from an axon with which it makes a synapse, or when current is artificially injected into a neuron during an experiment.

The starting point for the model is to assume that a nerve fibre is a leaky electrical cable. Current injected into the cable at one point will travel down the interior of the cable and leak out through the channels in the membrane.

Let us define a few quantities (see Fig. 15.5).

The interior of the fibre is filled with cytoplasm, which is a fair electrical conductor but has a significant resistance. The interior resistance of a length of fibre will be proportional to its length. We define r_i to be the resistance (in ohms) of a unit length of fibre. Now the resistance of an area of the membrane to current flow is determined by the number of passive channels in that area. The larger the area, the lower the resistance. We define r_m to be the resistance of a unit area of membrane.

Now consider a length of fibre between positions x_1 and x_2. Let the electrical potential of the interior of the fibre at point x_j $(j = 1, 2)$ be V_{i_j}. The potential difference between x_1 and x_2 is thus $\Delta V_i = V_{i_2} - V_{i_1}$. The resistance of the interior of the fibre between x_1 and x_2 is $r_i(x_2 - x_1) \equiv$

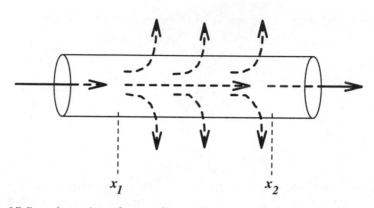

Figure 15.5   A section of nerve fibre. The arrows indicate the direction of current flow.

$r_i \Delta x$. By Ohm's law, the potential difference over the distance Δx must be equal to the current that flows between these two points multiplied by the resistance of this section of fibre. If we define positive current to be positive ions flowing in the direction of increasing x, then

$$\Delta V_i = -i_i r_i \Delta x. \tag{15.8}$$

Dividing through by Δx and taking the limit as $\Delta x \to 0$ gives

$$\frac{\partial V_i}{\partial x} = -i_i r_i. \tag{15.9}$$

We use partial derivatives since V_i is a function of both x and t.

Now if we assume that the fibre has a constant diameter and that the composition of the cytoplasm does not change with distance, the resistance r_i is independent of x. Taking the derivative of eqn (15.9) we thus obtain

$$x\frac{\partial^2 V_i}{\partial x^2} = -\frac{\partial i_i}{\partial x}r_i. \tag{15.10}$$

We now consider how the current i_i varies with position. Because the membrane is leaky, some current can enter or leave the fibre through the membrane. Let i_m be the current that leaves the membrane per unit length. Then, by a similar argument to that for voltage above, the change in current over a distance Δx is $\Delta i_i = i_{i_2} - i_{i_1}$. Since current flows in the $+x$ direction and is leaking out through the membrane, we expect $i_{i_2} < i_{i_1}$.

The membrane current over this distance is then $i_m \Delta x = i_{i_1} - i_{i_2} = -\Delta i_i$. In the limit as $\Delta x \to 0$, we get

$$i_m = -\frac{\partial i_i}{\partial x}. \tag{15.11}$$

Combining eqns (15.9) and (15.11) we obtain

$$\frac{\partial^2 V_i}{\partial x^2} = i_m r_i. \tag{15.12}$$

Now the membrane current i_m is composed of two parts: the current through the passive channels, which is the resistive part of the current, and the capacitive part, which is the current resulting from charge being deposited on either side of the membrane without actually flowing through it. From the definition of capacitance, $Q = CV$, and the fact that current is the rate of change of charge with time, $i = dQ/dt$, we can write

$$i_c = c_m \frac{\partial V}{\partial t} \tag{15.13}$$

where i_c is that part of the membrane current i_m due to the capacitance, c_m is the capacitance of the membrane in a unit length of fibre, and V is difference of the membrane potential from the resting potential. Note that V is *not* the same as V_i. In fact, if we define V_e to be the potential of the extracellular fluid and V_r to be the resting membrane potential, we have

$$V = V_i - V_e - V_r. \tag{15.14}$$

Finally, the resistive part of the membrane current, from Ohm's law, is

$$i_r = V/r_m \tag{15.15}$$

where r_m is the resistance of a unit length of membrane. Thus,

$$i_m = i_c + i + r = c_m \frac{\partial V}{\partial t} + V/r_m. \tag{15.16}$$

Now if we make a couple of additional (but reasonable) assumptions, we can tie all these equations together to get a partial differential equation for V. First, we assume that V_e is a constant. This means that we take the extracellular fluid to be a perfect conductor. This is not strictly true, but in practice there is usually much more of the extracellular fluid than there is of cytoplasm, so its resistance is much lower. In certain situations it is necessary to explicitly consider the resistance of the fluid, but usually taking V_e to be constant is a reasonable approximation.

Second, we also assume that V_r is a constant. Again, experimental measurements show this is reasonable.

If both V_e and V_r are constants, all derivatives of V_i will be the same as derivatives of V. We can make this substitution and combine eqns (15.12) and (15.16) to obtain

$$\lambda^2 \frac{\partial^2 V}{\partial x^2} - V - \tau \frac{\partial V}{\partial t} = 0 \qquad (15.17)$$

where $\lambda = \sqrt{r_m/r_i}$ and $\tau = r_m c_m$. This equation is known as the *cable equation*.

This equation is used in detailed modelling of single neurons or networks containing a small number of neurons. A formal, general solution to the cable equation can be obtained fairly easily using the technique of separation of variables. We assume that $V(x,t)$ can be expressed as a product of two functions $A(x)$ and $B(t)$: $V(x,t) = A(x)B(t)$. Making this substitution in eqn (15.17), and using subscript notation for partial derivatives ($V_t \equiv \partial V/\partial t$, $V_{xx} \equiv \partial^2 V/\partial x^2$, etc.), we have:

$$\lambda^2 A_{xx} B = AB + \tau A B_t. \qquad (15.18)$$

Dividing through by AB, we obtain

$$\lambda^2 \frac{A_{xx}}{A} = 1 + \tau \frac{B_t}{B}. \qquad (15.19)$$

Now, since the left-hand side is a function of x only and the right-hand side is a function of t only, the only way both sides can be equal for all values of x and t is if they both equal a constant k^2 (k may be a complex number, so by choosing the constant to be k^2, we are not excluding negative or complex values of the constant). We thus obtain two independent ordinary differential equations

$$\lambda^2 A_{xx} = k^2 A \qquad (15.20)$$
$$\tau B_t = (k^2 - 1)B \qquad (15.21)$$

Integrating, we obtain

$$A(x) = A_1 e^{kx/\lambda} + A_2 e^{-kx/\lambda} \qquad (15.22)$$
$$B(t) = B_0 e^{(k^2-1)t/\tau}. \qquad (15.23)$$

where B_0, A_1, and A_2 are constants.

One solution for $V(x,t)$ is then

$$V(x,t) = B_0 e^{(k^2-1)t/\tau}[A_1 e^{kx/\lambda} + A_2 e^{-kx/\lambda}]. \qquad (15.24)$$

Since eqn (15.17) is linear, any linear combination of solutions is also a solution, so the general solution is

$$V(x,t) = \int [e^{(k^2-1)t/\tau}(A_1 e^{kx/\lambda} + A_2 e^{-kx/\lambda})]K(k)dk \qquad (15.25)$$

where we have absorbed the constant B_0 into the constants A_1 and A_2. The function $K(k)$ is a *kernel*, which indicates which values of k are to appear in the integral, and in what proportion.

In order to obtain a particular solution to the cable equation, we must specify appropriate initial and boundary conditions. This will allow the constants A_1 and A_2 and the kernel $K(k)$ to be determined (in principle). In practice, of course, any but the simplest initial and boundary conditions require numerical solutions.

We will not delve any deeper into the intricacies of the cable equation, since we will not need it in most of our models. We can draw a couple of useful observations from it here, though, which will be useful later.[3]

First, consider the steady-state situation where the fibre has been subjected to a steady voltage distribution and allowed to come to equilibrium. In such a case, all time derivatives will be zero. We see from eqn (15.21) that we must have $k^2 = 1$, so that the solution will have the form

$$V(x,t) = A_1 e^{x/\lambda} + A_2 e^{-x/\lambda}. \qquad (15.26)$$

If the voltage is being held constant by an electrode inserted into the membrane at $x = 0$, we would not expect any exponential growth of the voltage, so the first term must be zero. The spatial distribution of voltage would then be

$$V(x,t) = A_2 e^{-x/\lambda}. \qquad (15.27)$$

In other words, we would expect a voltage pulse to decay exponentially with length constant $\lambda = \sqrt{r_m/r_i}$. If r_m, the membrane resistance, is high and r_i, the cytoplasmic resistance is low, the length constant is quite large, so that a voltage pulse would extend longer than in the converse case, where the cytoplasm offers more resistance and the membrane less.

Now consider the case where there is no change of V with x. In this case, from eqn (15.20), we see that $k^2 = 0$. The solution for V under these conditions is

$$V(x,t) = B_0 e^{-t/\tau}. \qquad (15.28)$$

We see that a uniform voltage pulse will decay exponentially with time constant $\tau = r_m c_m$. High membrane resistance and/or capacitance will cause the membrane to retain the voltage longer.

---

[3]Readers interested in a more comprehensive treatment of modelling using the cable equation are referred to early chapters in the book by Koch and Segev (1989).

Of course, these observations are only approximations for the more general case where V varies with both x and t, but they are useful guidelines for the behaviour of voltage pulses on a passive membrane. The significance of these observations lies in the fact that the dendrites and soma of a neuron will usually receive voltage pulses from a great many axons. These axons will have synapses at various places on the dendrites and soma, and will generate pulses at various times. In order for the recipient of all these diverse pulses to fire an action potential, it must sum up the pulses it receives and determine if the sum exceeds the threshold value required for an action potential to be generated (see below, when we discuss the action potential in more detail). If the synapses generating the pulses are too far apart, their effects cannot be summed because of the decay of voltage with distance—in order for separate pulses to add up to an appreciable value, the pulses must occur, roughly, within a distance λ of each other. Similarly, pulses that are separated in time by more than about τ will not add up either. This is one way the nervous system has of filtering out background noise generated by the sensory receptors. The only signals that will register are those that produce a set of pulses that are closely spaced in both space and time.

15.4   The action potential

The cable equation, discussed in the previous section, describes how electrical impulses are transmitted over short distances and times by the passive ion channels in the nerve membrane. Since the length constant λ is typically on the order of 1 mm and the time constant τ is of the order of 1 ms, passive conduction is clearly inadequate for long-distance communication, such as that required for the hands and feet to communicate with the spinal cord. Such impulses are transmitted by means of the action potential.

The precise details of the action potential will not figure prominently in any of the models we will consider in this book, so we will content ourselves with a brief description of how it works. The brevity of the treatment here should not mislead the reader into thinking that the elucidation of the details of how the action potential originates and propagates was a trivial problem. It required many years of research and resulted in the Nobel prize for Hodgkin and Huxley, the two researchers whose names have become synonymous with action potentials.

Only certain nerve fibres are able to support action potentials, since an action potential requires special *voltage-gated* ion channels to be present in the nerve membrane. Again, these channels come in a variety of forms, but for our purposes we can visualize them as of only two types: a sodium channel and a potassium channel. In a resting membrane, both types of channel are closed. When the membrane is depolarized (that is, the membrane potential is brought closer to zero), some of the sodium channels will open, allowing sodium ions to flow inwards across the membrane. Recall that a resting membrane has a potential of around −60 mV, and that sodium ions are in excess on the outside of the cell, so there is a strong tendency for sodium to enter the cell.

This depolarization also causes potassium channels to open, but more slowly than the sodium channels. The equilibrium potential for potassium is slightly more negative than the resting potential, usually around −75 mV. Because of this there is a tendency for potassium to flow out of the cell. There is also a higher conductance for the passive potassium channels than for the passive sodium channels, so in the early stages of depolarization, the outward potassium current is able to balance the inward sodium current. However, if depolarization continues to a certain level, called the *threshold*, the net current will become inward, since most of the voltage-gated sodium channels will open, dramatically increasing the conductance of sodium. Once this threshold (around −40 mV) is reached, the depolarization of the membrane becomes regenerative: more depolarization causes more sodium channels to open causing more depolarization and so on. The process continues until the membrane potential reaches the equilibrium potential for sodium, which is around +55 mV. By this time, the voltage-gated potassium channels have opened more fully, and the outward potassium current starts to redress the balance and restore the membrane potential to its resting value. The net result is a short spike in the membrane potential where it rises from −60 mV to +55 mV and falls back to −60 mV, all in the space of a few milliseconds (see Fig. 15.6).

The sodium channels are inactive for a brief period just after a spike, so that no matter how large a depolarization is applied to the membrane, another spike will not occur. This period is called the *refractory period* and sets an upper limit on the frequency with which action potentials can be generated.

The action potential's spike is transmitted down the nerve by means of passive membrane effects. The disturbance in the membrane potential is felt for a distance of approximately λ on either side of the spike. This will cause the membrane to depolarize to threshold level in both directions from the spike, but since the sodium channels on one side have just closed after a spike, they will not open again so soon. As a result, the spike is transmitted in only one direction down the nerve. The action potential continues down the axon until it arrives at a synapse with another neuron.

Besides doing much of the experimental work on the action potential, Hodgkin and Huxley also managed to construct a differential equation to describe the membrane potential as a function of distance and time. The Hodgkin–Huxley equation is a variant of the cable equation which takes account of the variable conductivity of sodium and potassium due to the

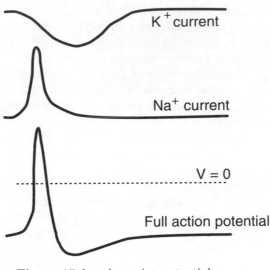

Figure 15.6   An action potential.

voltage-gated channels. The properties of this equation have amused many mathematicians, but as we will not need to use the equation in this book, we will not consider it further.

15.5 Synapses

Once an action potential reaches the end of an axon, it must attempt to communicate with another neuron. There are (at least) three ways in which this is done.

Firstly, the membranes of the two neurons (the axon of the first and that part of the second to which it is adjacent) may physically fuse to create a *gap junction*. In a gap junction, some of the ionic channels in the two membranes join up so that current can pass directly from one neuron to the other. Gap junctions are not common in mammals, although they do occur frequently in other animals.

Secondly, the two neurons may indirectly pass current from one to the other by means of an *ephaptic interaction*. Here the membranes of the two neurons remain distinct, but their close proximity causes currents passing through the membrane of one neuron to affect the currents in the neighbouring membrane. Ephaptic interactions can occur only in particularly dense concentrations of neurons.

The third and overwhelmingly the most common form of neural communication is the chemical synapse (Fig. 15.7). Here, the action potential

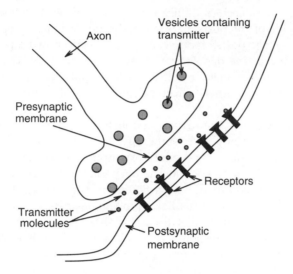

Figure 15.7   An action potential arriving at a synapse.

arriving at the end of the axon results in the release of little packets of a specialized molecule called a *neurotransmitter*. The axon (or *presynaptic membrane*) is separated from the recipient neuron (the *postsynaptic membrane*) by a gap called the *synaptic cleft*. The synaptic cleft is typically around 0.1 μm across. Neurotransmitter molecules diffuse across the cleft and arrive at the postsynaptic membrane where they attach to receptor sites. Depending on the types of transmitter and receptor, various things can happen to the recipient neuron. Some transmitters are primarily excitatory, so that they cause the membrane of the second neuron to depolarize. Other transmitters are inhibitory, increasing (*hyperpolarizing*) the membrane potential, thus making it harder for other, excitatory, transmitters to cause the neuron to fire.

A typical sequence of events in the transmission of information from one neuron to another is as follows. The membrane at the end of an axon contains special calcium channels. When the action potential arrives at the end of the axon, the resulting depolarization allows calcium into the axon. Meanwhile, neurotransmitter molecules have been synthesized by the cell and packaged into little spherical or ellipsoidal globules called *vesicles*. These vesicles hover near the presynaptic membrane awaiting the arrival of an action potential. The influx of calcium from the action potential triggers a chain of events that causes these vesicles to fuse with the inner surface of the presynaptic membrane, releasing their contents through the membrane and into the synaptic cleft.

The transmitter molecules diffuse across the cleft and seek out receptors on the outside of the postsynaptic membrane. Various receptors have different effects on the postsynaptic cell. Some receptors will open sodium channels, resulting in the depolarization of the membrane. Other receptors open potassium channels, resulting in hyperpolarization (inhibition) of the membrane. Still others affect calcium channels with a variety of side-effects.

The various effects of the arrival of the family of neurotransmitters are summed, both spatially and temporally, by the postsynaptic cell. If the combination of excitatory and inhibitory inputs (and other modulating effects) results in a depolarization at the beginning of the axon in this cell that is sufficient to generate an action potential, the cell will fire and the whole process will repeat itself further on in the network.

It should be apparent from this discussion that the geometry of the cell is vital in determining its response to a blizzard of impulses from other neurons. Most neurons have an intricate dendritic tree bringing in information from other neurons both far and near. Some of these dendrites will have excitatory synapses, other inhibitory. The relative placement of these synapses determines which ones will end up affecting the cell body, and, therefore, stand a chance of generating (or inhibiting) an action potential. An excitatory synapse that occurs upstream from an inhibitory synapse can be killed off if the inhibitory synapse is activated around the same time as the excitatory one, or it may be allowed through if the inhibitory synapse receives no (or a very small) stimulus.

This problem of geometry is one that most theoretical neural network models fail to consider. A typical theoretical neuron receives a large number of inputs, but these inputs are usually assumed to arrive all at the same time, so that they can simply be summed to determine if the net impulse exceeds the cell's threshold. Although, as we will see in subsequent chapters, networks composed of such simple neurons can perform some impressive feats which mimic real brains, little is known of how a network composed of neurons with particular geometries will work. One obvious reason for this lack of more realistic models is simply that they are very complicated; so complicated, in fact, that the construction and running of a realistic computer simulation of any reasonably sized network exceeds the capacity of most computers. However, with rapidly developing computer technology, more and better simulations are being done so that, within a few years, we may hope to see genuine progress in this area.

The chemical synapse is so common in neural networks because it offers immense flexibility. Just as the biochemistry of DNA allows the storage and management of vast quantities of complex information, and the biochemistry of the immune system allows the body to cope with a bewildering array of foreign invaders, so the biochemistry of the neural system allows a wide range of complex stimuli, memories, and instructions to be processed in a subtle and controlled manner.

15.6 Modelling the brain

A prospective modeller of the human brain, or any other neural network, is faced with an embarrassment of possibilities. There are many subsystems in the brain for which a model could be built. For those interested in highly detailed models, where as much of the biology of the real neuron is included as possible, there are models, usually of fairly small networks, where such things as separate ion channels and neural geometry and timing are considered in detail. Models have been constructed for separate components of the brain, such as the olfactory bulb (which governs the sense of smell), various aspects of the visual system (object recognition, colour vision and binocular vision, to name a few), the auditory system (including speech recognition), the hippocampus (believed to be important in the formation of memories), the motor system (responsible for muscular movement), and so on. More general, psychological models have constructed networks that mimic the conditioned response (as, for example, with Pavlov's dog, which was taught to expect food whenever a bell was rung, so that after some training, the dog would salivate when the bell was rung even if no food was present), concept representation, problem solving, and so on.

In a book of this size, which is not devoted exclusively to neural network models, it would be folly to attempt a comprehensive survey of what has been done, let alone what is possible. As such, we will concentrate mainly on models of memory. Such models have the advantage that there are many simple examples which do not require a detailed knowledge of the anatomy of the brain. These models are also fairly easy to program, giving the reader the satisfaction of watching a network composed of only a few simple neurons learn to recognize and classify sets of patterns.

These models, because of their simplicity, have the disadvantage that they are not particularly realistic. As mentioned above, most network models assume a neuron to be essentially a geometric point which receives a number of inputs and, depending on the sum of the inputs, generates an output. As well, because of the limitations on the size of computer memory and speed, it is not possible to simulate a network with more than a few thousand cells, although the human brain contains many orders of magnitude more than this. Even though the models show promise in displaying many of the attributes of human memory, we cannot tell if the same behaviour will occur in a network which is much larger, or, even if the behaviour does occur, whether the network can function in a reasonable time.

Even within the single field of memory, however, we cannot do justice to all the models which have been proposed. We have tried to concentrate on those models that illustrate the main principles of memory modelling while at the same time are easy to understand and to program. This means that several important classes of models will not be covered in this book. In an attempt not to slight the researchers concerned, I will briefly mention these models here, and give some references so that interested readers can pursue them elsewhere.

The chapters in this part of the book are concerned mainly with networks whose neurons exist in one of two discrete states: firing or quiescent. Real neurons express the intensity of a stimulus, not by varying the amplitude of their action potentials, but by varying the frequency. Thus, instead of analysing a network by examining the response of each neuron at a discrete set of times, as the models we will consider here will do, we could define an activity variable $x_i(t)$ for neuron i at time t, which measures the frequency of firing of that neuron. If the activity variable is assumed to be a continuous function of time, the dynamics of the network can then be described by a system of differential equations in the variables x_i. This is the approach of Stephen Grossberg and his collaborators, who, since the 1960s, have been producing models of neural networks designed to explain many of the brain's functions, including memory and vision. Grossberg's work is not easy to penetrate for a newcomer to neural modelling, since it tends to assume a level of sophistication in both neuroanatomy and mathematics that are rarely found in one reader. Those interested in studying Grossberg and coworkers' models will find the book by Daniel Levine (1991) a good starting point, since it does not assume a high level of mathematical knowledge, and contains numerous references to Grossberg's original papers. A somewhat more advanced treatment is the collection of papers edited by Grossberg (1988).

Models of associative memory (the association of a particular response with a particular input pattern) have been devised by Teuvo Kohonen. Kohonen's models tend to be more rigorously mathematical than those we will consider in this book. Recently, Kohonen has applied his models to the recognition of human speech. Interested readers may consult the books by Kohonen (1977, 1984) and the article by Kohonen (1988).

Several other models of memory, some of which make use of data on higher structures within the brain, may be found in the book by Byrne and Berry (1989).

16

Memory

16.1 Introduction

How does the brain store its past experiences? It would be reasonable to think that there is a strong analogy between the human brain and a modern digital computer. After all, both systems are composed of a large number of units (neurons in the brain, bits in a computer), which communicate with each other electrically, have two main states (firing and quiescent in the brain, binary 1 and 0 in the computer) and can store enormous amounts of information which can be retrieved more or less at random (you can think of widely different topics in quick succession, and a computer's RAM— random access memory— can be accessed in any location).

However, the analogy is not a good one. Firstly, there is the difference in speed. Present-day (early 1990s) computers have cycle times (the time required to perform the shortest instruction) in the nanosecond (10^{-9} second) range, while it takes several milliseconds (10^{-3} seconds) for one neuron to send an action potential to another.

Secondly, anyone who has used computers for more than playing games will realize that computers do well at things that human brains do badly or slowly, and vice versa. For example, very few people can quickly multiply two three-digit numbers in their heads, let alone cope with highly repetitive and complex calculations, such as calculating the determinant of a large matrix or the numerical solution of a differential equation. Given an algorithm, it is simple to program a computer to do these things. However, most people find it relatively easy to remember the faces and names of several hundred people, and are able to recognize these faces in various lighting conditions, from various angles and with various amounts of distortion, as when the person wears a hat, grows a moustache or puts on makeup. Such a task is beyond a computer, at least at present.

Third, most computers have a single central processing unit, or CPU, which means that they can only do one thing at a time. Such computers are called *serial* computers because they can only handle algorithms that have a single instruction at each step. Serial computers are adequate for problems where the result of each calculation is needed for the next step.

Parallel computers, which contain more than one processor, are capable of doing several things at once (one job per processor). Tasks which can be accomplished by several independent calculations are more efficiently done with a parallel algorithm. A simple example is the addition of two matrices. The same operation must be performed on each location in the matrix, and none of the elements is needed to calculate any of the other elements. Although parallel computers are relatively rare at the moment, it is likely that they will become increasingly common and more powerful over the next few years.

It is fairly obvious from what is known of the circuitry of the brain that it is a highly parallel computer. Its parallel nature largely compensates for the relative lethargy of its electronics, so that it is able to outstrip a digital serial computer in tasks involving such things as pattern recognition and motor control of the body. Of course, the brain must have a serial component as well, since you must be able to think your way through a problem one step at a time.

One main reason for the differences between a digital computer and the brain is that the first computers were designed to do things that are difficult for the brain, so that such things as elementary arithmetic functions were built in as primitive operations. Most computer programs used in everyday life are based ultimately on arithmetic. Financial programs such as spreadsheets, databases for storing and retrieving information and even graphics used in computer games and other, more academic, applications are all implemented by calculating sums and differences to determine where a given bit of information is stored and how it should be altered.

The brain, however, is the product of evolution and we would therefore expect it to be 'custom-designed' to solve evolutionary problems. The main such problem is staying alive long enough to reproduce, so the brain will have survival functions such as evasion of predators, location of food, and the reproductive drive as its 'primitive operations'. It should not be surprising that the brain is better at observing and reacting to stimuli from the environment than it is at solving equations or storing lists of names and numbers.

The final difference between computers and brains that we shall consider here bears directly on the topic of this chapter. A computer's memory consists of some electric or magnetic medium (a silicon chip or magnetic disk or tape) in which information is stored by the electrical or magnetic state of a crystal of silicon or iron oxide. The connections between these storage locations are provided by the active computer circuits. There are no 'connections' between sites on a floppy disk, for example. The information stored there cannot be accessed unless it is read by the computer.

From what is known about memory in the brain, it appears that the memories are stored as an integral part of the brain. In other words, there is no part of the brain which is reserved as a memory storage area with no other function—you do not have a 'disk drive' in your head! Since neurons are constantly altering their states between active and passive, memories cannot be stored as states of neurons. Rather, they seem to be stored as a pattern of strengths of connections between cells. The synapses joining the axon of one cell to the dendrites of other cells can be strengthened (or possibly weakened) by the perception of some phenomenon (seeing a face or smelling an aroma, for example). This change in the synaptic connection can be permanent (or at least very long-lasting). A pattern of such changes in synaptic strengths constitutes a memory.

This chapter will survey what is known on the biological side about memory. There are still large gaps in our knowledge, so that very little can stated with certainty. There is no detailed overall view of what happens in the brain when something is learned. The experiments are still at a stage where we can say that a certain part of the brain is required for a certain type of learning to occur. Other experiments have established that certain patterns of stimulation of neurons in certain areas of the brain cause particular changes in firing thresholds of certain synapses. A comprehensive, though somewhat technical, survey of the current knowledge in memory research is given in the book by Dudai (1989). Some of the experiments discussed in this chapter are covered by Kandel and Schwartz (1985).

This relatively primitive state of affairs has been both a boon and a bane to theorists. Because little is known for sure on the biological side, many theorists have not attempted to constrain their models to fit many biological details. Some models propose simple networks of neurons whose only connection with biology is that they sum inputs from other neurons and fire if this sum exceeds a threshold. Other models try to include more of what is known from experiments, but trying to build a truly biological simulation of memory is virtually impossible due to the lack of data.

In such a situation, the main value of modelling is that it can show the sorts of behaviours that various types of networks can produce. It is to be hoped that, when a model produces behaviour that is similar to that observed in a real network, some of the assumptions that have gone into the model may prove to be true of the biological system as well. Most of the models presented in this section of the book should be interpreted in this way.

16.2 Habituation and sensitization

The ability to learn seems to have appeared at an early stage in the evolution of animals. Although it is obvious that the higher animals all have the capacity to learn—your pet dog or cat can learn its name, and parrots can pick up fragments of speech, although it is doubtful that they understand what they are saying—it may come as a surprise to discover that even invertebrates such as fruit flies and sea slugs have a limited ability to learn as well. This is fortunate from the researcher's point of view, since the neural networks in these 'lower' animals are considerably simpler than the mammalian brain. They offer, therefore, the opportunity to discover how memory works in a system that is much easier to manipulate.

The sort of learning that these creatures exhibit is, of course, nothing as sophisticated as learning their names (assuming that scientists name their experimental sea slugs). There are three types of learning that practically any animal can do: habituation, sensitization, and conditioning. As humans show these forms of learning as well, it is perhaps easiest to describe them in terms with which readers are familiar from their own experience.

Habituation occurs when you are subjected to a repetitive stimulus whose effect on you is neither good nor bad. You usually notice the stimulus when it first occurs, but eventually you 'tune it out' so that you are no longer of conscious of it, even though it is still occurring. Some everyday examples are the ticking of a clock and the feel of your clothes on your skin. You will notice the ticking of a clock if someone brings a clock into the room and sets in on a table near you, but after a few minutes you become accustomed to the noise and no longer notice it. Similarly, when you put your clothes on in the morning, you are initially conscious of the different feel they have, but after you have worn them for a few minutes, you tune out the sensation (assuming that the clothes fit properly so that they do not produce uncomfortable or painful sensations—in such a case you do *not* ignore the feelings; you would change your clothes or adjust them so that they feel more comfortable).

Most animals display habituation to some degree. The sea slug, for example, has a gill and a siphon protruding from its back which it will withdraw for safekeeping if they are touched, rather like a land snail withdraws into its shell if it is disturbed. If the gill or siphon is repeatedly touched, however, this reflex action eventually disappears, so that the gill and siphon remain where they are. Since the touch is a neutral stimulus it poses no threat, so there is no point in responding to it.

Sensitization is essentially the opposite of habituation. If a particularly harmful or noxious stimulus is received, this can cause the animal to be more, rather than less, receptive to subsequent stimuli. In the case of the sea slug, for example, delivering a painful shock to the tail causes the gill-siphon withdrawal reflex to occur with a lighter touch than normal. It is as if the animal senses that it is in danger so that the slightest disturbance in its surroundings will cause it to withdraw its gill and siphon for safety.

You may have experienced a similar feeling if you have ever been in a situation that you perceive as dangerous. Many people report 'heightened senses' in such situations.

The effects of habituation and sensitization can last for days or even weeks, so that some form of long-term alteration seems to have been made in the neural system. Experiments on the cellular and molecular level have discovered the apparent biochemical sequence of events that causes these phenomena.

Consider habituation first. Recall from Chapter 15 that, when an action potential reaches the synapse at the end of the axon, it causes some calcium channels to open in the presynaptic membrane, allowing calcium ions to come into the cell. These ions start a chain of events leading to the release of transmitter molecules into the synaptic cleft. If some way could be found to reduce the amount of calcium entering the cell, this would reduce the amount of transmitter released which, in turn, would reduce the effect on the postsynaptic membrane. If this reduction proceeded far enough, the postsynaptic cell would no longer receive enough transmitter to depolarize the membrane far enough to produce an action potential. The signal carried by the sensory neuron would not propagate any further, so that the stimulus that caused the action potential in the sensory neuron would never be registered. Repeated action potentials from a neutral stimulus seem to cause many of the calcium channels in the presynaptic membrane to close so that the postsynaptic signal gets weaker and the neural network becomes habituated to the stimulus. Fig. 16.1 illustrates the process in the marine snail *Aplysia*.

Sensitization is a bit more complicated. In the case of *Aplysia*, for example, a shock to the tail can cause sensitization of the gill–siphon system (see Fig. 16.2). The sensory signal from the tail connects to the sensory signal from the siphon through other neurons, called *facilitatory interneurons*. These interneurons make synapses with the incoming signals from the siphon right at the presynaptic membrane—this is a so-called axo-axonic synapse, since one axon makes a synapse directly on another axon, rather than on a dendrite or cell body, as is more usual. The interneurons use special transmitter substances to affect the events in the presynaptic terminal of the sensory cell. Recall that an action potential is initiated by the opening of sodium channels and stopped by the subsequent opening of potassium channels which repolarize the membrane. In the presynaptic terminal, the repolarization of the membrane also closes the calcium channels which, in turn, shuts down the release of transmitter into the synaptic cleft. The facilitatory interneurons, through an involved sequence of steps, delay the opening of the potassium channels in the presynaptic membrane of the sensory axon, which means that the calcium channels remain open longer, thus releasing more transmitter and enhancing the signal delivered to the postsynaptic membrane.

These studies show that habituation and sensitization involve changing the connection strength between two neurons. In both cases the sensory

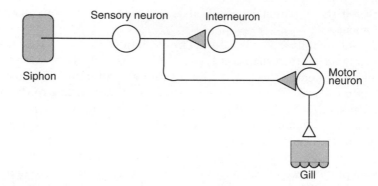

Figure 16.1   Habituation in *Aplysia*. Stimulating the siphon excites the sensory neuron which in turn stimulates the motor neuron in the gill, both directly and via the interneuron. Repeated stimulation of the siphon causes less transmitter to be released from the shaded synapses, reducing the stimulation of the gill.

neuron delivers the same magnitude of signal to its presynaptic terminal, but experience has modified the way this signal is handled. In habituation, the signal is attenuated, while in sensitization it is enhanced. In the terminology that will be used frequently in the following chapters, we say that the *synaptic weight* between the two neurons has been changed.

The experiments on habituation and sensitization confirm a hypothesis made in 1949 by Donald Hebb in his book *The Organization of Behavior* in which he proposed that memory is stored in the brain, not by altering the states of neurons, but by changing the strengths of the connections between them. This hypothesis has been at the heart of virtually every theoretical neural network model of memory that has been constructed.

16.3   Conditioning and associative learning

Habituation and sensitization may be classified as *non-associative learning* since they require a response to only a single stimulus. Of more interest to network modellers is *associative learning* in which the relation between two (or more) stimuli is learned. In psychology, this phenomenon has been known as *classical conditioning*, and has become famous through the nineteenth-century experiments of Pavlov.

Although 'Pavlov's dog' has become a cliché these days, the experiment itself is a good example of associative learning. A hungry dog is trained

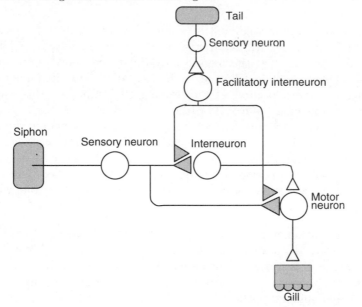

Figure 16.2 Sensitization in *Aplysia*. Delivering a shock to the tail causes the facilitatory interneuron to influence the shaded synapses in a way that prolongs the stimulation of the gill so that the siphon–gill pathway is sensitized.

by the experimenter ringing a bell shortly before each time that food is provided. After several training sessions, the dog associates the sound of the bell with the appearance of food, so that whenever the bell is rung the dog begins to salivate even before any food is given to it. This represents a change in the behaviour pattern of the dog, since before the experiment, the sound of the bell would have no effect on the dog.

Classical conditioning is used or experienced frequently by humans. Many language learning methods are based on associative learning: the student is given lists of foreign words with their English equivalents and made to study the lists over and over again until the mention of the foreign word elicits the corresponding English word as a response (or vice versa). Advertising companies are well aware of classical conditioning. Most advertisements in the media contain music or images that have no explicit relation to the product being sold, but these sounds or images become linked with the product in the mind of the potential customer. If the images are pleasurable, it is hoped that this will enhance the product in the mind of the viewer.

Returning to the sea slug, we find that it can be conditioned as well. In addition to the gill and siphon, an *Aplysia* has another structure called the mantle. Touching the mantle will cause the gill and siphon to be withdrawn as well. Under ordinary circumstances, if the mantle is repeatedly touched, the withdrawal reflex will habituate, just as with touching the siphon. To condition the sea slug, the mantle is touched and shortly afterwards, a painful electric shock is delivered to the tail. When the siphon is touched, however, no shock occurs. After training the animal in this way, it is found that touching the mantle without delivering any shock to the tail is much more likely to cause the gill to withdraw than touching the siphon. The training can be reversed so that the tail shock follows touching the siphon and no shock follows touching the mantle. In this case, the *Aplysia* is conditioned to expect a shock after its siphon is touched, and is much more likely to withdraw the gill when the siphon is touched than when the mantle is touched.

This conditioning only works in one direction. That is, if the tail shock is given *before* the stimulus to the mantle or siphon, no relation between the two stimuli is learned. The animal is only capable of learning that an otherwise innocuous event (touching its siphon or mantle) means that a potentially dangerous event (the tail shock) is about to occur, and not the other way around.

A model has been proposed to explain classical conditioning, including the temporal dependence of the two events (Fig. 16.3). The model is a more involved version of that for sensitization. In the case of *Aplysia* conditioned to expect a shock in the tail after its mantle is touched, but not after the siphon is touched, the synapses from the mantle to the motor neurons causing the gill to retract have fired just before the shock is delivered to the tail. This results in the sensitization caused by the tail shock to be enhanced. The molecular mechanism responsible begins with extra calcium channels being opened by the initial touch to the mantle. The impulse arriving from the tail shock combined with the influx of calcium ions triggers a cascade of interactions involving several proteins and other molecules which ultimately results in the potassium channels remaining open longer, causing more transmitter to be released to the postsynaptic neuron. Although the details of the model differ from that proposed for sensitization, both models require a change in the synaptic weights in the network.

Classical conditioning has also been induced in the fruit fly *Drosophila*. Flies were given the choice of two pleasurable (to the flies) aromas. Flies that chose one aroma encountered an electric shock, while flies that chose the other aroma encountered no harmful effect. After a training session, it was found that flies given a choice of the two aromas usually chose the one for which no shock was given during training—the flies had learned that one aroma led to a dangerous situation and therefore avoided it.

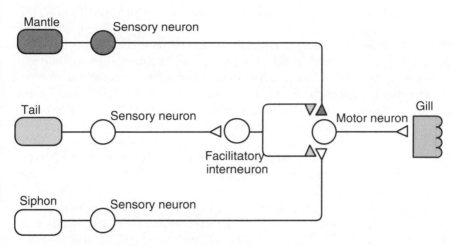

Figure 16.3   Conditioning in *Aplysia*. The animal is trained to expect a tail shock after a touch to its mantle, but not after a touch to its siphon. The synaptic weight at the shaded synapse is increased.

16.4   Long-term memory

The examples of biological memory given above are capable of inducing changing in the synaptic weights that last for several days or in some cases, weeks. However, many memories will persist for much longer than this; in some cases, many decades.

The mechanisms given above to explain habituation, sensitization, and conditioning cannot give rise, on their own, to long-term memory. All of these mechanisms require changes in the structure of proteins caused by varying concentrations of ions (usually calcium). Despite the complexity of the molecules involved, these interactions are nothing more than reversible chemical reactions, so that the changes induced in protein structure are not permanent. As well, the protein molecules themselves have limited lifetimes, which are rarely longer than a few weeks.

One mechanism postulated to explain long-term memory is that of regenerative molecular cascades. An idea along these lines was proposed by Francis Crick (1984). Suppose there is a protein X which consists of two subunits X_1 and X_2, each of which can exist in either an unmodified form or a modified form. The protein X can act to enhance a synaptic weight only if both its subunits are modified. A learning session will, through mechanisms similar to those discussed in the preceding section, modify molecules of X so that a short-term memory is activated. Because the modification of the subunits of X is reversible, some of these units will, in time, revert to their unmodified state. If this were allowed to continue, the synaptic weight would gradually decay and the memory would be lost. However, the existence of another protein Y is assumed which can modify one subunit of X only if the other subunit is already in the modified state. Thus the protein Y can maintain a memory if one exists but, since it cannot change a totally unmodified X molecule, it cannot generate memories on its own.

This model suffers from two drawbacks. The first is that there is no experimental evidence that such a mechanism exists, although this could be only temporary, of course. The second objection is that the regenerative cascade will prolong memory only as long as there are some partially modified X molecules around. Since all proteins have a limited lifespan, eventually all the X molecules will decay and, despite the efforts of Y, the memory will be lost.

Another model for long-term memory which has received much more attention is that of alteration in genome expression. Here, the idea is that the acquisition of a short-term memory triggers changes in the way in which the neuron's DNA is expressed, so that new proteins, or at least differing combinations of existing proteins, are synthesized.

There has been experimental evidence since the 1960s that drugs taken during a training session could block the acquisition of long-term memory without affecting short-term memory. Since that time, it has been discovered that these drugs specifically inhibited protein synthesis in general, so it appears that some sort of gene expression is necessary for a short-term memory to be converted into a long-term memory. It is still not clear which genes are involved, or exactly what is happening as a result of this protein synthesis.

Finally, there is some evidence that the structure of a neuron itself can be changed in a learning session. For example, many dendrites have small knob-like protrusions called *spines*, which are favoured as sites for synapses. Changes in the size and shape of spines have been observed after learning.

The architecture of an entire network can change as well. If the nerve to some part of the body is severed, that part of the brain which used to control that part will often turn its attention to controlling neighbouring parts of the body. For example, if a nerve to one of the fingers is severed, the brain region formerly in control of that finger starts to control the other fingers on the same hand, indicating that new connections between existing neurons have been formed (or at least strengthened).

16.5 Models of memory

The lack of an overall experimental view of the function of memory means that theoretical models have, at the moment, very few constraints. The main features of biological memory on which there is more or less universal agreement are as follows:

1. Memory is distributed over large groups of neurons—it is not stored at particular sites like a computer memory.

2. The acquisition of a memory involves changes the strengths of contacts (the synaptic weights) between neurons.

3. Presentation of part of a pattern that has been stored can result in the reconstruction of the remainder of the pattern, or the generation of a memorized response to that pattern.

Most theoretical models of memory tend to ignore the finer details of the biochemical changes in neurons. In many models, a neuron is considered to be a 'black box' which performs the task of summing up its inputs and producing an output (action potential) if this sum exceeds a certain value (the threshold). The biological details of the summation and resultant firing are ignored.

Other models attempt to incorporate more biological detail by, for example, using the cable equation (described in Chapter 15) to calculate the propagation of impulses from the synapse on a dendrite to the rest of the neuron and perform the summation explicitly.

A general rule in neural network modelling is that the more realistic you make the neurons, the smaller the network which you can model. This is due to limits on computer memory and computing time. A simulation involving explicit calculation of the membrane potentials involves numerical procedures for solving the cable equation, or its discretized form used in models where the neurons is broken up into compartments. The space and time required to process any model containing more than a few thousand such neurons is prohibitive. Even networks consisting of simpler neurons can take large amounts of time to train.

We shall begin our study of neural network models in the next chapter by examining the early model of McCulloch and Pitts. Although this model is not really a model of memory, its effect on all subsequent neural modelling has been so profound that no survey would be complete without considering it. The McCulloch–Pitts model assumes simple, point-like neurons that sum their inputs and fire if their threshold is exceeded. The model is important because it demonstrates that networks of such simple components can compute virtually any logical function. Since the ability to reason is based ultimately upon making simple binary decisions, the McCulloch–Pitts model lays the groundwork for a theory of the brain.

The McCulloch–Pitts network cannot learn to recognize patterns without actually changing either the number of neurons in the network or the connections between them. No allowance is made for plasticity, that is, the ability to modify the strength of an interaction between two neurons. Although this idea was suggested by Donald Hebb in 1949, one of the first quantitative treatments of variable synaptic weights was the perceptron theory of Rosenblatt and, following on from Rosenblatt's work, the work of Minsky and Papert in the 1960s. We will examine some of the predictions of perceptron theory. In particular, we will see one of the first networks with variable synaptic weights that can actually learn to recognize various patterns.

Although perceptrons looked promising as models for the brain, Minsky and Papert showed that many relatively simple patterns could not be learned easily, if at all, by a perceptron, no matter how large it is or how long it is trained. This dampened interest in network models for several years, but with the emergence of new network architectures (and faster computers), the subject enjoyed a renaissance in the 1970s and 1980s. The general area of neural network theory involving nets of simple point neurons connected together with variable-strength synapses has been dubbed *connectionism*. A few of the methods and results of connectionist theory will be described in Chapter 19. The issue of the relevance of such models to biological brains has been, to a certain extent, forgotten in the excitement over connectionism, because such networks have proven very useful when applied to computer science. Artificial neural networks applied to computer circuitry have allowed the development of 'intelligent' robots that can recognize objects, navigate their way through mazes, read printed text or handwriting, and so on. Although many of these tasks are also activities that real animals can learn, it is still uncertain how closely the neural circuits used in human brains parallel those used in computers. Still, it is tempting to think that, because the inspiration for these new computers came originally from biology, there must be some similarity in the methods that the two systems use.

Following our excursion into connectionism, we examine a model that is based on the same idea we saw used in modelling the origin of life: spin glasses. The motivation for such a model is similar to that encountered in the origin of life problem: we have a collection of interacting units (individual nucleotides from RNA or DNA in one case, neurons in the other) in which we wish to store a large number of stable patterns (stable RNA sequences in one case, memories in the other). We know that a spin glass has numerous stable minima in its energy function for any given set of interactions between its units. A spin glass memory, then, works by choosing the interactions between neurons (the synaptic weights) in such a way that the desired stable patterns (memories) can be stored.

Despite being an elegant idea, the spin glass brain, if we may call it that, suffers from the same lack of biological realism as most other network models. However, in the absence of experimental data, it is best to consider as many options as we can, and the spin glass model is a strong contender, since it reproduces many of the features of biological memory with which other models have difficulties.

We shall return, after this, to examine another model from connectionist camp: unsupervised learning. All the models treated prior to this chapter have had a teacher: some external guide that instructs the network as to its proper response to each input pattern. The nets in these supervised scenarios learn by comparing their output to the desired output and correcting their synaptic weights accordingly. However, animals frequently must discover features of the world for themselves, without being taught. The competitive learning algorithm provides a method by which a network can learn to classify various inputs into several categories, based on common features it detects. Again, the obvious practical applications of such networks in the computer industry have overshadowed their biological value to a certain extent, but the models do mimic many of the processes involved in discovering the world for yourself.

Our final model invokes the theory of evolution. Some of the ideas from Darwin's theory of evolution are applied to neural networks in an attempt to introduce some of the internal structure of neurons into a model. The brain is envisioned as a collection of nearly identical subnetworks, each of which has a certain ability to recognize a pattern or perform a function. Those networks that perform best are selected and propagate their structures to other, less 'fit' networks, thus gradually improving the ability of the brain as a whole to perform certain tasks. Although the model makes use of much of the current neurophysiological data, there are several assumptions made that have, as yet, no experimental foundation.

The reader may be worried by the fact that none of the models presented in this section are truly biological. Every one of them makes some assumptions that are almost certainly not to be found in a real brain. However, the value in considering such models, indeed in model building in general, is to discover what is needed to obtain certain behaviour from a system constructed out of elements that conform, as far as possible, to those features of real neural networks that are universally acknowledged. Although it is unlikely that any of the models considered here will turn out to be *the* model of human and animal memory, it is to be hoped that by studying them we will gain some insight into what features a correct model will ultimately have.

17

The McCulloch–Pitts neural net

17.1 Introduction

One of the earliest purely theoretical treatments of a neural network was
that of Warren McCulloch and Walter Pitts (1943). The original paper
is quite forbidding to the modern reader, since it uses the terminology of
formal logic, something which is not often taught in undergraduate courses,
even those in mathematics. Despite the abstract notation, however, the
basic ideas in McCulloch and Pitts' paper are quite simple. Considering the
state of the art when the paper was published (long before the widespread
use of computers to which we have become accustomed) its ideas are ahead
of its time, and the paper deserves its reputation as one of the classic papers
of theoretical biology.[1]

The McCulloch–Pitts (MP) neuron does not attempt to model accurately the biological details of real neurons. Rather, it concentrates on a
few of the fundamental properties of neurons and sets out to show that,
using these properties, it is possible to construct a neural net that can perform essentially any logical function. Unlike later models of neural systems,
the MP neural net cannot learn; indeed the neurons and their interconnec-
tions are assumed to be unchangeable. The goal of MP theory is not to
explain how learning occurs. To quote from the original paper:

> ...for nets undergoing [learning], we can substitute equivalent
> fictitious nets composed of neurons whose connections and thresh-
> olds are unaltered. But one point must be made clear: neither
> of us conceives the formal equivalence to be a factual expla-
> nation. *Per contra!*—we regard ... learning as an enduring
> change which can survive sleep, anaesthesia, convulsions and
> coma. The importance of the formal equivalence lies in this:

---

[1] For those who cannot locate the original 1943 reference, the paper has been reprinted
in McCulloch and Pitts (1990). Regrettably, the reprint suffers from a large number
of typographical errors not present in the original. These errors occur mainly in the
mathematical notation, which makes an already abstract paper even more difficult to
read.

that the alterations actually underlying facilitation, extinction and learning in no way affect the conclusions which follow from the formal treatment of the activity of nervous nets, and the relations of the corresponding propositions remain those of the logic of propositions.

In other words, it is important to show that a neural network can be constructed to respond correctly to a stimulus before looking for a mechanism by which the net might learn the response pattern.

17.2 Logic

Although we do not wish to get too deeply into the theory of logical calculus[2], a few of the basic terms will make MP nets easier to understand. These terms should be familiar already to anyone who has studied introductory computer science.

Logic concerns *statements* which have certain *values*. The logic used by MP is *two-valued logic*, meaning that a statement can take on only one of two values, usually *true* or *false*. Other forms of logic allow more values, but we will not be concerned with those forms here.

Statements can be combined with several *operators* to produce compound statements. The operators are those common from computer terminology: *not, and, or, equals*. These operators are either *binary* operators (that is, they take two operands) or *unary* operators (which take one operand).

The definitions of the operators are as follows:

NOT The NOT operator is a unary operator which reverses the value of its operand. Thus NOT(TRUE) = FALSE and NOT(FALSE) = TRUE.

AND AND is a binary operator which is true only if both its operands are true. Thus (TRUE) AND (TRUE) = TRUE; (FALSE) AND (TRUE) = FALSE, and so on.

OR OR is a binary operator which is true if either of its operands is true.

EQUALS EQUALS is a binary operator which is true if both of its operands have the same value. Note that the logical statement (EXPRESSION 1) EQUALS (EXPRESSION 2) is not the same type of

---

[2]Bertrand Russell once commented that, after writing the three volumes of the *Principia Mathematica* (with Whitehead), in which mathematics is given a rigorous foundation in logic, his mind had, in effect, burned out. We would not wish such a fate on any reader of this book!

statement as the algebraic assignment 'Let $x = 6$.' The equals operator in the first case does not alter either of its operands—it is a comparison operator. The expression 'Let $x = 6$' assigns the value 6 to the variable x, thus possibly changing the value of x. This distinction is well known to computer programmers as all computer languages use different symbols for the two operators. In Pascal, for example, the assignment operator is := while the equality test is just =. The first operator is used to assign values to variables while the second operator is used in 'if' statements to test if two variables or expressions have the same value.

The effects of these operators are often represented in a *truth table*:

Op 1	Op 2	NOT (Op 1)	(Op 1) AND (Op 2)
TRUE	TRUE	FALSE	TRUE
FALSE	TRUE	TRUE	FALSE
TRUE	FALSE	FALSE	FALSE
FALSE	FALSE	TRUE	FALSE

Op 1	Op 2	(Op 1) OR (Op 2)	(Op 1) EQUALS (Op 2)
TRUE	TRUE	TRUE	TRUE
FALSE	TRUE	TRUE	FALSE
TRUE	FALSE	TRUE	FALSE
FALSE	FALSE	FALSE	TRUE

To save writing, operands are usually represented by single letters, such as X and Y, and the two values are usually represented by the assignments TRUE = 1 and FALSE = 0. The truth table above can be rewritten using this notation:

X	Y	NOT X	X AND Y	X OR Y	X EQUALS Y
1	1	0	1	1	1
0	1	1	0	1	0
1	0	0	0	1	0
0	0	1	0	0	1

In addition, there is another logical operator commonly used: the IMPLIES operator. This is also a binary operator, although its operands are usually a bit more complex than those of the operators just mentioned. An example of IMPLIES would be the statement: ((X EQUALS Y) AND (Y EQUALS Z)) IMPLIES (X EQUALS Z) Although this statement may read like an English sentence, it may be interpreted in several ways. One way is just to read it as it stands. In that case it is a true statement. Algebraically, it states that if $x = y$ and $y = z$ then we must have $x = z$, which is true. However, remember that the left-hand operand of IMPLIES, namely ((X EQUALS Y) AND (Y EQUALS Z)), is a logical statement, and may be TRUE or FALSE. In particular, if (X EQUALS Y) is TRUE and (Y EQUALS Z) is FALSE, then ((X EQUALS Y) AND (Y EQUALS Z)) is FALSE. The implication may then be drawn that the right-hand operand is FALSE as well, that is, that (X EQUALS Z) is FALSE. Relations such as this are used in certain artificial intelligence languages (such as PRO-LOG) to allow computers to make inferences from a database of facts and relations among them.

Compound statements formed by applying operators to simple statements can also be either true or false. The value of a compound statement depends on the values of the statements of which it is composed and the operators used to combine them.

For example, a few statements in English are:

1. The Earth is flat. (False)

2. Dundee is in Scotland. (True)

3. Beethoven composed nine symphonies. (True)

Compound statements consisting of the above statements combined by operators are:

1. (The Earth is flat) AND (Dundee is in Scotland)

2. (NOT (The Earth is flat)) AND (Beethoven composed 9 symphonies)

3. (The Earth is flat) OR (Dundee is in Scotland)

The first of these compound statements is false, because the AND operator requires both of its operands to be true in order for the compound statement to be true. The second compound statement is true, since NOT turns a false statement into a true one (and vice versa), so both operands of the AND are now true. The last statement is true, since the OR operator requires only one of its operands to be true in order for the compound statement to be true.

Any compound statement, no matter how complex, that contains only these operators can be evaluated by applying the rules in this table. For example, the statement (A OR ((B AND (NOT C)) OR (A EQUALS (B OR C)))) in the case when A = 0, B = 1, C = 0 can be evaluated by working from the innermost brackets to the outermost:

1. (0 OR ((1 AND (NOT 0)) OR (0 EQUALS (1 OR 0))))

2. (0 OR ((1 AND 1) OR (0 EQUALS 1)))

3. (0 OR (1 OR 0))

4. (0 OR 1)

5. (1)

Thus the compound statement is true.

17.3   Constructing neural nets

The neuron envisaged by McCulloch and Pitts is a simple device to which may be connected any number of excitatory synapses, but only one inhibitory synapse. Each excitatory synapse delivers a unit impulse to the neuron. If the neuron receives a number of excitatory impulses greater than or equal to its *threshold* θ, the neuron will fire. In the simplest version of the model, an inhibitory impulse completely neutralizes all excitatory impulses received at the same time. However, McCulloch and Pitts show that even if this assumption is relaxed so that an inhibitory impulse merely raises the threshold of the neuron rather than shutting it down completely, their results still hold.

Signals are provided to the network by a layer of input neurons. These neurons receive no input from any other neurons in the network, but are assumed to be externally stimulated, rather like our brains are provided with input by impulses provided by our five senses. These input signals are then processed by the internal neurons of the net until one or more output signals are generated. The main idea of McCulloch and Pitts' paper is to show that a net can be constructed which will calculate virtually any logical function composed of the operators defined in the last section.

The MP network is a *synchronous network*, which means that each neuron may only fire at regular discrete time intervals. A neuron that fires at time t, where t is an integer, transmits an impulse down its axon and all its branches. This impulse is received by all neurons on which the axon makes synapses. Each neuron then sums its inputs, checks to see if an inhibitory impulse has been received and, if the sum equals or exceeds the threshold and no inhibition has been received, fires at the next time interval, $t + 1$.

MP networks deal with particular types of logical expressions called *temporal propositional expressions* or TPEs. For the most part, a TPE is a logical statement composed of elementary logical statements combined by one of the operators listed in the last section. However, there is one other logical operation we must consider before we can define a TPE properly.

Remember that an MP network is synchronous, so that at each time t each neuron in the network has a definite state which we can call $N_i(t)$.

Here the subscript i refers to the neuron, so that if the net contains n neurons, $i = 1, \ldots, n$. Since each neuron is either firing or not firing, $N_i(t)$ is a binary function, with values of either 0 or 1. Starting at $t = 0$, we can describe the entire life history of neuron i by listing its values of $N_i(t)$ for $t = 0, 1, 2, \ldots$. In particular, if we know the state of the neuron at time t, we can define a unary logical operator PREV which, when applied to $N_i(t)$, gives $N_i(t-1)$, the state of the neuron at the previous time step:

$$\text{PREV } (N_i(t)) = N_i(t-1). \tag{17.1}$$

Note that this is a genuine logical operator, since it has only two possible values; TRUE or 1 if the neuron was firing at time $t-1$ and FALSE or 0 if it was not.

We may now define a TPE. In general a TPE is defined recursively by the statements:

1. An elementary logical statement S is a TPE. In the context of the MP neural net, an elementary logical statement would be the state of a neuron at a particular time, that is, $N_i(t)$.

2. If S_1 and S_2 are TPEs with the same time argument (that is, they represent states of neurons at the same time step), then any of the following statements are also TPEs: PREV S_1; S_1 AND S_2; S_1 OR S_2, and S_1 AND (NOT S_2). No other combinations of TPEs are allowed.

It should be noted that each of the operations defined in the second part of the definition of a TPE imply a forward step in time. This is because the implementation of each of these operations in a neural net involves combining the outputs of two neurons into a single value, which can be done only by passing these outputs through some sort of processor, which, in a neural net, must be another neuron. Introducing another neuron means advancing one time step. The examples below will clarify this point.

McCulloch and Pitts show the following three results in their paper:

1. Every network composed of MP neurons can be expressed as a TPE, provided that this network does not have any circular paths in it. A circular path in a neural net is a chain of neurons connected together by synapses in such a way that if you start at any one of the neurons in the chain and follow the synapses from each neuron to the next, you will eventually arrive back at the neuron from which you started. Beginning at neuron A, you may trace a path such as $A \to B \to C \to D \to A$.

2. It is possible to construct a network without circular paths which will calculate any TPE.

3. Any logical statement S constructed of elementary statements $N_i(t - k)$ (where k is an integer) by means of the operators NOT, AND, OR, EQUALS, and IMPLIES is a TPE if and only if the expression is FALSE or 0 when all the elementary statements $N_i(t-k)$ are FALSE or 0.

To examine these statements in more depth, it will be helpful if we consider some specific networks. We will assume that each neuron has a threshold of 2 units, so that two or more excitatory inputs (and, of course, no inhibitory input) are required for a neuron to fire.

Let us begin by seeing how the basic logical operators can be represented as neural networks.

The AND operator is shown in Fig. 17.1. The two input neurons are shown on the left. Each of these neurons makes a single excitatory synapse onto the third neuron, whose output produces the output of the net. Since the threshold of the third neuron is 2, it will only fire if both input neurons fire, so that the output of neuron 3 is the AND of the outputs of neurons 1 and 2.

Note however, that this network takes one time step to produce its output, so that the output of neuron 3 at time t, that is, $N_3(t)$ is actually the AND of the outputs of neurons 1 and 2 at time $t - 1$, so that

$$N_3(t) = N_1(t - 1) \text{ AND } N_2(t - 1). \qquad (17.2)$$

We can write this using the PREV operator:

$$N_3(t) = (\text{ PREV } N_1(t)) \text{ AND } (\text{ PREV } N_2(t)) \qquad (17.3)$$

or equivalently as:

$$N_3(t) = \text{ PREV } (N_1(t)) \text{ AND } N_2(t)). \qquad (17.4)$$

Since we have written an expression for the net entirely in terms of the operators allowed in the definition of a TPE, we see that this net can indeed be represented by a TPE.

The net shown in Fig. 17.2 implements the OR operator. Since the threshold of neuron 3 is two inputs, it will fire if either neuron 1 or neuron 2 is active, in which case neuron 3 will receive exactly two excitatory impulses, or if both neurons 1 and 2 are active, in which case neuron 3 will receive four inputs. In terms of the basic logical operations this net can be written

$$N_3(t) = \text{ PREV } (N_1(t)) \text{ OR } N_2(t)). \qquad (17.5)$$

The PREV operator on its own can be represented by the net shown in Fig. 17.3. Since neuron 1 makes two excitatory contacts with neuron

2, the state of neuron 2 at time t will be exactly the same as the state of neuron 1 at time $t - 1$, so that this net represents the TPE

$$N_2(t) = \text{PREV } N_1(t). \tag{17.6}$$

The final operation allowed in a TPE is the AND NOT operator. The net shown in figure 17.4 implements the TPE

$$N_3(t) = \text{PREV } (N_1(t) \text{ AND NOT } N_2(t)). \tag{17.7}$$

Neuron 3 will never fire if neuron 2 has fired, since neuron 2 inhibits neuron 3 and if any inhibition is received by a neuron all excitatory input is cancelled. Thus neuron 3 will only fire if neuron 1 fires and neuron 2 does not.

With these preliminary examples behind us, we can return to a more general examination of the three properties of MP nets given above.

To demonstrate the first claim, we observe that the state of any neuron in the net at time t (except for one of the input neurons) is determined by the state of the other neurons in the net at time $t - 1$. Therefore we can write, for any neuron i:

$$N_i(t) = \text{PREV } \{\text{State of net at time } t\}. \tag{17.8}$$

Now in order for neuron i to fire at time t, it must receive a number of excitatory inputs equal to or greater than its threshold θ_i, and no inhibitory inputs. Consider how we can ensure that enough excitatory inputs are received. Any given neuron i may receive varying numbers of synapses from any or all of the other neurons in the net. In the examples given above, the net implementing the AND operator receives only a single input from each of two neurons, while in the net representing the OR operator, each input neuron sends two inputs into the output neuron. In the general case, we can make a list of all possible combinations of inputs into neuron i that will cause it to fire. For the AND net, there is only one such combination: both neurons 1 and 2 must fire. For the OR net, there are three combinations: neuron 1 alone, neuron 2 alone or both neurons 1 and 2. If any one of these combinations is realized, neuron 3 will fire.

Having made our list of acceptable combinations, we can write a logical statement indicating that neuron i will fire if combination 1 is realized OR if combination 2 is realized OR ....

Each of these combinations is a requirement that a certain set of neurons must fire. As a logical statement, this can be written 'for all neurons N_j in the combination, where j is a member of the set C of neuron indices representing those neurons in the combination, we must have $N_{j1}(t)$ AND $N_{j2}(t)$ AND ... AND N_{jn}, where the subscripts run through

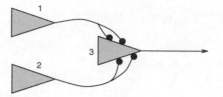

Figure 17.1   The AND operator. $N_3(t) = N_1(t-1)$ AND $N_2(t-1)$.

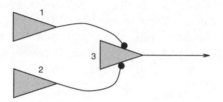

Figure 17.2   The OR operator. $N_3(t) = N_1(t-1)$ OR $N_2(t-1)$.

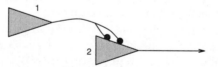

Figure 17.3   The PREV operator. $N_2(t) = N_1(t-1)$.

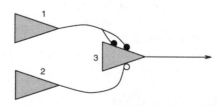

Figure 17.4   The AND NOT operator. $N_3(t) = N_1(t-1)$ AND NOT $N_2(t-1)$. The filled circles are excitatory synapses and the open circle is an inhibitory synapse.

all the neurons in the combination. This is just a fancy way of saying that all neurons in the particular combination must fire. We have written it this way because we need to show that the condition can be written using elementary logical operators.

To include the condition that no inhibitory input be received, we make another list of all neurons that have inhibitory synapses with the target neuron i. Since we require that none of these inputs be active, we have the logical condition (NOT input 1) AND (NOT input 2) AND .... Each of these inputs is given by the state of the neuron from which the signal comes so that each input can be written as $N_j(t)$, where neuron j is one of the neurons that makes an inhibitory synapse onto neuron i.

In order for neuron i to fire, we must ensure that both conditions above are met: sufficient excitatory input and no inhibitory input. Thus we take the AND of these two conditions. Overall, we have

$$N_i(t) = \text{PREV} \{\text{Sufficient excitatory input} \;\; \text{AND} \;\; \text{No inhibitory input}\}.$$
(17.9)

In general, the various neuron states that appear in this expression will be a mixture of the states of some of the input neurons (which have no predecessors) and of other, internal neurons in the net. Each of these internal neurons has a state that is, in turn, determined by the state of the net at the previous time step. However, since we have assumed that the net contains no circular or cyclic paths, if we trace the history of the net back far enough we must eventually come to a time when the only signals in the net are those of the input neurons. By replacing each internal neuron state in eqn (17.9) by an expression in terms of the previous time step, we can ultimately produce an expression for $N_i(t)$ that is entirely in terms of the states of the input neurons at some earlier time. Since all the operations we have used in doing this are acceptable operations according to the definition of a TPE, any network without circular paths can be expressed as a TPE.

The second claim, that any TPE can be represented as a neural network, should be fairly obvious since we have shown how to represent all the basic TPE operations in network form above. Any more complex TPE must be built up recursively of simpler TPEs, since by the definition of a TPE this is the only way a TPE can be formed. Ultimately, any TPE must be reducible to components consisting solely of the simplest operations.

This technique of successive reduction of a TPE is the best way to construct a net that will calculate any TPE. As an example, suppose we want to build a net that will compute the following TPE:

$$N_4(t) = (N_1(t-1) \text{ AND } (N_2(t-2) \text{ OR } N_3(t-2))) \text{ AND } (\text{ NOT } N_1(t-2)).$$
(17.10)

The best way to begin is to eliminate the time delays by using the PREV operator. We get

$$N_4(t) \quad = \quad \text{PREV } (N_1(t) \text{ AND PREV } (N_2(t) \text{ OR } N_3(t))$$
$$\text{AND NOT (PREV } N_1(t))). \tag{17.11}$$

Now we have reduced the expression to a combination of the elementary operations for which we already have networks written down. We start at the innermost network and work our way outwards. The innermost block is PREV $(N_2(t) \text{ OR } N_3(t))$. Since the result of this calculation does not synapse directly on the output neuron, we must introduce an intermediate neuron, say neuron 5, to compute the result. The first part of the network looks as shown in Fig. 17.5.

Now the output from neuron 5 must be combined with the output of neuron 1 to produce the left-hand operand of the final AND, that is, we must compute PREV $(N_1(t) \text{ AND } N_5(t))$. We can use the standard network for the AND operator given above to obtain the next stage of the network, in Fig. 17.6. Again, this requires the introduction of an intermediate neuron, neuron 6.

Now we deal with the right-hand operand of the final AND, namely NOT PREV $N_1(t)$. The innermost object here is PREV $N_1(t)$, for which we have a network ready. Adding this to the already formed network involves creating another intermediate neuron, neuron 7 (Fig. 17.7).

Finally, we can combine the outputs of neurons 6 and 7 using the AND NOT network model to obtain the complete network (Fig. 17.8).

The third claim above gives a set of rules by which you can determine if a logical expression is a TPE and, therefore, whether it can be evaluated by an MP neural net. Probably the most useful condition to check is whether, if no input neurons are firing, the expected output is zero. The simplest example of a logical expression that is not a TPE is $N_2(t) = \text{NOT } N_1(t-1)$. In this case, if neuron 1 is quiescent, the expected output is that neuron 2 should fire. This condition could only be achieved if neuron 2 had a threshold of zero, but even in this case the NOT function could not be realized, since neuron 2 would always be firing, regardless of its input.

17.3.1   Hot and cold receptors in the skin

The discussion up to now has been abstract in the extreme. To demonstrate that simple biological systems exist that can be explained using the MP model, there is an excellent example given by McCulloch and Pitts themselves in their original paper.

There is a simple experiment you can try for yourself that illustrates the system we are about to model. If you touch a cold object, such as an ice cube, very briefly and then remove it, you will experience a sensation

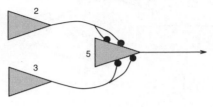

Figure 17.5

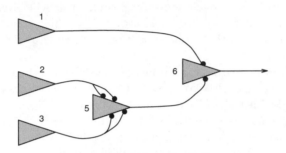

Figure 17.6

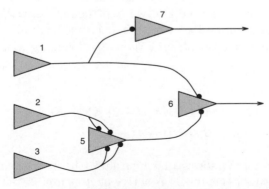

Figure 17.7

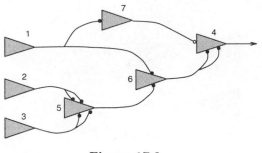

Figure 17.8

of heat rather than cold. You may have had this experience by accident when you unexpectedly touch something cold. You will often jerk your hand away as if it had been burnt. However, if you place your hand on a cold object and keep it there, the sensation you feel is undeniably one of cold with no hint of heat.

It is known from anatomical studies of the skin that there are different receptors for heat and cold. We may think of these receptors as the input neurons in an MP net. Let N_1 be a heat receptor and N_2 a cold receptor. Suppose further that we have two output neurons: N_3 and N_4. If N_3 fires, the network has concluded that heat is being felt, while if N_4 fires, the network believes it is in contact with something cold.

We require a network which will cause N_3 to fire if N_2 fires only briefly and then stops (corresponding to your brief contact with a cold object) or if N_1 fires (corresponding to a touch on a genuinely hot object), but will result in N_4 firing if N_2 fires continuously. We may formulate these requirements a bit more precisely if we assume that a 'brief' contact means that N_2 fires for only one time interval and then stops, while continuous contact results in N_2 firing for more than one time interval.

At first thought, you might write down the following equations for N_3 and N_4:

$$N_3(t) \;=\; N_1(t-1) \text{ OR } (N_2(t-2) \text{ AND NOT } N_2(t-1)) \quad (17.12)$$
$$N_4(t) \;=\; N_2(t-2) \text{ AND } N_2(t-1). \quad\quad\quad\quad\quad (17.13)$$

The equation for N_3 states that neuron 3 (the heat signal) will fire if either the heat sensor (neuron 1) is active or if neuron 2 (the cold sensor) fired two time intervals ago, but then immediately shut off. The equation for N_4 states that the cold signal will fire if the cold sensor is on for two time intervals in a row.

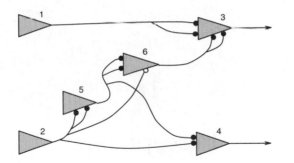

Figure 17.9   Network modelling hot and cold skin receptors. Filled circles are excitatory synapses, open circle is an inhibitory synapse.

So far, so good. But consider how the time intervals accumulate in the first expression. The signal from neuron 2 at time $t-2$ must be advanced by one time interval and combined with the signal at time $t-1$ using the AND NOT operator. However, the result of this operator must be advanced one time step since it requires an intermediate neuron to do the calculation. Thus we are already at time t and we have not yet included the signal from neuron 1 at time $t-1$. Thus we cannot produce a single result by time t as required. In order to correct this problem we must regress the times in the first expression by one interval to obtain:

$$N_3(t) \;=\; N_1(t-1) \text{ OR } (N_2(t-3) \text{ AND NOT } N_2(t-2)) \quad (17.14)$$
$$N_4(t) \;=\; N_2(t-2) \text{ AND } N_2(t-1). \quad\quad\quad\quad (17.15)$$

We may now construct a net that implements these equations. This may be done by the same step by step procedure as was used for the last example. We leave this as an exercise for the reader and present the finished network in Fig. 17.9.

17.4   Conclusion

The work of McCulloch and Pitts is a milestone in the theory of brain function, since it demonstrates that networks composed of simple binary threshold devices such as the basic neurons in their model are capable of calculating virtually any logical function. The ideas in the MP model, together with Hebb's 1949 hypothesis concerning the role of modification of synaptic weights in learning, have formed the foundations of virtually every neural network model since that time, as the models we examine in the next few chapters will demonstrate.

18

Perceptrons

18.1 Introduction

One of the more mathematically rigorous treatments of a neural network is that of Minsky and Papert, originally published in 1969, but republished with an epilogue in 1988. Minsky and Papert's theory deals with an object called a *perceptron* originally proposed by Rosenblatt (1962). On one level, perceptrons can be thought of as purely algebraic objects about which rigorous theorems can be stated and proved. Indeed, Minsky and Papert's book deals with perceptrons, for the most part, in this way. However, the properties of perceptrons make them relevant to the study of real neurons, at least on a simple level.

'Perceptrons', to quote Minsky and Papert, 'make decisions—determine whether or not an event fits a certain "pattern"—by adding up evidence obtained from many small experiments. This clear and simple concept is important because most, and perhaps all, more complicated machines for making decisions share a little of this character. Until we understand it very thoroughly, we can expect to have trouble with more advanced ideas.'

To get a feel for what a perceptron is before we plunge into a more detailed and quantitative explanation, envision a rectangular sheet of paper on the desk (or some convenient surface) in front of you. Suppose this paper has some figure or collection of figures drawn on it. Now, if someone else comes along and looks over your shoulder, he may ask you a question about the drawing on the paper, such as 'Is the drawing a single unbroken curve?' or 'Is that a picture of your mother?'. It is up to you to answer 'Yes' or 'No' to the question, that is, you are expected to produce only a binary reply. In this frivolous example, you are acting as a perceptron, since a perceptron is a device which, when asked a question about some input, is able to answer yes or no.

In the first part of this chapter, we will see how to construct perceptrons which are tailor-made to answer specific questions. However, it would be much more interesting and useful if we could start with some arbitrarily constructed perceptron and train it to give the correct answer to a specific question. We will see that the Perceptron Learning Theorem allows us to do just that.

18.2   Constructing a perceptron

A *perceptron* consists of three main parts (see Fig. 18.1):

1. An input field or *retina* R which will serve as the universal set. For a particular pattern on the retina a subset X of R will contains points that are 'on', with the remainder of the points in the retina being 'off'. For example, if the pattern is a horizontal line, the set X will contain those points defining the line. Points will have value 1 if they are 'on' and 0 if they are 'off'.

2. A set of functions $\phi_i(X)$ which receive inputs from some of the points on the retina. Each function is independent of all the others, both with respect to which points of R it samples and with respect to the calculation it performs on them. Each of these functions may be thought of as a neuron, since it receives input from many sources and produces a single output.

3. An integrating function Ω which receives input from all the ϕ_is and produces a single output, which we call $\psi(X)$. This final object ψ is the object of the whole calculation: the value of ψ determines if a certain condition is true or false.

Borrowing a bit of terminology from the theory of logic, we can call $\psi(X)$ a *predicate*, that is, a function with only two possible values, true or false, determined by the choice of X.

In summary, then, a perceptron is essentially a single-layer neural network designed to decide the truth or otherwise of a single question. This question must refer to some property of the set X of points chosen from the retina R.

The sorts of questions we have in mind are usually fairly simple geometric properties of X, such as: Is X a square? or Does X have an odd number of points? Saying that the geometric properties are simple, however, does not necessarily imply that the set of functions we need to define for calculating the predicate are easy to find.

How, in general, do we test a predicate? In keeping with the structure of a biological neuron, we define $\psi(X)$ to be a threshold function similar to that used in the McCulloch–Pitts model:

$$\psi(X) = 1 \text{ if and only if } \sum_{i=1}^{n} \alpha_i \phi_i(X) > \theta \tag{18.1}$$

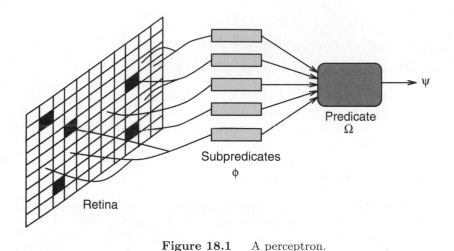

Figure 18.1   A perceptron.

where α_i are weights used to determine how important a particular function ϕ_i is to the predicate ψ and θ is the threshold level. For now, you can think of the α_is as constants, though as we will see later, it is possible to work out a scheme for modifying the weights which will allow the neural net to 'learn' to recognize patterns. This formula is just saying that the outputs from the n neurons making up the net are summed, with weighting factors, to produce a decision about whether a particular property is true or not.

Since we will be using the condition 'OneThing = 1 if and only if AnotherThing is true', it is convenient if we define a special notation for this condition. Writing

$$A = \lceil B \rceil \tag{18.2}$$

means '$A = 1$ if B is true and $A = 0$ otherwise'. Thus the definition of $\psi(X)$ above can be rewritten:

$$\psi(X) = \left\lceil \sum_{i=1}^{n} \alpha_i \phi_i(X) > \theta \right\rceil . \tag{18.3}$$

The functions $\phi_i(X)$ are predicates in their own right, which depend on the points x_j in the retina. Since the ϕ_is are used to make up a larger predicate ψ, we will call them *subpredicates*. As an example, one of the simplest subpredicates tests if a point x_i is in the set X, that is, whether $x_i = 1$:

$$\phi_i(X) = \lceil x_i = 1 \rceil. \tag{18.4}$$

Since x_i can have only the two values 0 and 1, this equation would usually be written in the simpler form

$$\phi_i(X) = x_i. \tag{18.5}$$

A set of these subpredicates covering all points in the retina R can be used to see if the total number of points in X, written $|X|$, is larger than some constant, say m. In this case the predicate $\psi(X)$ is true if the condition $|X| > m$ is true. Since[1] $\phi_i(X) = 1$ if $x_i \in X$ and zero if $x_i \notin X$, the number of elements in X is just the sum of the ϕ_is, so

$$\psi(X) = \left\lceil \sum_{i=1}^{N} \phi_i(X) > m \right\rceil. \tag{18.6}$$

In this case all the weights are 1 and $\theta = m$.

As you might guess from this example, the real challenge in constructing a perceptron to test a particular predicate ψ is to figure out how to express the subpredicates $\phi_i(X)$ in terms of the individual points x_i. The catch is that the final form for the predicate ψ *must* be in the form of a linear threshold function. In the previous example, this was fairly easy to do, but consider the (seemingly) almost identical problem of testing whether $|X| = m$. In principle, this is a trivial problem: all we have to do is count up the number of points in the retina that are 'on' and compare this with m. However, putting into linear threshold form is not quite so easy.

Before we see the solution to the problem of counting the number of elements in X, we need to introduce the concept of *order* of a perceptron. In the example above, we defined $\phi_i = x_i$, so that each of the ϕ_is depends only on a single point in the retina. We could picture such a subpredicate ϕ_i as a neuron with only one synapse that receives only a single input. However, it is possible to define ϕ_i in such a way that it receives input from more than one point, just a neuron usually has more than a single input. The order of the predicate ψ is the largest number of inputs that a *single* subpredicate ϕ_i in the sum receives. Thus the order of $\psi(X) = \lceil |X| > m \rceil$ above is 1, since all the ϕ_is in the sum depend on only one point.

It turns out that we can write any nth order predicate ψ as a sum of subpredicates of orders $k \in \{0, \ldots, n\}$, where a subpredicate of order k will be a product of k x_is. That is, we can rewrite the predicate ψ as:

---

[1]For those unfamiliar with set notation, the statement $x_i \in X$ means 'the point x_i is in the set X. Similarly, $x_i \notin X$ means x_i is not in the set X.

$$\psi = \left[\alpha_0 + \sum_i \alpha_i x_i + \sum_{i<j} \alpha_{ij} x_i x_j + \ldots + \sum_{i<j<\ldots<m} \alpha_{ij\ldots m} x_i x_j \ldots x_m > 0 \right]$$

$$(18.7)$$

where the last sum contains terms with n x_is in them.

Note that we have rewritten the predicate so that the threshold is always zero. We have done this by introducing the term α_0 on the left of the inequality sign. This term may be thought of as a 'zeroth order subpredicate'. In reality it is simply the negative of the threshold:

$$\alpha_0 = -\theta. \qquad (18.8)$$

In terms of neurons, you may think of α_0 as an input that is always on: it is an innate property of the neuron, which does not require any external input from other neurons.

To construct a perceptron capable of deciding the predicate $\psi(X) = \lceil |X| = m \rceil$, we need some of the subpredicates to be order 2. (This can be proved rigorously, but that is beyond our scope here. The interested reader is referred to Minsky and Papert (1988).) An order 2 subpredicate can be defined by

$$\phi_{ij} = x_i x_j \qquad (18.9)$$

which means that $\phi_{ij} = 1$ only if both x_i and x_j are in X. The analogy with neural systems becomes a little strained at this point, but you can think of an input from a point not in X as an absolute inhibitor, so that any neuron that receives an input from such a point will not fire.

Armed with order 1 and order 2 subpredicates, we can now construct our predicate $\psi(X) = \lceil |X| = m \rceil$. We observe, as above, that

$$\sum_{i=1}^{N} x_i = |X| \qquad (18.10)$$

and further that

$$\sum_{i<j} x_i x_j = |X|(|X| - 1)/2 \qquad (18.11)$$

where the sum here is a double sum over all i and j such that $i < j$. The result follows because the terms in the sum are 1 only if both x_i and x_j are in X. Thus this sum must be the number of ways of choosing 2 points from $|X|$ points, which is as shown.

We can invert these two equations to obtain

$$|X| = \sum_{i=1}^{N} x_i \qquad (18.12)$$

and

$$|X|^2 = 2\sum_{i<j} x_i x_j + |X| = 2\sum_{i<j} x_i x_j + \sum_{i=1}^{N} x_i. \qquad (18.13)$$

Now we observe that (recall that $|X|$ and m are integers) the only way the inequality

$$-(|X| - m)^2 > -1 \qquad (18.14)$$

can be satisfied is if $|X| = m$. Expanding the binomial and substituting for $|X|$ from above, we get

$$(1 - m^2) + (2m - 1)\sum_{i=1}^{N} x_i + (-2)\sum_{i<j} x_i x_j > 0 \qquad (18.15)$$

which is in linear threshold form. The weights of all the order 1 subpredicates are $(2m - 1)$ and the weights of all the order 2 subpredicates are -2. The zeroth order weight is $\alpha_0 = 1 - m^2$.

Thus a perceptron capable of testing whether the number of points in a pattern is a certain number must receive inputs from all points in the retina singly and in pairs. For a retina with 100 points this requires $100 + 100\times99/2 = 5050$ neurons. However, a perceptron which determines only if the number of points in the pattern is greater than a certain number requires only 100 neurons. Clearly the difference between order 1 and order 2 perceptrons is substantial. In terms of computational efficiency, an order 2 perceptron takes a time proportional (roughly) to N^2 to do a calculation, while an order 1 perceptron takes a time proportional to N.

There are usually many different ways of defining predicates to resolve a question. For example, to test whether the number of points in a set is equal to some number m, we could also have used the fact that the only way that the inequality

$$-(|X| - m)^4 > -1 \qquad (18.16)$$

could be satisfied is that $|X| = m$ and then worked out representations for the powers of $|X|$ up to the fourth in terms of sums of products of the points x_i. As you might expect, this leads to an order 4 predicate which will require neurons that have up to 4 inputs. Such a scheme is horribly inefficient, of course, and is not recommended.

Returning to the order 2 predicate ψ above, though, we noted at the time that all the order 1 subpredicates (the x_is in the sum) had the same weight, as did all the order 2 subpredicates (the $x_i x_j$ terms). It turns out that this is a special case of a more general principle.

18.3   Group invariance

Many of the questions that can be asked of a perceptron have answers that do not change if the points on the retina are transformed in some simple way. For example, the predicate $\psi(X) = \lceil |X| = m \rceil$ considered in the previous section will still have the same answer if the points in the retina are permuted or translated (moved as a block in one direction). If the transformation is a *group*, in the mathematical sense of the word, then we can show that predicate can be expressed in a particularly simple form.

For those unfamiliar with the mathematical definition of a group, we will review the definition here.[2]

To define a group we need (i) a set of objects and (ii) an operation which can be applied to members of the set. For example, we may define the set to be a collection of retinal states, such as the set of all states in which 10 of the points are 'on' and the rest 'off'. The operation may be, for example, a permutation of the retinal points.

The combination of the set and the operation is a group if the following conditions are true:

1. The set must be *closed* under the operation. This means that whenever the operation is applied to any member of the set, another member of the same set is generated. In the case of the permutation operation applied to the set of retinal states with 10 firing cells, this condition is satisfied since rearranging the cells does not change the number of cells that are on, so any rearrangement will always yield a retinal configuration with 10 firing cells.

2. There is an identity operation, that is, one that leaves all members of the set unchanged. In the case of the permutation, if we just leave all the cells in the same place we have an identity permutation.

3. There is an inverse operation for every operation, that is, there is an operation which will restore the original set element if applied to the element obtained after its initial transformation. For a permutation, we may define the inverse operation to be the permutation which restores the original configuration of the retina after an initial

---

[2]We will not need any more from group theory than this definition, so if you haven't studied groups before, don't panic.

permutation has been applied. For example, if the original permutation interchanged the elements as follows: $1 \to 2$, $2 \to 4$, $4 \to 3$, and $3 \to 1$ with all other cells remaining in the same place, the inverse permutation would be: $1 \to 3$, $3 \to 4$, $4 \to 2$, and $2 \to 1$. That is, we reverse each interchange in the original permutation, starting with the last and working our way back to the first.

Many simple transformations of the retinal points are group transformations. For example, the translation operation, where the entire retina is shifted rigidly by a given amount horizontally and vertically, is a group, as the reader is invited to show. We will now investigate the significance of groups in perceptron theory.

Picture one such group (the permutation group is a good one to use) and now consider what happens to the inputs received by the various neurons when this group is applied to the retina. If you consider the neurons used in the order 2 predicate $\psi(X) = \lceil |X| = m \rceil$ from the previous section, then permuting the points on the retina will also permute the order 1 subpredicates $\phi_i = x_i$ among themselves. However, it will not change the members in this set of order 1 subpredicates: all the ϕ_is that were there before the permutation will still be there afterwards. Another way of looking at it is that all you have done is connect the neurons to different points on the retina. Each neuron will receive input from a different retinal point, but all the retinal points will still be transmitting input to some neuron, and all neurons will still be receiving input from some retinal cell.

Now consider the order 2 subpredicates $\phi_{ij} = x_i x_j$. Permuting the retinal points will permute these subpredicates in a similar sort of way. Each order 2 neuron will be receiving input from two, possibly different, retinal points, and all the retinal points will still be projecting onto some order 2 neuron.

Further, the order 1 and order 2 neuron sets are disjoint under this operation: permuting the points will not cause any of the order 2 neurons to only receive one input, or any of the order 1 neurons to start receiving 2 inputs. The two sets of order 1 and order 2 neurons form two separate subsets that mix only within themselves and not between them.

These conditions are what are required for the two subsets of neurons to be *equivalence classes* under the group operation of permuting the points on the retina. The name equivalence class comes from the fact that the members of one such class are equivalent to each other under this transformation, since the transformation affects them all in the same way.

Minsky and Papert's *group invariance theorem* states that if you define a group operation and find that for the set of subpredicates you happen to be using in your perceptron that this set splits into one or more equivalence classes under this operation, then it is possible to find a representation of the perceptron where the weights are the same within each equivalence class. This is exactly what happened in the perceptron above where all the order 1 subpredicates had weights of $(2m - 1)$ and all the order 2 subpredicates had weights of -2.

It should be noted here that the group invariance theorem only says that it is *possible* to find such a representation of the predicate; it does *not* say that *all* representations of a predicate will actually have this form. When we come to study how perceptrons can be taught the form for a predicate, we will see that it is highly unlikely that such a neat form for a predicate will be found.

18.4   Abilities of perceptrons

18.4.1   Finite and infinite order

What sorts of things can perceptrons do? Minsky and Papert have been viewed as pessimistic about the abilities of the perceptron, since they show in their book that there are many fairly basic sorts of perceptual tasks that perceptrons either cannot perform, or else can perform only with great difficulty. However, most of the critics of the perceptron model have not managed to produce alternative models which are demonstrably better in a full-scale problem. Certainly some of the more popular alternative theories, such as back propagation (to be described in the next chapter), rely almost entirely on computer simulations of small systems and avoid the thorny problem of how their models behave when the system gets larger.

We will examine some of these alternative theories in later chapters. To begin, we will examine how perceptrons can be made to perform some simple geometric tasks. To introduce these methods, we must examine small systems ('toy systems', as Minsky and Papert call them) in order to make the technique clear. However, even though perceptrons may seem to cope well with such systems, we must always ask: 'Will such a system work efficiently when the system is scaled up to a realistic size?'

We have already introduced the concept of the order of a predicate: essentially it is a measure of the largest number of points which a single neuron must sample. We will now draw a distinction between predicates of finite and infinite order. Predicates of finite order do not change their order as the size $|R|$ of the retina increases. The predicates we examined above for comparing the size of a set $|X|$ to some fixed number m all had finite order since to test the predicate $\psi = \lceil |X| > m \rceil$ we needed only order 1 subpredicates, while to test $\psi = \lceil |X| = m \rceil$, we needed order 1 and 2 subpredicates.

A predicate of infinite order does not mean that we need infinite order predicates for finitely sized retinas; rather it means that the order of the predicate increases with the size of the retina. The rate of increase may be linear, exponential or even faster. Since most infinite order predicates require not only a subpredicate with the highest order, but subpredicates of all lower orders as well, they are much more complicated and inefficient than finite order predicates.

18.4.2 Parity

One example of a predicate with an infinite order is the so-called *parity* predicate:

$$\psi_{PARITY} = \lceil |X| \text{ is an odd number}\rceil. \tag{18.17}$$

Since the proof that ψ_{PARITY} has infinite order is fairly straightforward, and also illustrates the use of group invariance, we will outline it here.

Suppose ψ_{PARITY} has order K, so that we can write it in the form

$$\psi_{PARITY} = \left\lceil \sum_i \alpha_i \phi_i > 0 \right\rceil \tag{18.18}$$

where all the ϕ_is consist of products of K or fewer x_is. Now if we apply the permutation operation to the retina we won't change the value of ψ_{PARITY} since all we are doing is rearranging the points, not changing their number. Also, under this transformation, all subpredicates ϕ_i belonging to a single order k will transform among themselves, but no ϕ_is of different order will be interchanged. Thus the sets of ϕ_is of each order form equivalence classes under this transformation, so by the group invariance theorem above, there must exist a form for the predicate in which all ϕ_is in each class have the same coefficient α_i. We can therefore write

$$\psi_{PARITY} = \left\lceil \alpha_1 \sum x_i + \alpha_2 \sum x_i x_j + \ldots + \alpha_K \sum x_i x_j \ldots x_K > 0 \right\rceil \tag{18.19}$$

where the last sum contains terms with K x_is.

Now, we can use the same sort of argument that we used in deriving the form for the predicate $\lceil |X| = m \rceil$. Consider one of the sums in the above equation, say the one with order k. Each term of this sum contains k x_is and will only be non-zero if all the x_is are in the set X, i.e. if $x_i = 1$ for all i. The number of such terms is just the number of ways of choosing k points from the set X, which is the binomial coefficient $\begin{pmatrix} |X| \\ k \end{pmatrix}$. Written out in terms of factorials, this is

$$\begin{pmatrix} |X| \\ k \end{pmatrix} = \frac{|X|(|X| - 1)\ldots(|X| - k + 1)}{k!} \tag{18.20}$$

which is a polynomial of degree k in $|X|$. (Since we know from above that $|X| = \sum x_i$ is a first order term, we see that this is indeed an order k term.)

Thus the predicate ψ_{PARITY} can be written as a polynomial of degree K in $|X|$. If this predicate is to correctly distinguish between even and odd values of $|X|$, then we must have

$$\psi_{PARITY} \begin{cases} > 0 & \text{if } |X| \text{ is odd} \\ \leq 0 & \text{if } |X| \text{ is even} \end{cases} \tag{18.21}$$

For such a predicate to work on all sets X chosen from some retina of size $|R|$, the polynomial would have to change direction at least $|R| - 1$ times (that is, it has at least $|R| - 1$ points with a horizontal tangent). Only polynomials with degree at least $|R|$ can do this, so the order of ψ_{PARITY} must be at least $|R|$. QED.

Since polynomials of degree N that change direction $N - 1$ times must contain terms of all degrees, it follows that the predicate ψ_{PARITY} contains subpredicates of all orders. In fact, Minsky and Papert show that it contains *all* terms $x_i x_j \ldots x_k$ of all orders from 1 up to $|R|$. This means that the number of subpredicates that must be computed to test for parity is $\sum_{k=1}^{|R|} \binom{|R|}{k} = 2^{|R|} - 1$, where the sum is evaluated by using the binomial theorem on $(1 + 1)^{|R|}$. In this case, the time required to determine if a set contains an even or an odd number of points increases exponentially with the size of the retina. For any realistically sized retina, this method of determining parity is not to be recommended. For a retina containing 100 points, around $2^{100} \approx 10^{30}$ calculations need to be done: a prospect that would bring even a supercomputer to its knees.

Another fairly basic geometric property that has infinite order is *connectedness*. A set X on a retina R is connected if it is possible visit all points in X by starting at any point in X and moving from one point to another without ever leaving X. This is just a fancy way of saying that there are no parts of X isolated from any other parts. For example, any single solid figures (like a square or a circle) are connected, but two non-intersecting line segments, or a hollow circle with a dot in the middle are not.

18.4.3   Image transformations

People have the ability to recognize shapes even after they have been distorted in various ways. For example, you can probably still read this book if you move it a few inches to the left or right, if you rotate it by any amount about an axis perpendicular to the page (even turning the book upside down shouldn't confuse you too much) or if you move the book nearer or further away from you, thus changing the size of the letters in your field of view. These are the basic image transformations of translation, rotation and scaling. How do perceptrons fare under these transformations?

Let us consider translations. A translation is a group operation, since it is closed (any two translations simply give another translation), has an inverse (just reverse the translation and move the object back to where it started) and an identity operation (don't move the object at all). If we can find a set of subpredicates that have equivalence classes that are invariant under the translation operation, we can construct predicates out of these subpredicates that are translation invariant.

First of all, order 1 predicates that deal only with questions of the relative number of points in a set X, such as $\lceil |X| > m \rceil$, are invariant under translation, since merely shifting the points by a fixed distance has no effect on the number of points present. We can invert the argument, though, and notice that all single points must lie in the same equivalence class of the translation operation. Why? Because there is always *some* translation which will map any point into any other point. Of course it is not possible to arbitrarily rearrange the points in any single translation (that would require a permutation), but if we wanted to map x_i into x_j for any values of i and j there is always at least one translation that will do it. In such a translation, it may not be possible to simultaneously map x_k into x_l, but there will be some other translation that will allow this mapping. Thus all single points can be mapped into each other by some translation and therefore all lie in the same equivalence class. Thus any translation-invariant predicate containing first order terms can have only a single coefficient α_1 for all of them, by the group invariance theorem.

There is an important point to notice here. We have stated that a translation invariant order 1 predicate will consist of order 1 subpredicates that all have the same coefficient. If such a predicate evaluates to 'true' for two different figures, this does *not* necessarily mean the two figures are merely shifted versions of each other. To see this all you need to remember is that the same predicate is invariant under permutation, and a translation is just a special case of a permutation. Since all order 1 predicates invariant under permutation are also invariant under translation, there is no way, using such predicates, you can distinguish between patterns that have been permuted in general and those that have been merely translated.

For order two terms, we must work out which pairs of points can be mapped into each other under some arbitrary translation. Since translations do not allow any rotations or distortions of distance, only pairs of points that are the same distance apart and have the same orientation can be mapped into each other. Thus each set of points satisfying these conditions forms one equivalence class of the translation operation, and will therefore have the same coefficient in the predicate. Using this observation, we can split a pattern up into its 'geometric spectrum', as Minsky

and Papert call it. We will use the following notation to count the number
of pairs in each equivalence class. The number of points is $n_{x,y}$, where x
is the difference in horizontal location of the two points measured relative
to the left-most of the two points (so that $x \geq 0$) and y is the difference in
vertical location of the two points. y is measured relative to the left-most
of the two points if $x > 0$, otherwise, if $x = 0$, y is the distance from the
lower to the upper point, so that $y \geq 0$ if $x = 0$.

   For example, consider the figure

```
         *
       *****
         *
```

This figure has a geometric spectrum as follows:

x	y	$n_{x,y}$
0	1	2
1	−1	2
1	0	4
1	1	2
1	2	1
2	−1	1
2	0	3
2	1	2
3	0	2
3	1	1
4	0	1

   The sum of all the $n_{x,y}$s for any figure with $|X|$ points should equal
the total number of pairs of points, which is $|X|(|X| - 1)/2$. For the figure
above, $|X| = 7$, so there are 21 pairs of points. For this figure, a translation
invariant predicate of order 2 would have the form

$$\psi(X) = \alpha_1 |X| + \alpha_{0,1} n_{0,1} + \ldots + \alpha_{4,0} n_{4,0}. \qquad (18.22)$$

   Since we know the values of all the $n_{x,y}$s we can substitute these in to
get

$$
\begin{aligned}
\psi(X) \ = \ & 7\alpha_1 + 2\alpha_{0,1} + 2\alpha_{1,-1} + 4\alpha_{1,0} + 2\alpha_{1,1} + \alpha_{1,2} + \alpha_{2,-1} + 3\alpha_{2,0} \\
& +2\alpha_{2,1} + 2\alpha_{3,0} + \alpha_{3,1} + \alpha_{4,0} \qquad (18.23)
\end{aligned}
$$

   We could extend this argument to higher orders in the same way. For
order 3, we list all the distinct configurations of 3 points that can occur in

a pattern—each of these forms one equivalence class under translation, so each of them will have a constant coefficient in a predicate of order 3. To construct such a predicate for a particular pattern, we count the number of each of these configurations that occurs in the figure and place one term for each configuration in the predicate.

Just as with the order 1 case, the fact that an order 2 translation invariant predicate returns 'true' for two different patterns is no guarantee that the two patterns are translations of each other. Any two patterns with the same geometric spectrum, that is, the same numbers of each of the possible configurations of pairs of points, will always give the same result with such a predicate. For example, the two figures

$$***\qquad\qquad\qquad *$$
$$*\qquad\qquad\qquad ***$$

have identical spectra and cannot be distinguished by any order 2 translation invariant perceptron. (They can, however, be separated by an order 3 or higher perceptron.) Thus to produce a predicate capable of recognizing a fairly complex shape, such as a printed letter, a high-order predicate is required.

There are a number of other similar geometric applications of lower-order perceptrons which are treated by Minsky and Papert, but they do not really add anything to the basic idea of using the perceptron to detect certain types of patterns. One major aspect of perceptron theory that we have not yet considered, however, is that of learning. To this we now turn.

18.5 Perceptron learning

So far, we have considered the perceptron only as a feature detector which must be preprogrammed for every pattern which we expect it to encounter. We have not determined the coefficients α_i for the subpredicates in many cases explicitly—rather, we have shown how the group invariance theorem can be used to reduce the number of different coefficients we need to find and have then left the matter hanging.

Indeed, if we had to determine the coefficients by hand for every situation, perceptrons would be very cumbersome to use. They would also be unsatisfactory models of any real neural system, since one of the most remarkable things about the biological brain is that it can learn.

We will now consider the so-called *perceptron convergence theorem* or *perceptron learning theorem* which gives an algorithm for determining the coefficients α_i for a particular predicate $\psi(X) = \lceil \sum \alpha_i \phi_i > 0 \rceil$ in any case where a solution exists. The latter condition is an important one to remember, since it is not always possible to decide the truth of a predicate with the given set ϕ_i of subpredicates. We have already seen examples of this where the predicate ψ is of infinite order. In the case of ψ_{PARITY} for example, if we are dealing with a retina of 100 points and propose an order 2 predicate model, there is no way we can choose the coefficients α_i to give us a working ψ_{PARITY}.

Assuming that a solution exists, what do we need to do to find it? First, we must specify the set of subpredicates that we shall be using, that is, we must specify the set of ϕ_is. For ease of notation, we can think of this set as a vector $\Phi = [\phi_0, \phi_1, \phi_2, \ldots, \phi_N]$, where there are $N + 1$ subpredicates (of any order) in our predicate ψ. (The subpredicate ϕ_0 is the zeroth order subpredicate, which is always 1.) We can also represent the coefficients α_i as a vector $A = [\alpha_0, \alpha_1, \alpha_2, \ldots, \alpha_N]$. With this notation, we can now write the predicate ψ as a scalar product:

$$\psi(X) = \lceil A \cdot \Phi(X) > 0 \rceil. \tag{18.24}$$

This predicate will be required to answer some specific question about the set X. That is, once we specify the set X, we will know in advance what answer we *want* $\psi(X)$ to give. Since $\psi(X)$ is a binary function, we can divide the set of all possible patterns X on the retina R into two subsets: T, the set of all patterns for which $\psi(X)$ should return 'true', and F, the set of all patterns for which $\psi(X)$ should return 'false'.

We can start things off by guessing some values for the coefficients of A. Then we can input a series of patterns X to the perceptron and watch what it produces as its answer for each pattern. If it gives the right answer (that is, 'true' when $X \in T$ and 'false' when $X \in F$) then things are going well and we don't want to change the coefficients. If it makes a mistake, though, we would like to change some or all of the α_is to improve its future performance.

How do we choose the new values? First, suppose the perceptron responded 'true' when it should have said 'false'. In this case, the coefficients are too large, since $A \cdot \Phi > 0$ when we should have $A \cdot \Phi < 0$. We should decrease the values of the coefficients, but in what manner? Decreasing them at random is obviously a bad move. One observation to make is that only those coefficients corresponding to subpredicates that were 'on' (that is, equal to 1) when the mistake was made can have anything to do with the value of $A \cdot \Phi$, since all the other subpredicates are zero. We could try subtracting something from all those α_is whose corresponding ϕ_is were non-zero when the mistake was made. In a similar fashion, if the perceptron responded 'false' when it should have said 'true', we can add something to the α_is corresponding to those ϕ_is that were non-zero.

We still don't know how much to add or subtract. In the absence of anything to bias our choice we might as well add or subtract the same amount to each α_i. Thus we arrive at the procedure: if the perceptron gives the wrong answer, add or subtract a multiple of Φ to A.

If a solution exists, it will be a vector A^* with the property that

$$A^* \cdot \Phi(X) > 0 \text{ if } X \in T \tag{18.25}$$

and

$$A^* \cdot \Phi(X) \leq 0 \text{ if } X \in F. \tag{18.26}$$

When we come, in a moment, to state and prove the convergence theorem, it will be more convenient if we take A^* and Φ to be unit vectors. This will mean abandoning the convenience of assuming all our coefficients to be integers, but it doesn't really change anything in the theory. Since the components of Φ are the individual subpredicates ϕ_i, each of which is either zero or one, all that is required to convert Φ to a unit vector is to count up the number n of non-zero ϕ_is and divide the vector by $\sqrt{n}$. To distinguish between the vector Φ, whose components are the usual zeroes and ones, and the unit vector, we will denote the unit vector by $\hat{\Phi}$. We have therefore:

$$\hat{\Phi} = \frac{\Phi}{\sqrt{n}}. \tag{18.27}$$

Because of the nature of the algorithm, we do not require A to be a unit vector.

The algorithm we will use is then:

1. Choose initial values A_0.

2. Choose a pattern X.

3. Apply the perceptron to X.

4. If the answer is correct, return to step 2. Otherwise, if the answer is true when it should have been false, generate the value of A at step $t+1$ from the value at step t using the formula $A_{t+1} = A_t - \hat{\Phi}$. If the answer is false when it should have been true then $A_{t+1} = A_t + \hat{\Phi}$.

Note that step 4 can actually be condensed a bit. If we replace all the $\hat{\Phi}$ vectors in the case where the required answer is false by their negatives, then we can require that the perceptron answer 'true' to all patterns.

One thing that is missing from this algorithm is a termination condition. There are various criteria that might be used. If you are certain that a solution exists, then, since (as we will see in a minute) the algorithm is guaranteed to converge to the solution if it exists, you can let the algorithm run for a certain number of cycles and then test all the patterns in the two sets T and F to see if the answers generated by the perceptron are all correct. If not, keep going.

In the (more likely) case where you are not sure whether a solution exists for your choice of Φ, you may need to apply some sort of convergence test. For example, you could test the value of $|A_{t+1} - A_t|$ and stop the algorithm when this drops below some predefined error tolerance. This technique will not work, of course, if the algorithm is not converging. In such cases, it is advisable to check the value of A every so many cycles to see what is happening. It is possible that the values of A are diverging, in which case the program will eventually crash when an overflow occurs. A nastier possibility is that A has settled into some sort of oscillation, in which case the algorithm will never stop, since convergence will never be obtained and the values of A will always remain within acceptable limits as far as the computer is concerned. To guard against such possibilities it is always wise to put an upper bound on the number of iterations.

The statement and proof of the convergence theorem now follow.

Perceptron Convergence Theorem: Assume that the vectors $\hat{\Phi}$ for which the perceptron was to have answered 'false' have been replaced by their negatives, so that the perceptron is required to answer 'true' for all patterns. If a unit vector A^* exists such that $A^* \cdot \hat{\Phi} > 0$ for all patterns, then the algorithm above will converge to a solution in a finite number of steps.

Note that the theorem says that a solution will be obtained (if it exists) in a *finite* number of steps. This is *not* an asymptotic algorithm, like most iterative algorithms in numerical analysis, for example. You *will* get an *exact* answer after a finite amount of time.

Now to prove the convergence theorem. Since the correct vector A^* satisfies the condition $A^* \cdot \hat{\Phi} > 0$ for all patterns, and there are a finite number of patterns, this scalar product must have a minimum value, say δ. That is, we can write

$$A^* \cdot \hat{\Phi} \geq \delta > 0. \tag{18.28}$$

We can define the 'angle' β between the current vector of coefficients A and the solution vector A^* in terms of a scalar product:

$$\cos \beta = \frac{A^* \cdot A}{|A^*||A|} = \frac{A^* \cdot A}{|A|}. \tag{18.29}$$

(Recall A^* is a unit vector, so $|A^*| = 1$.) Now A^* is only one of the possible solution vectors—in general there will be a cone (or, more properly, a hypercone, since we are dealing with higher dimensional spaces) of vectors that will all satisfy the required conditions. All that is required for the algorithm to converge is for A to come close enough to A^*, or in other words, for β to approach zero so that $\cos \beta$ will come close enough to 1.

Let us derive recurrence relations for the numerator and denominator of this expression to see how they change with successive iterations of the algorithm. The numerator gives:

$$\begin{aligned} A^* \cdot A_{t+1} &= A^* \cdot (A_t + \hat{\Phi}) \\ &= A^* \cdot A_t + A^* \cdot \hat{\Phi} \\ &\geq A^* \cdot A_t + \delta \end{aligned}$$

or, extending the argument n times:

$$A^* \cdot A_n \geq n\delta. \tag{18.30}$$

Now the denominator gives:

$$\begin{aligned} |A_{t+1}|^2 &= (A_t + \hat{\Phi}) \cdot (A_t + \hat{\Phi}) \\ &= |A_t|^2 + 2A_t \cdot \hat{\Phi} + |\hat{\Phi}|^2 \\ &< |A_t|^2 + 1 \end{aligned}$$

where the last inequality follows from the fact that $2A_t \cdot \hat{\Phi} < 0$, since the perceptron made a mistake on iteration t, and that $|\hat{\Phi}|^2 = 1$ since $\hat{\Phi}$ is a unit vector. After the nth application of this procedure we have

$$|A_n|^2 < n. \tag{18.31}$$

We now have a lower bound on the numerator and an upper bound on the denominator. We can combine the two to obtain

$$\cos \beta > \frac{n\delta}{\sqrt{n}}. \tag{18.32}$$

The right-hand side must exceed 1 after N applications of the correction step (that is, after the perceptron has made N mistakes) as soon as

$$N > \frac{1}{\delta^2}. \tag{18.33}$$

Hence the algorithm must converge in fewer than N steps.

You might think that this proof also gives you an idea of how long the algorithm will take to converge, since N is expressed in terms of δ, which is the minimum of $A^* \cdot \hat{\Phi}$. But this doesn't help you much unless you know A^* which, of course, you don't.

Another problem with this algorithm is that it tells you that a correct answer will be found after a finite number of *incorrect* responses have been given by the perceptron. However, as the weight vector A gets closer to

correct vector, fewer mistakes are made, so that the convergence does seem
to be approximately asymptotic if the test patterns are generated randomly.
One way around this problem is to run through the complete set of patterns
in each training cycle. To avoid bias in the learning pattern, the order in
which these patterns are presented should be varied in each cycle.

18.6   Limitations of the perceptron

The perceptron is the first major neural network model in which learning is possible by variation of the synaptic weights. Given the explosion
of research papers and industrial applications of this principle that have
occurred since the perceptron model was proposed, you may think that
Rosenblatt's and Minsky and Papert's work would have been hailed as a
major advance in brain theory, to say nothing of computer science. In fact,
nothing of the kind happened at the time. Immediately after the publica-
tion of Minsky and Papert's book, very little further research into neural
networks took place. The blame for this relative lethargy has been laid
at the feet of Minsky and Papert themselves, for they are not optimistic
that perceptrons of low order can be constructed to solve any predicates
which answer 'interesting' questions; questions like 'Is that a picture of your
mother?' rather than 'boring' questions like 'Are there more than 100 dots
on this piece of paper?'. This pessimism stems mainly from the fact that
perceptrons designed to answer interesting questions seem to need large, if
not infinite, order to succeed. Minsky and Papert recognize that the class
of neural network they have treated in their book is restricted, in that it
consists of only a single layer of processors between the input layer and
the single output neuron, but they speculate that even if you increase the
complexity of the network by introducing additional layers, adding more
output neurons, and so on, you will still not achieve an efficient network
for answering interesting questions.

The workers of the Parallel Distributed Processing (PDP) group, whose
back propagation model we will consider in Chapter 19, claim to have
overcome the problems that Minsky and Papert found so depressing in their
study of perceptrons. As we shall see, the PDP model, which introduces
just those modifications which Minsky and Papert predicted would have no
appreciable effect, does seem to allow calculation of some of the predicates
which require an infinite order perceptron. However, the amount of training
required to produce these results is often disproportionately large compared
to the significance of the result obtained. With faster computers, however,
this limitation is becoming less noticeable. The improvements in computer
technology have, unfortunately, tended to obscure the fact that models that
require thousands of training steps to recognize simple patterns cannot be
realistic models of biological memory. The speed of the brain remains the

same despite the improvement in the speed of the machines which it has
designed.

19

Connectionism

19.1 Introduction

Minsky and Papert's work on perceptrons (Chapter 18) is widely regarded as having put a wet blanket on research into neural networks for many years, since it shows that perceptrons are severely limited in the sorts of predicates they could handle efficiently. The perceptron theorems, however, apply specifically to networks with an input layer (the retina), a single 'hidden' layer (the subpredicates) and an output layer (the single predicate ψ). The weights from the input layer to the layer of subpredicates are fixed, so the only adaptable parts of a perceptron are the weights from the hidden layer to the output cell. Minsky and Papert hypothesized, but did not prove, that adding more hidden layers would not lead to any improvement in the performance of the network.

In the late 1970s and early 1980s, interest began to revive in network models. Since that time, there has been a dramatic increase in the amount of work done in the subject. This has probably been due largely to the advances in computer technology in the 1980s, especially in the area of parallel processing. More powerful computers mean that it is possible to run network simulations much more quickly, making it easier to test models of perception and learning. What used to take hours or days can now be done in minutes. At the same time, neural network theory has found a new application in the design of parallel computer systems. Research into 'neural computers', of course, has no need to restrict itself to biologically realistic models, and so will not concern us in this book. It is important, however, to realize that many research papers published in the area of neural networks are concerned more with developing computer systems than with explaining how the brain works.

The 'new' neural network theory of parallel computation, both in brains and computers, has been dubbed *connectionism*. There are many books, papers, and journals concerned almost exclusively with network theory, but a two-volume set of books (Rumelhart and McClelland, 1986) has become known as the 'Connectionist's Bible', since it was written by a group of researchers who were the prime movers in the new network movement.

The books' title (*Parallel Distributed Processing* or PDP for short) has also become the name of the research group, though the term 'connectionism' seems to be more widely used. Since we will refer to these books frequently in this chapter, we will call them PDP to save space.

How much has this flurry of activity accomplished? This seems to be largely a matter of opinion. Reading the chapters in PDP, one comes away with the impression that the models therein stand a good chance of being the beginnings of the definitive theory of brain function. The authors of PDP feel that they have overcome many of the limitations of perceptrons, in that they have constructed networks that seem able to learn many predicates that low order perceptrons could not.

Minsky and Papert, however, in their epilogue to the original *Perceptrons* book (1988) criticize PDP at length. Their arguments refer mainly to the generalized delta rule, which will be described in this chapter, but the general criticism applies to connectionism as a whole. The PDP authors, say Minsky and Papert, consider only very simple networks and do not consider what would happen if their methods were to be applied to problems with a large number of neurons. The implication is that such models would run into the same problems as perceptrons. If that is the case, then the PDP approach is no better at producing a model of the brain than the perceptron approach; indeed, the two methods might just be variants of a common theme.

One difficulty the objective reader faces in trying to reconcile perceptrons and connectionism is that the approaches taken by their respective authors are very different. Minsky and Papert take a rigorous, mathematical approach to their subject, while the PDP authors tend to rely more on heuristic argument and computer simulation. Both approaches have their merits and drawbacks. A mathematical approach leaves the reader with a greater feeling of confidence in the conclusions, but it is very difficult, if not impossible, to produce mathematical proofs for any but the simplest systems. What Minsky and Papert show in their book is that many of these simple systems *must* be computationally inefficient, but they can do no more than speculate that such inefficiency is a common feature of all networks, no matter what their architecture.

The PDP approach, relying as it does on computer simulations, cannot say much of anything that is both general and certain. Doing a set of simulations on a particular system allows you to say with a fair degree of certainty how such a system will behave, but it is difficult and dangerous to extend the behaviour of one system to another system with a different architecture, or even to the same system applied to a different problem.

The moral is that both approaches have contributions to make to the theory, provided that their limitations are recognized and accepted. It is unlikely that a complete mathematical analysis of any 'real-life' size

neural network is possible, but then it is also unlikely that a full computer
simulation of such a network could be run within a reasonable time (such
as a few days).

One other problem that frequently gets overlooked in neural network
discussions is: How biologically realistic are these models? Perceptrons,
although they incorporate the idea of a threshold function for determining
neural output, and allow learning through adjustable weights, were not
proposed primarily as brain models. Minsky and Papert's analysis seems
concerned mainly with the subject for its own sake and its application to
computer science.

The PDP approach is intended to propose models of real psychological
and biological phenomena. The second volume of PDP is concerned with
such models. However, the authors admit that many of the assumptions
they have made have little support in the neurobiological literature, though
they have avoided making assumptions that are contradicted by data. This
is not so much a criticism of the PDP approach as it is a comment on
the lack of hard experimental data on just how real neural systems work.
Despite decades of work in the area, no one can yet say precisely what
happens on the neural or molecular level when people interpret what they
see or when they memorize something.

Although the lack of data can be frustrating, such a state of affairs
affords a great opportunity for theorists. By exploring the behaviour of
neural networks on a computer, they can discover what architectures allow
various aspects of perception and cognition to occur. If the assumptions
and results are not supported by the available data, they can provide directions in which experimentalists can search. In turn, the data from new
experiments can constrain and redirect the modellers' efforts.

The PDP models, then, should not be taken as theoretical descriptions
of what is already known experimentally. Rather, they are models of how
the brain *might* work at the neural level.

19.2   The delta rule

We will examine a PDP model, proposed by Rumelhart *et al.* (1986),
that is superficially similar to the perceptron. The network consists of an
input layer or retina, an arbitrary number of inner or hidden layers, and
an output layer which may be regarded as the response of the net to the
pattern injected into the input layer (see Fig. 19.1). Each of these layers
may contain any number of neurons. Thus, unlike the perceptron, the
output of the net may be a pattern over several neurons rather than just a
single neuron which is either on or off.

Each neuron in each layer may be connected to any neuron in any
higher layer, but lateral connections (between neurons in the same layer)

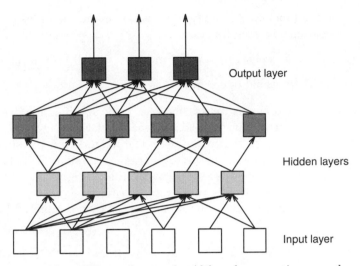

Figure 19.1 A multilayered network. Although connections are shown only between neurons in adjacent layers, any neuron may be connected to any other neuron in any higher layer.

and backward connections (from the output towards the input) are not allowed. Such a net is called a *feed-forward* net. Each of these connections is assigned a weight. The input received by a cell is the weighted sum of signals from all cells that have connections to it. If this input exceeds the threshold for the cell, the cell produces an output signal that feeds into all cells in higher layers with which it connects. Signals are propagated from layer to layer until they reach the output layer, where the final set of signals is recorded as the response of the net.

To make these notions definite, we need a bit of notation.

- Layers will be numbered from layer 1 (the input layer) up to layer N (the output layer).

- n_i = the number of cells in layer i.

- $i_{i,j}$ = the input received by cell j in layer i.

- $o_{i,j}$ = the output from cell j in layer i. For a classical neuron, the output will be 0 if the cell does not fire and 1 if it does. However, we will see that in order for the delta rule to work, the output must be a differentiable function of the input to the cell. The output function of a classical neuron is a step function and therefore does not satisfy this requirement. We will therefore take

$$o_{i,j} = f(i_{i,j}) \tag{19.1}$$

where the function f must be differentiable and be a reasonable approximation to a step function.

- $w_{k,m;i,j}$ = the weight *from* cell j in layer i *to* cell m in layer k.

- $\theta_{i,j}$ = the threshold of cell j in layer i.

In practice, the only quantities that need to be specified in advance are the $o_{1,j}$s, that is, the output signals from the input layer (layer 1). This is the pattern that is presented to the net. The weights and thresholds can be given random values at the start of a training session. The delta rule which we will consider below is used to adjust these weights and thresholds until the net responds correctly to all input patterns.

The input to any cell above the input layer is then calculated from the relation:

$$i_{i,j} = \sum_{k=1}^{i-1} \sum_{m=1}^{n_k} w_{i,j;k,m} o_{k,m} - \theta_{i,j}. \tag{19.2}$$

The outer sum adds in contributions from all layers below layer i. The inner sum adds in all the signals from the cells in layer k. The output from cell i, j is then calculated from the relation $o_{i,j} = f(i_{i,j})$ as mentioned above. To calculate the output of the net, this formula would be applied, in order, to all cells $j \in \{1, \ldots, n_i\}$ in all layers $i \in \{2, \ldots, N\}$.

To produce a differentiable output function, we need a function $f(x)$ which is asymptotically zero for large, negative x and asymptotically one for large positive values of x. The PDP authors use the sigmoid function:

$$o_{i,j} = f(i_{i,j}) = \frac{1}{1 + e^{-i_{i,j}}}. \tag{19.3}$$

Since $0 < o_{i,j} < 1$, it could be interpreted as a probability of the neuron firing, although this is not the interpretation used by PDP. Rather, the value of $o_{i,j}$ is taken to be the strength of the output signal generated by the cell. In this sense it may seem that the neuron is not behaving classically at all, since such a cell will not generate an all-or-none impulse. However, the strength of a nerve impulse can be conveyed by the frequency of the action potentials. The value of $o_{i,j}$ could be interpreted as the fraction of maximum frequency produced by the cell. Such a graded response is actually more realistic than a step function if $o_{i,j}$ is interpreted in this way, since no natural system can respond with the precision of a discontinuous function.

19.3   Training the net

The net can be trained by a similar sort of learning rule to that used in the perceptron. A series of patterns is presented to the net and each allowed to generate a response. The desired response is compared with the observed output, and corrections are made to the weights in an attempt to improve the performance of the net.

One problem that nets with hidden layers faced initially was that there was no obvious way to update the weights on connections to the hidden layers, since there was no 'desired response' from a hidden layer with which to compare its output. To see how this problem was solved, we first consider the training rule for weights on connections leading directly into the output layer.

In the perceptron, we used a simple rule: correct only those weights on connections that are active for a given pattern, and make all corrections the same size. In a PDP net, though, there is no clear-cut distinction between an active and an inactive line, since the output of a cell is not a step function. Thus we will get different strength responses from each line and we can't expect any line to have a zero-strength signal.

An easier way to proceed is to define some measure of the error the net has made in responding to a particular pattern and see if we can find an algorithm for reducing this error. The severity of an error in perception can, of course, depend on the context in which the error is made. For example, if you mistake a red light for a green light when you are in the middle of heavy traffic, you could get yourself killed, but if you mistake a red light for a green light at 4 a.m. on a deserted road, it is unlikely that it will make any difference. However, for the purposes of a simple model, we need a simple error gauge. One of the simplest is the sum of squares of the differences between the required and observed output values for each cell in the output layer. Let $r_{N,j}$ be the required response from cell j in layer N (recall layer N is the output layer). Then the error in the response to a single pattern is

$$E(pattern) = \sum_{j=1}^{n_N} (r_{N,j} - o_{N,j})^2. \tag{19.4}$$

Now if we concentrate on reducing this error without considering what changes this is making on the net's response to other patterns, we have no guarantee that the changes we make in the weights will improve the net's performance overall. Thus what we really want to reduce is the total error:

$$E(total) = \sum_{all\ patterns} E(pattern). \tag{19.5}$$

We are assuming that there is a finite number of patterns to which the net is expected to respond.

Since we want to reduce E by changing the weights, we can consider the error to be a function of the weights. We can then use a gradient descent method to minimize E by taking small steps for each weight.

The gradient descent method is a generalization of the method for locating the minimum of a function, $g(x)$ say, of one variable. Since the minimum of a continuous function occurs at a value x_0 such that its derivative $g'(x_0) = 0$, the value of $g'(x)$ is a rough indication of how far from the minimum you are for a given value of x. If $g'(x) > 0$, you are moving away from the minimum, since the function is increasing, so you should decrease x. Similarly, if $g'(x) < 0$, you should increase x. Thus the amount Δx by which x should be changed at each step is roughly proportional to $-g'(x)$, and we can write

$$\Delta x = -Kg'(x) \qquad (19.6)$$

where K is a positive constant. The trick is to choose K to be the right size. If K is too large, you can overshoot the minimum and end up on the other side. In fact, for some values of K the sequence of values may oscillate forever, or even diverge. On the other hand, if you take K to be too small, the procedure can take a very long time to converge.

The thorniest problem with gradient descent methods is that of local minima. In the case of the PDP net, we want the global minimum of the error function. Since E depends on all the weights in a non-linear way (recall that the outputs $o_{N,j}$ are non-linear functions of the outputs from lower layers) it is likely to have many local minima in addition to the global one. If K in eqn (19.6) (or its equivalent in the multidimensional problem) is chosen to be too small, the procedure can easily get trapped inside one of these local minima. This will usually result in the net responding correctly to some of the patterns but not to all of them. You can always get out of a local minimum (assuming that you haven't settled right to the bottom of it so that all the derivatives are zero) by choosing a larger value for K, but again you risk the possibility of overshooting the global minimum.

One consolation with the PDP net problem is that you can always tell when you have found the global minimum, since the net will respond correctly to all input patterns. If you obtain a solution where this is not the case, you have found a local minimum and should run the training session again, possibly with a larger step size.

In the multidimensional case, we should adjust each weight $w_{N,j;k,m}$ by an amount proportional to the gradient of E with respect to that weight, that is:

$$\Delta w_{N,j;k,m} \propto -\frac{\partial E}{\partial w_{N,j;k,m}}. \qquad (19.7)$$

Using the chain rule for derivatives, we have

$$\frac{\partial E}{\partial w_{N,j;k,m}} = \frac{\partial E}{\partial o_{N,j}} \frac{\partial o_{N,j}}{\partial w_{N,j;k,m}}. \qquad (19.8)$$

Note that, although E depends on all the output values, there is only one output value $o_{N,j}$ that depends on the particular weight $w_{N,j;k,m}$[1], so there is only one term in the chain rule expansion.

Now we have expressions for E in terms of $o_{N,j}$ (eqn (19.4)) and for $o_{N,j}$ in terms of $w_{N,j;k,m}$ (eqns (19.2) and (19.3)), so we can evaluate both derivatives. Doing the calculations we find:

$$\frac{\partial E}{\partial o_{N,j}} = -(r_{N,j} - o_{N,j}) \qquad (19.9)$$

and

$$\frac{\partial o_{N,j}}{\partial w_{N,j;k,m}} = o_{N,j}(1 - o_{N,j})o_{k,m}. \qquad (19.10)$$

Combining all these factors, we find that the change in weight should be

$$\Delta w_{N,j;k,m} = \eta(r_{N,j} - o_{N,j})o_{N,j}(1 - o_{N,j})o_{k,m} \qquad (19.11)$$

where η is a positive constant of proportionality, often called the *learning rate*, since its magnitude determines the size of the steps taken in each learning cycle.

This equation applies only to the weights for connections into the output layer. It cannot be used for hidden layers, since we do not know the values of the $r_{i,j}$s for any hidden layer elements. However, we can do a bit more algebra to derive a formula that is valid for any weight in any layer, hidden or not.

We start from the same point by assuming that the weight change must be proportional to the gradient of the error with respect to the weight in question:

$$\Delta w_{i,j;k,m} \propto -\frac{\partial E}{\partial w_{i,j;k,m}}. \qquad (19.12)$$

Using the chain rule, we can split this into factors arising from (i) the change in the error due to change in the input into cell i, j and (ii) the change in the input to cell i, j due to the change in the weight $w_{i,j;k,m}$:

$$\frac{\partial E}{\partial w_{i,j;k,m}} = \frac{\partial E}{\partial i_{i,j}} \frac{\partial i_{i,j}}{\partial w_{i,j;k,m}}. \qquad (19.13)$$

Again, since cell i, j is the only cell that depends on the weight $w_{i,j;k,m}$, there is only one term in the chain rule expansion of the derivative.

From eqn (19.2), the second factor in eqn (19.13) is

$$\frac{\partial i_{i,j}}{\partial w_{i,j;k,m}} = o_{k,m} \qquad (19.14)$$

---

[1]See eqns (19.2) and (19.3).

We will use a shorthand notation for the first derivative:

$$\delta_{i,j} \equiv -\frac{\partial E}{\partial i_{i,j}} \qquad (19.15)$$

so we can write

$$\Delta w_{i,j;k,m} = \eta \delta_{i,j} o_{k,m} \qquad (19.16)$$

where η is the learning rate, as defined in eqn (19.11).

We still need to find a value for $\delta_{i,j}$. We can use the chain rule to split this term again:

$$\delta_{i,j} = -\frac{\partial E}{\partial i_{i,j}} = -\frac{\partial E}{\partial o_{i,j}} \frac{\partial o_{i,j}}{\partial i_{i,j}} \qquad (19.17)$$

The second factor can be evaluated from eqn (19.3):

$$\frac{\partial o_{i,j}}{\partial i_{i,j}} = \frac{e^{-i}}{(1 + e^{-i})^2} = o_{i,j}(1 - o_{i,j}). \qquad (19.18)$$

The first factor in eqn (19.17) is the rate of change of error E with respect to the output from cell i, j where, in general, this cell is in a hidden layer. Since we don't know directly how the error depends on hidden cell parameters, it may seem that we are just going around in circles. However, we can use the chain rule once again (this is the last time!). This time, however, we bring into play those levels that are closer to the output layer than layer i. In a general feed-forward net, the output from a cell in layer i can connect to any cell in layers $i+1$ through to the output layer N. We can use an inductive approach to finding the values of the $\delta_{i,j}$s. We know how to calculate $\delta_{N,j}$, since we have explicit formulas relating E to $o_{N,j}$ and $o_{N,j}$ to $i_{N,j}$. We can write, for the output layer:

$$\delta_{N,j} = -\frac{\partial E}{\partial i_{N,j}} = (r_{N,j} - o_{N,j}) o_{N,j}(1 - o_{N,j}). \qquad (19.19)$$

We now assume that we have calculated all δs from layer N down to layer $i+1$, and we wish to find the set of $\delta_{i,j}$s for layer i. The only things we need to complete our calculation are the values of $\partial E/\partial o_{i,j}$. Since the output from cell i, j can affect the inputs of all cells in layers $i + 1$ to N, we can use the chain rule to write

$$\frac{\partial E}{\partial o_{i,j}} = \sum_{q=i+1}^{N} \sum_{r=1}^{n_q} \frac{\partial E}{\partial i_{q,r}} \frac{\partial i_{q,r}}{\partial o_{i,j}} \qquad (19.20)$$

$$= -\sum_{q=i+1}^{N} \sum_{r=1}^{n_q} \delta_{q,r} w_{q,r;i,j}. \qquad (19.21)$$

We have thus managed to express $\delta_{i,j}$ in terms of the δ values for layers *higher* than layer i, which we have already calculated. Combining all the above results, we have the expression for the change of a weight leading into a hidden layer:

$$\Delta w_{i,j;k,m} = \eta o_{k,m} o_{i,j}(1 - o_{i,j})\delta_{i,j} \qquad (19.22)$$

where

$$\delta_{i,j} = \sum_{q=i+1}^{N} \sum_{r=1}^{n_q} \delta_{q,r} w_{q,r;i,j}. \qquad (19.23)$$

Just for completeness, we repeat the formula (19.11) for correcting the weights leading into the output layer:

$$\Delta w_{N,j;k,m} = \eta o_{k,m} \delta_{N,j} \qquad (19.24)$$

where

$$\delta_{N,j} = o_{N,j}(1 - o_{N,j})(r_{N,j} - o_{N,j}). \qquad (19.25)$$

To apply this rule, you begin by updating the weights into the output layer using formula (19.24), then work backwards one layer at a time applying the recursive formula (19.22) until all weights have been updated. Since this method involves propagating the corrections to the weights backwards through the net, from output layer to input layer, it is often called the *back propagation* method. The full name for the overall method of training a net is the *generalized delta rule with back propagation*.

One final detail needs to be addressed. We mentioned earlier that the threshold for each neuron was generated randomly when the net is initialized, and updated along with the weights. How is this done?

If we refer back to eqn (19.2), we see that the input to a cell is determined by summing the weighted outputs of those cells that make synapses on the cell under consideration, followed by subtracting off the threshold value $\theta_{i,j}$. We can consider this threshold value to be an input from another cell, one that is separate from the cells that have been explicitly included in the network. If this special cell is assumed to fire at all times (it is always 'on', so to speak), then the threshold value $\theta_{i,j}$ is just the weight from this special cell to cell j in layer i, and can be altered just like any other weight. Since every cell above the input layer is assumed to have a variable threshold, the special cell must be assigned a position in the input layer so that it can affect all cells in the net. A convenient way of doing this is to define cell number 0 in the input layer to be this special 'threshold cell',[2] and assume that it has connections to all other cells in the network (except those in the input layer).

---

[2]Sometimes called a *bias* cell.

If this is done, the thresholds of the cells in the output layer can be altered in each learning cycle using eqn (19.24), with $k = 1$ and $m = 0$. In this case the weight $w_{N,j;1,0}$ is just the negative of the threshold $\theta_{N,j}$ (negative, since the threshold is subtracted in eqn (19.2) rather than added as all other contributions are), and the output $o_{1,0} \equiv 1$, since the threshold cell always fires. We have then:

$$\Delta\theta_{N,j} = -\eta\delta_{N,j} \tag{19.26}$$

where

$$\delta_{N,j} = o_{N,j}(1 - o_{N,j})(r_{N,j} - o_{N,j}). \tag{19.27}$$

To change the thresholds of cells in the hidden layers, we may use eqn (19.22), again with $k = 1$ and $m = 0$, with the same reasoning as above:

$$\Delta\theta_{i,j} = -\eta o_{i,j}(1 - o_{i,j})\delta_{i,j} \tag{19.28}$$

where

$$\delta_{i,j} = \sum_{q=i+1}^{N} \sum_{r=1}^{n_q} \delta_{q,r} w_{q,r;i,j}. \tag{19.29}$$

19.4 Training a multilayer net

To illustrate the theory, let us consider a simple multilayer net designed to solve the so-called exclusive-or (or XOR) problem. The net is to accept two input signals and produce a single output signal which implements the XOR logical function. We can define the XOR function using a truth table (see Chapter 17):

Input 1	Input 2	XOR
TRUE	TRUE	FALSE
TRUE	FALSE	TRUE
FALSE	TRUE	TRUE
FALSE	FALSE	FALSE

That is, the XOR of two inputs is true (the output neuron fires) if and only if just one of the input neurons fires.

The XOR function is a special case of the parity function which we considered in the chapter on perceptrons, since the output neuron will fire if an odd number (one) of input neurons fire and remain silent if an even number (zero or two) of input neurons fire. As we mentioned in the previous chapter, a perceptron which calculates the parity function must be of infinite order, that is, the highest-order subpredicate increases without limit as the size of the retina increases.

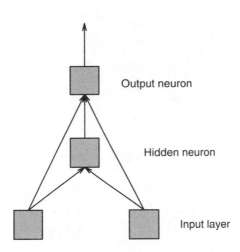

Output neuron

Hidden neuron

Input layer

Figure 19.2   A network used to solve the XOR problem.

A network used by the PDP group for calculating the XOR of two inputs is shown in Fig. 19.2. The input layer contains two neurons, there is a single hidden layer containing one neuron and a single output neuron. In this model, the two input neurons and the hidden neuron make direct connections with the output neuron. In addition, the two input neurons connect with the hidden neuron.

The network is trained by repeatedly presenting the four possible input patterns (in random order) to the input neurons, allowing the network to generate its output for each pattern, and then training it using the back propagation algorithm. The changes in the three weights for connections to the output neuron can be calculated directly using eqn (19.24), and the changes to the two weights leading to the hidden neuron can then be calculated using eqn (19.22).

Notice that although this network may look like a perceptron in that there is a retina (the two input neurons) a subpredicate (the hidden neuron) and a final predicate (the output neuron), it is not a perceptron because (i) the weights connecting the input layer to the hidden neuron are allowed to vary and (ii) there are direct connections from the input layer to the output layer.

The PDP group reports that the solution shown in Fig. 19.3 was reached after 558 presentations of the four patterns (a total of 2232 learning cycles).[3] The solution shows that the hidden neuron and the output

---

[3]The author used his own version of a delta rule program to train this net and found that it usually required significantly more learning cycles before a solution was found.

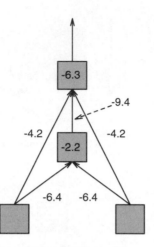

Figure 19.3   A solution of the XOR problem with negative thresholds. Weights are shown adjacent to connections between neurons; thresholds are shown on the neuron body.

neuron attained negative thresholds, and that all of the weights were negative. If you trace through the network by hand for each of the four inputs, you will find that the network does indeed produce the desired output for each one. For example, given the input where neuron 1 in the input layer fires and neuron 2 does not, we require the output neuron to fire. Let us trace through the network to see what happens.

The hidden neuron will receive an input of −6.4, which does not exceed its threshold of −2.2, so it will not fire. The output neuron therefore receives a total input of −4.2, which exceeds its threshold of −6.3, so it will fire, as required. That the net generates the correct behaviour for the other three input patterns may be verified in a similar manner.

Despite the fact that this network solves the XOR problem, does it actually represent a biologically plausible solution? The fact that both neurons above the input layer have negative thresholds means that they will always fire unless they are turned off by inhibition from other neurons. In fact, in the network shown in Fig. 19.3, the hidden neuron will only fire when neither of the input neurons fires, that is, when it receives no input at all. Although there are many circumstances in which biological neurons fire continuously without external stimuli, the existence of such neurons in a network designed to recognize patterns is a bit dubious.

A wide spread of solutions is also possible.

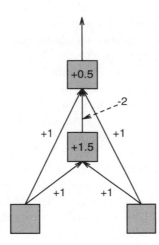

Figure 19.4 A solution of the XOR problem with positive thresholds.

However, the solution in Fig. 19.3 is not the only solution with the same network architecture. Figure 19.4 shows a different solution in which both neurons have positive thresholds.[4] This solution is much more biologically plausible.

The existence of two solutions for the same problem in the same network architecture raises the question of just how many solutions there are. This is a question that is difficult to answer, since there are no rigorous mathematical theorems about existence and uniqueness of solutions in PDP theory. We pointed out the problems with local minima in the energy space when we introduced the gradient descent method above. Unfortunately, there is no sure-fire way of avoiding these problems, although we can take some comfort from the fact that we can always tell if we obtained a correct answer simply by testing the net's response to each of the input patterns.

The PDP authors claim that local minima occur only rarely, and are fairly easy to escape by jolting the parameters a bit and then retraining the network. However, they have only treated small-scale problems. It is likely that increasing the size of the network and the complexity of the problem it is supposed to solve will also increase the number of local minima and

---

[4]The reader who wishes to refer to the PDP article from which these figures were taken should be cautioned that the PDP authors refer to *thresholds* of neurons in one figure (with the same meaning as we are using) and *biases* in the other figure. The PDP authors define a bias to be the negative of a threshold. Merely glancing at the two figures without studying the accompanying captions and text will not reveal this.

non-biological solutions, and the difficulty of detecting and escaping from them.

Another problem with multilayered networks is the length of time required to train them. We mentioned above that the XOR problem is a special case of the more general parity problem: given N inputs with some subset of them firing, determine if the number n of firing input neurons is even or odd. Minsky and Papert showed that on the order of 2^N calculations are needed for a perceptron to solve this problem. The PDP authors found that networks with N inputs required N hidden units (all in the same layer) and a single output to solve the parity problem. However, for the case of a network with four input cells (hence $2^4 = 16$ possible input patterns) the network required 2825 presentations of *each* pattern (a total of 45 200 training cycles) before the net could correctly determine the parity of its input lines. This net takes more than 20 times as many training cycles as the XOR net. If this is an indication of the rate of growth of the training time required for the parity problem, we are certainly no better off with a multilayer net than we were with a perceptron.

It is perhaps the enormous number of training sessions required by these nets that causes the greatest concern when we attempt to use them as models for biological systems. The neurons in the human brain can communicate with each other in the space of a few milliseconds at best. Each training cycle, when applied to a real person or animal, requires not only impressing a pattern on the network which is to learn the task at hand, but also the sensory processing, muscle coordination and so on which must accompany each cycle. If even the simplest task took thousands of repetitions to learn, humans would be incapable of doing much more than a sea slug. This drawback is frequently overlooked because these neural network models are run on modern computers with circuitry that is capable of working more than a million times faster than the human brain. It is precisely this fact which makes neural network models useful, since neural network algorithms make computers appear intelligent. The term 'artificial intelligence', as applied to these models when they are used in a computer, has, perhaps, an unintentional connotation. The intelligence shown by computers is based on methods that are far too inefficient for use in 'real' intelligence.

However, we must not be too negative in our assessment of such models, lest we run the risk of dampening research initiative in the area.[5] These models do show the ability to learn patterns by adjusting synaptic weights in a network that is at least superficially biological. The challenge to future researchers is to retain the biologically relevant features, but to improve the efficiency of the networks.

---

[5]There really isn't much chance of that!

20

Attractor neural networks

20.1 Introduction

Up to now, the memory models we have considered have been what we might call 'single-pass' networks. Once a set of patterns has been learned, only a single pass through the network is required to produce a response when an input is presented. A perceptron, having only one layer, essentially requires only a single computation to produce an answer of 'true' or 'false'. A PDP network with hidden units may require several computations, but only one sweep of the net from the input layer to the output layer is needed before a response is generated.

An *attractor neural network* is similar to the nets we have already considered in that it can be trained to respond in certain ways to a set of patterns, but differs in that retrieval of a pattern is an iterative process, rather than a one-shot calculation. Such networks have the ability to reconstruct an entire pattern from fragments of the original, a feature called *associative memory*. We have all experienced this effect in everyday life; for example, you may see a person who resembles someone you know, although the person doesn't look exactly like your friend. Certain things, such as hair colour, eye colour, height, build, and so on, may remind you of your friend, and these factors serve as a fragment of an overall pattern which contains a more complete picture of the person you know. Your mind will use these fragments to iteratively build up a larger part of the complete picture. Probably the first thing to be reconstructed is a complete image of your friend's face, changing the features from those of the person who resembled your friend to the features your friend actually has. From there, you may start to remember other things about your friend, such as things he says or does, good times you have spent together, arguments you have had, and so on. Each of these memories is retrieved because they are *associated* with another memory that has just been retrieved, except for the first occurrence of a memory of your friend which was triggered by seeing the other person in the street.

In such an associative chain of memories, it is also common to make errors. You might remember your friend as having a certain shade of blue eyes whereas the true shade is quite different. Later in the chain of memories you might recall that your friend said something on a particular occasion, when, in fact, it was someone else who was there at the same time. The chance of making such errors depends to a large extent on how vivid your memories of these events are. If someone is holding a knife to your throat you are more likely to remember details of that event than you are of going to the shop to buy a litre of milk (assuming that the former event happens to you rarely and the latter is a common occurrence). Thus a memory is more likely to be correctly recalled if it dominates your pattern of thinking.

Attractor neural networks (ANNs for short) attempt to model these sorts of events in a network that is at least superficially biological. The theory of the ANN has been developed largely by physicists, so the language and concepts used may not be familiar to those without a physics background. As this book does not assume such a background, we cannot develop the theory of the ANN to any great depth, but we can get a good feel for how the models work, and how biologically realistic they are.

A brief outline of how an ANN works may be useful before we consider the details below. The network is constructed of the same type of neuron which we have used in all our models so far: a simple point object which sums its inputs and fires if the inputs exceed the threshold of the neuron. Memories are stored in the network either by specifying a set of synaptic weights in advance, or by a learning procedure similar to those we have used in the preceding chapters.

Assuming the net has the correct weights stored, it can be used to retrieve memories by presenting a pattern to the net and then waiting for it to decide on its response. Unlike the perceptron and PDP nets, all neurons in an ANN are on the same level: they serve as input, output, and intermediate units during the course of a calculation. Starting with the input pattern, which is a set of signals presented to the entire net, not just to one layer, the neurons will send signals to each other over several time cycles, changing their firing patterns in the process. Eventually, the net will usually settle into a stable pattern of activity, where the same neurons are firing from one cycle to the next. When (if) this happens, the net has converged on a stable activity state, and this stable state may be taken as the net's 'response' to the input pattern. In other words, imposing a particular pattern of excitation on the net as an initial condition causes the net to follow a dynamic path and settle on some stable fixed pattern of activity. This pattern is the net's version of a memory that has been recalled by the input pattern.

ANNs originated with two main contributions: a paper published by Little (1974) and one by Hopfield (1982). Most of what has been done in the area since those times can be traced back to one or the other of these papers. A good overview of the subject can be found in the book by Daniel J. Amit

(1989). Amit's book attempts to present the theory of the ANN in a way that is accessible to those with about the same mathematical background as readers of this book are assumed to have, and limited exposure to biology or physics, although those readers with limited exposure to physics will find it heavy going. It also contains a comprehensive set of references.

20.2 The basic models

Both the Little and Hopfield models use a minimal neuron as their unit of calculation. Unfortunately, each paper on the subject seems to have invented its own notation for the various quantities. We will attempt to follow the notation used in Amit's book as far as possible.

A network is composed of N neurons all of which can potentially be linked by synapses in both directions. The synaptic strength *from* neuron j *to* neuron i is defined to be J_{ij}. Positive values of the Js correspond to excitatory synapses, negative to inhibitory synapses. The larger the magnitude of J, the stronger the connection. Neurons are assumed never to make synapses on themselves, so $J_{ii} \equiv 0$ for all i.

A neuron is assumed to be in one of two states: firing or not firing. The state of neuron i is given by a variable σ_i which is 1 if the neuron is firing and 0 if it is not. Most of the analyses of ANNs are easier to do if the state of the neuron is represented by $+1$ or -1 rather than 1 or 0. To accomplish this, a new variable S_i is defined as

$$S_i \equiv 2\sigma_i - 1. \tag{20.1}$$

The input received by a neuron over a certain time period is the sum of its inputs from all other neurons, weighted by the corresponding synaptic strengths. Defining U_i to be the input received by neuron i, we have

$$U_i = \frac{1}{2} \sum_{j=1}^{N} J_{ij}(S_i + 1). \tag{20.2}$$

Note that the term with $j = i$ is automatically excluded from this sum since $J_{ii} = 0$. This convention saves us the trouble of having to explicitly state that each such sum excludes the self-synapse term.

The response of neuron i after receiving this input depends on which form of the model we are considering. Before we go any further, we will stop and consider our options.

Synchronous or asynchronous? Little's model assumes a so-called *synchronous* updating rule for the net. In his model, the neurons are given the chance to change their state at regular clock intervals, so that the entire net could change its character all at once. In this model, the state of the neuron at clock tick $n + 1$, $S(n + 1)$, depends only on the states of the neurons at tick n.

In Hopfield's model, the updating is *asynchronous*. Here, only one neuron is updated at a time, so that the overall state of the net can change only gradually. In a simulation, a neuron is chosen at random from the set of all N neurons. The input as given by eqn (20.2) for the current state of the net is calculated and the response of the neuron (by methods to be given below) is determined. This new state of the neuron is then used in all future calculations of the behaviour of other neurons in the net, until that neuron is chosen again.

Is there any noise? The perceptron and PDP models we have considered in the preceding chapters assume that neurons have a precise threshold response: if the sum of the inputs to a neuron exceeds the threshold, the neuron will fire. In reality, of course, the effect of an action potential on the postsynaptic neuron can vary somewhat, due to varying amounts of neurotransmitter that are released, background chemical and electrical interference and so on. The models offer the option of considering either 'clean' nets without such effects, or 'noisy' nets where some account is taken of these fluctuations. Originally, Little's model incorporated noise effects while Hopfield's model did not.

In Hopfield's model, there is assumed to be no noise, so the updating rule is simply

$$S_i = \operatorname{sgn}\left(U_i - T_i\right) \tag{20.3}$$

where T_i is the threshold for neuron i, U_i is the input as given by eqn (20.2) and the sign function returns the sign of its argument:

$$\operatorname{sgn}\left(x\right) = \begin{cases} +1 & \text{if } x > 0 \\ -1 & \text{if } x \leq 0 \end{cases} \tag{20.4}$$

A typical simulation using a Hopfield net would begin by assigning values to the synaptic strengths J_{ij} (which we will consider below) and to the states of the neurons S_i. Then neurons are chosen randomly, one at a time, and the updating rule (20.3) applied to each one. The process continues until we decide to stop.

To simulate Little's synchronous model without noise, we would set up the net as for the Hopfield simulation. Instead of choosing neurons one at a time, we update the entire net using rule (20.3). Note that two sets of S_is will need to be stored, since only the old values of S_i are to be used to generate *all* the new states of the net.

If we introduce noise into the model, the updating rule (20.3) becomes a probabilistic rule rather than the deterministic one used in the Hopfield model. The assumption made in Little's model is that the actual change in the membrane potential of neuron i produced by the action potentials arriving from other neurons is normally distributed[1] with a mean $\bar{U}_i$ given by eqn (20.2):

$$\bar{U}_i = \frac{1}{2} \sum_{j=1}^{N} J_{ij}(S_i + 1). \qquad (20.5)$$

The variance depends on the effects mentioned above (variation in neurotransmitter released, background electrical and chemical noise, and so on). If we represent this variance by δ^2, then the probability density for the actual change in membrane potential U_i received by cell i is

$$P(U_i) = \frac{1}{\sqrt{2\pi\delta^2}} \exp\left[-\frac{(U_i - \bar{U}_i)^2}{2\delta^2}\right]. \qquad (20.6)$$

Now the probability that the neuron will fire is the probability that its potential U_i exceeds the threshold T_i, which is the integral of the density (20.6) over the region $U_i > T_i$. This is the quantity that can be found in tables of the normal distribution. We have:

$$Prob(S_i = 1) = \int_{T_i}^{\infty} P(U_i)dU_i = \frac{1}{2}\left[1 + \text{erf}\left(\frac{\bar{U}_i - T_i}{\sqrt{2}\delta}\right)\right] \qquad (20.7)$$

where erf (x) is the *error function*:

$$\text{erf}(x) \equiv \frac{2}{\sqrt{\pi}} \int_{x}^{\infty} e^{-t^2} dt. \qquad (20.8)$$

Since the neuron must be either firing or not firing, the probability that the neuron will be in the non-firing state is

$$Prob(S_i = -1) = 1 - Prob(S_i = 1) = \frac{1}{2}\left[1 - \text{erf}\left(\frac{\bar{U}_i - T_i}{\sqrt{2}\delta}\right)\right]. \qquad (20.9)$$

Using the fact that the error function is odd, so that erf $(-x) = -$ erf (x), we can combine the two probabilities into a single equation, where $Prob(S_i)$ is to be interpreted as the probability that the state of neuron i after receiving its input will be S_i. We have

$$Prob(S_i) = \frac{1}{2}\left[1 + \text{erf}\left(\frac{S_i(\bar{U}_i - T_i)}{\sqrt{2}\delta}\right)\right]. \qquad (20.10)$$

A reasonable approximation to the error function is

$$\frac{1}{2}(1 - \text{erf}(x)) \approx \frac{1}{1 + e^x}. \qquad (20.11)$$

---

[1]See Appendix B for a discussion of the normal distribution.

Applying this approximation to eqn (20.10), we obtain a form which is more amenable to calculation:

$$Prob(S_i) \approx \frac{\exp(\beta h_i S_i)}{\exp(\beta h_i S_i) + \exp(-\beta h_i S_i)} = \frac{1}{2}[1 + \tanh(\beta h_i S_i)] \quad (20.12)$$

where $h_i = \bar{U}_i - T_i$, $\beta = 1/(\sqrt{2}\delta)$, and the hyperbolic tangent, $\tanh x$ is defined as

$$\tanh x \equiv \frac{e^x - e^{-x}}{e^x + e^{-x}}. \quad (20.13)$$

Note that $\tanh x$ tends to -1 as x tends to negative infinity, and to $+1$ as x tends to positive infinity. Thus, as we would expect, if the input received by the neuron is much below threshold, the probability of the neuron firing tends to zero, and if the input is much greater than threshold, the neuron is almost certain to fire.

To incorporate noise into either Little's or Hopfield's model, we replace the deterministic eqn (20.3) by a step which calculates the probability of the neuron firing according to eqn (20.12). This can be done by generating a random number r between 0 and 1 and comparing r to $Prob(S_i = +1)$. If $r < Prob(S_i = +1)$, then $S_i = 1$, otherwise $S_i = 0$.

20.3   Determining the synaptic weights

One of the main differences between an ANN and the perceptron-like networks we have considered up to now is that an ANN is a dynamical system: once the geometry of the network is specified and initial conditions given, the net will continue to evolve without any further input. The network may settle into a stable pattern or enter into some other form of behaviour, but the neural activity will never cease. Whereas, in a perceptron or PDP model, we feed an input pattern into the input layer of the net and wait for an answer to be produced in the output layer, in an ANN we must examine the state of the net after some time to determine the state at which the net has arrived, if any.

If the net is started off with some pattern of activity that is close to the pattern that was learned, then the learned pattern should emerge after the net has gone through several cycles of updating by one of the rules given in the previous section. For example, a net of 4 neurons could be taught the pattern $[-1, 1, 1, -1]$, which means that the first and fourth neurons are not firing and the second and third neurons are. Then if the net is started off in the state $[1, 1, 1, -1]$ and allowed to go through several cycles of updating, hopefully it will converge on the learned state: $[-1, 1, 1, -1]$. If this state is dynamically stable, the net will remain in that pattern of activity forever (in a noiseless model). If more than one pattern has been memorized, the net will converge on one of the memorized patterns, usually the pattern closest to the initial state. The problem is to determine the values of the synaptic weights J_{ij} which will make the desired patterns stable states in the net's dynamics.

20.3.1 Symmetric weights

As mentioned above, there are two methods by which the synaptic weights J_{ij} may be determined for a net which is to memorize a set of patterns. One method is a generalization of the perceptron learning rule, which we will get to later. However, the most common procedure is the one used by Hopfield in his original model. The idea is very loosely based on the Hebb rule that a synapse which fires during the learning of a pattern is strengthened relative to those synapses that do not fire. Suppose we have a net of N neurons which is to learn the pattern given by $[\xi_1, \xi_2, \ldots, \xi_N]$, where $\xi_i = \pm 1$ depending on whether neuron i is to be firing or not. If this is the first pattern which the net is to learn, we would begin by setting all the synaptic weights to zero: $J_{ij} = 0$ for all i and j.

The Hopfield prescription for the change in the weight J_{ij} when this pattern is added to the net's repertoire is

$$\Delta J_{ij} = \frac{1}{N} \xi_i \xi_j \tag{20.14}$$

with the usual condition that $\Delta J_{ii} = 0$, since neurons do not make synapses on themselves.

If a total of p patterns are to memorized by the net, the overall synaptic weight between neurons i and j is the sum of all these changes, so

$$J_{ij} = \frac{1}{N} \sum_{\mu=1}^{p} \xi_i^\mu \xi_j^\mu \tag{20.15}$$

where ξ_i^μ is the state of the ith neuron in the μth pattern.

Equation (20.15) implies that the synaptic weights are symmetric ($J_{ij} = J_{ji}$). Biologically, this implies that every pair of neurons has a synapse in both directions, and that these synapses are of equal strength. There is absolutely no justification for this assumption, and this fact has been the main criticism of the model by neurobiologists. Since the assumption is so non-biological, why is it made? The answer seems to be that if the weights are *not* symmetric, it is very difficult to do much analysis on the model without resorting to computer simulations. This, in itself, is not a particularly good reason to make the assumption. However, in this case, work has been done to investigate how far the conclusions obtained from the symmetric model extend to cases where the weights are not symmetric. The general conclusion is that the nets become somewhat less efficient at storing and retrieving patterns, but not drastically so.

The form of the weights also implies that a synapse is strengthened if both of the neurons that it connects do *not* fire in a given pattern, and that the synapse is weakened if one fires but the other does not. Again, there is no biological evidence for either of these assumptions. In fact there is some evidence that inactive synapses do not change at all. Studies have shown that if these assumptions are relaxed somewhat, the net is still capable of storing and retrieving patterns, though with reduced efficiency.

Despite the extra work that has been done on ANN models in attempts to make them more realistic, one cannot get away from the fact that they are not biologically plausible models from the very beginning. The studies referred to in the last couple of paragraphs assume that the weights are first constructed according to eqn (20.15) and *then* perturbed to remove some of the symmetry. In a biological network, of course, the weights are *never* symmetric, so the whole scheme of learning is different. The value of ANN models is not as a theory of how learning takes place in a brain; rather they show the structure that a network may have after learning has taken place. The idea that a retrieved memory is a persistent state of activity in a network rather than a single set of output values which is read once and then discarded (as assumed by the perceptron and PDP models, for example) does seem closer to reality. When we recall something, the memory is not just there for a split second and then gone; it remains for quite some time, and can affect our future thought patterns.

20.3.2   Training the net

A somewhat more realistic approach to determining the weights is to generalize the perceptron learning algorithm (see Chapter 18).

Suppose the net is currently in the state μ, which is one of the patterns it is supposed to learn. Then the firing pattern of the net at the current time is given by the vector $[\xi_1^\mu, \xi_2^\mu, \ldots, \xi_N^\mu]$ and the current state of neuron i is ξ_i^μ. Now in order that this pattern be stable, each neuron must remain in the same state in the next time cycle. That is, if neuron i is currently firing, we must have

$$\sum_{j=1}^{N} J_{ij}\xi_i^\mu \xi_j^\mu > T_i \qquad (20.16)$$

where T_i is the threshold of neuron i. The inequality is reversed if neuron i is not firing.

If we have p patterns, all of which are to be stable attractors, the same condition must hold for all patterns.

Now focus on one particular neuron, say neuron i. This neuron must respond correctly according to inequality (20.16) (or its reverse for a non-firing neuron) for all p patterns. Thus neuron i on its own behaves exactly like a perceptron. A net of N such neurons is, in effect, a collection of N perceptrons. Since the weights J_{ij} are independent for each neuron (here we are not assuming that the weights must be symmetric), the perceptron learning theorem can be applied to each neuron separately to work out the values of the weights.

The formal correspondence between the notation of this chapter and that of Chapter 18 is:

$$J_{ij} \quad \rightarrow \quad A_j \tag{20.17}$$
$$\xi_i^\mu \xi_j^\mu \quad \rightarrow \quad \phi_j \tag{20.18}$$

The quantity $\xi_i^\mu \xi_j^\mu$ thus plays the role of the subpredicate in perceptron theory.

The algorithm for training the net then proceeds analogously to the perceptron learning algorithm.

1. Choose a random set of initial values for the J_{ij}s.

2. Choose one of the patterns to be learned.

3. For neuron i, $i = 1, \ldots, N$, test to see if its response is correct according to relation (20.16). If so, leave it alone. If not, then change J_{ij}, for $j = 1, \ldots, N$, $j \neq i$, by adding $\xi_i^\mu \xi_j^\mu$.

4. Repeat from step 2 until convergence is obtained (or until you get tired of waiting, in which case a solution probably doesn't exist).

Just as with perceptron theory, we cannot guarantee that a solution will exist. However, it can be shown that if the number of patterns to be learned is small enough, a solution always exists. There are theoretical limits on the number of patterns that can be memorized, though if you want to try learning more patterns than this, it may still be possible.

The proof that this algorithm works is similar to that for a single perceptron, so we will not dwell on it here. Details can be found in the paper by Gardner (1988).

20.4 Dynamics and attractors

The reader may have noticed that the same symbol J_{ij} is used here for the synaptic weights as was used in Chapter 4 for the interaction between two bases in a primitive RNA molecule when we were considering the spin glass model of the origin of life. This is not a coincidence, since both the origin of life model and the ANN model had their origins in the same area of physics: the theory of magnetism. In magnetic theory, J_{ij} represents the strength of the interaction between two atomic or molecular 'spins' S_i and S_j, and the overall state of a system is determined by minimizing an energy function given by

$$E = -\frac{1}{2} \sum_{i \neq j} J_{ij} S_i S_j. \qquad (20.19)$$

In the origin of life model, a spin represents a particular type of base in an RNA molecule. In the ANN model, it represents the state (firing or not firing) of a neuron.

In the origin of life model, the energy E was used to determine the probability of survival of the various sequences of RNA molecules that had formed in the last generation—the lower a molecule's energy, the greater its chance of survival. In this way, the energy E determined the dynamics of the molecular population, since those molecules with a lower energy would tend to increase their numbers at the expense of those with a higher energy. We will see that the same energy function determines the dynamics of an ANN as well.

Another feature of the energy function that makes it particularly attractive as a model of the origin of life is that it has a large number of local minima, providing a large assortment of relatively stable molecular sequences. This feature is also attractive for a model of memory, since if each local minimum corresponds to a memorized pattern, the presence of many minima means a high capacity for memorized patterns.

To see how the energy function (20.19) determines the dynamics of an ANN, consider first the noiseless Hopfield model. Recall the rule (20.3) for determining the state of a Hopfield neuron: the state S_k of neuron k is determined by comparing the total input to neuron k with its threshold T_k. Assuming that the state of the neuron changes, let us calculate the change ΔE in the energy that results from the change. Neuron k appears in two places in the energy: in the factors S_i and S_j (when $i = k$ or $j = k$ in the sum). The change in E will result from terms containing S_k only. If S_k changes, then it will simply change its sign: $S_k \rightarrow -S_k$. The resulting change in E will be:

$$\Delta E = S_k \sum_{j=1}^{N} J_{kj} S_j + S_k \sum_{j=1}^{N} J_{jk} S_j. \qquad (20.20)$$

Now consider the first term. Using the relation between the 'spin' variables S_i and the actual neuronal state variables σ_i given by eqn (20.1), we have for this term:

$$S_k \sum_{j=1}^{N} J_{kj} S_j = S_k \left(2 \sum_{j=1}^{N} J_{kj} \sigma_j - \sum_{j=1}^{N} J_{kj} \right). \qquad (20.21)$$

Using relation (20.2), we have

$$S_k \sum_{j=1}^{N} J_{kj} S_j = S_k \left(2U_k - \sum_{j=1}^{N} J_{kj} \right) \qquad (20.22)$$

where U_k is the total input into neuron k.

If neuron k receives input, on average, from half the other neurons, then its average input level will be $\bar{U}_k = \frac{1}{2} \sum_{j=1}^{N} J_{kj}$, so we can write

$$S_k \sum_{j=1}^{N} J_{kj} S_j = 2S_k \left(U_k - \bar{U}_k \right). \qquad (20.23)$$

It turns out that the largest number of patterns can be stored in a network where the average input to each neuron is the same as the threshold, that is, $\bar{U}_k = T_k$. If we are dealing with a network where this condition holds, then we have

$$S_k \sum_{j=1}^{N} J_{kj} S_j = 2S_k \left(U_k - T_k \right). \qquad (20.24)$$

Now, if neuron k has just changed sign, then using eqn (20.3), we must have $S_k = -\text{sgn}\,(U_k - T_k)$, so that the right hand side in eqn (20.24) is always negative.

In a general network, the matrix element J_{kj} has no correlation with element J_{jk}, so we cannot guarantee that the second term in eqn (20.20) is also negative. However, if the synaptic weights are symmetric, then $J_{kj} = J_{jk}$ and the two terms on the right-hand side of eqn (20.20) are identical. In such a case, whenever a neuron changes state, the energy is lowered. Thus, for this special case, we can guarantee that the net will converge on one of the minima of the energy function.

Of course, we had to impose some biologically unrealistic conditions to arrive at this condition. In a real neural network, it is unlikely that the synaptic weights will be symmetric, just as it is unlikely that the average input on each neuron will be equal to that neuron's threshold potential. However, several analytic and numerical studies have been done which indicate that these conditions can be violated to a certain degree without removing the net's ability to converge onto one of its stored memories. In a completely general network, though, this is far from certain, and such nets can exhibit oscillatory or even chaotic behaviour.

A similar analysis can be done for the synchronous Little model, and it is found that the energy function plays a similar role. However, with synchronous dynamics, it is possible for the network to oscillate even if the synaptic weights are symmetric.

To discuss the dynamics of a noisy network, we need to understand a fair bit about thermodynamics. Since such a background is not assumed of the reader, we will not enter into any details of noisy dynamics. The energy function can now be used to calculate a probability of the net being in any given state, and it is found that the lower the energy of a state, the higher the probability that the system will be found in that state. Thus the energy still governs the dynamics of the system, although its effects are statistical, rather than absolute, in the presence of noise.

20.5   Network capacity

How many patterns can a network of a given size hold? In order to answer this question, we need to define a bit more precisely the problem we are trying to solve. For example, when we say that the net has 'memorized' a pattern, are we requiring that it can recall the entire pattern perfectly, or would we be satisfied with, say 90 per cent of the initial pattern? What restrictions are we placing on the synaptic weights? Are we requiring them to be symmetric, or are we determining them by using the learning theorem described above?

Let us begin by considering a Hopfield network like that used in the last section. It has symmetric synaptic weights, and each neuron has a threshold equal to its average input. In such a case, the asynchronous updating rule (20.3) becomes

$$S_i \;=\; \text{sgn}\,(U_i - T_i) \tag{20.25}$$

$$=\; \text{sgn}\left(\frac{1}{2} \sum_{j=1}^{N} J_{ij}(S_j + 1) - T_i \right) \tag{20.26}$$

$$=\; \text{sgn}\left(\frac{1}{2} \sum_{j=1}^{N} J_{ij} S_j \right) \tag{20.27}$$

where we have used the condition $\sum_{j=1}^{N} J_{ij} = 2T_i$, obtained from the condition that each neuron's threshold T_i is equal to its average input.

Now suppose such a net has had p patterns stored in it by specifying the synaptic weights according to eqn (20.15). The state of neuron i is *stable* in this network if it retains its value from one update to the next. In order for an entire pattern to be stable, all neurons must remain in the same state once they are placed in the state corresponding to the pattern. The condition for neuron i to remain in the same state is

$$S_i I_i > 0 \qquad (20.28)$$

where

$$I_i \equiv \sum_{j=1}^{N} J_{ij} S_j = \frac{1}{N} \sum_{j=1,(j \neq i)}^{N} \sum_{\mu=1}^{p} \xi_i^\mu \xi_j^\mu S_j \qquad (20.29)$$

is the input to neuron i. As before, ξ_i^μ is the state of neuron i in pattern μ.

The condition (20.28) says that the input to neuron i must have the same sign as its current state, so that no change in state will take place.

Now let us investigate the stability of a particular neuron. Suppose that pattern 1 has been imposed on the net. Since all the other neurons in the net are in states dictated by pattern 1, we have $S_j = \xi_j^1$ for all j. Then neuron 1 will have value ξ_1^1 and the input to neuron 1 will be

$$I_1 = \frac{1}{N} \sum_{j=1,(j \neq i)}^{N} \sum_{\mu=1}^{p} \xi_1^\mu \xi_j^\mu \xi_j^1. \qquad (20.30)$$

Now the quantity $S_i I_i = \xi_1^1 I_1$ for neuron 1, and is given by

$$\xi_1^1 I_1 = \xi_1^1 \frac{1}{N} \sum_{j=1,(j \neq i)}^{N} \sum_{\mu=1}^{p} \xi_1^\mu \xi_j^\mu \xi_j^1. \qquad (20.31)$$

If we split the sum over patterns (μ) to isolate the term $\mu = 1$, we get

$$\xi_1^1 I_1 = \xi_1^1 \frac{1}{N} \sum_{j=1,(j \neq i)}^{N} \xi_1^1 \xi_j^1 \xi_j^1 + \xi_1^1 \frac{1}{N} \sum_{j=1,(j \neq i)}^{N} \sum_{\mu=2}^{p} \xi_1^\mu \xi_j^\mu \xi_j^1. \qquad (20.32)$$

Now, since $\xi_j^1 = \pm 1$, the first term gives merely $(N-1)/N$, so we have

$$\xi_1^1 I_1 = \frac{N-1}{N} + \xi_1^1 \frac{1}{N} \sum_{j=1,(j \neq i)}^{N} \sum_{\mu=2}^{p} \xi_1^\mu \xi_j^\mu \xi_j^1. \qquad (20.33)$$

For large nets $(N-1)/N \approx 1$, so the question of stability reduces to asking if the second term ever gets more negative than -1. The second term is a sum of the product of four quantities, all of which are $+1$ or -1. There are $(N-1)(p-1)$ terms in the sum, so if most of the terms are -1, the sum could certainly become significantly negative. However, if we are dealing with random patterns, there should be no correlation between the states of a given neuron in two different patterns. Thus we would expect the terms in the sum to be $+1$ or -1 with equal probability. Adding up such a sequence of terms is known in the theory of stochastic processes as taking a *random walk* in one dimension. Random walks have been studied in detail and it is known that the root mean square distance from the origin of a walk of n steps is $\sqrt{n}$. In our case, the walk has $(N-1)(p-1) \approx Np$ steps, so the sum, on average, will have a magnitude of $\sqrt{Np}$. The second term therefore has a magnitude of $\sqrt{p/N}$.

We see that if $p \ll N$, the second term will be much less than 1 in magnitude, and the state of the neuron is stable. Since there was nothing special about neuron 1 or pattern 1 in the above argument, this is a demonstration that all patterns are stable, provided that we don't try to store too many patterns in the net.

But how many is too many? Instead of being happy with a vague statement like 'the second term has a magnitude of approximately $\sqrt{p/N}$', we might ask for the probability that the second term is greater than -1. Again, from the theory of random walks, the distance from the origin after n steps with values $+1$ or -1 follows a normal distribution with zero mean and variance n. Thus the variance of the second term in eqn (20.33) is p/N. The probability that any single neuron is stable is then

$$Prob(\xi_1^1 I_i > 0) \quad = \quad Prob(\text{second term } > -1) \tag{20.34}$$

$$= \quad \frac{1}{2}[1 + \text{ erf } (\sqrt{N/2p})] \tag{20.35}$$

where the error function erf (x) was defined in eqn (20.8).

We would still expect that, in order for all patterns to be recalled correctly, N would have to be considerably larger than p. If we assume this, we can use the approximation to the error function for small arguments, which is

$$\text{erf } (x) \approx 1 - \frac{1}{\sqrt{\pi}x}e^{-x^2}. \tag{20.36}$$

Using this approximation, we obtain

$$Prob(\xi_1^1 I_i > 0) \approx 1 - \sqrt{\frac{p}{2\pi N}}e^{-N/2p}. \tag{20.37}$$

This is the probability for a single neuron to be stable, but a random pattern contains N such neurons. To find the total probability that a pattern is stable, we must raise this single probability to the Nth power:

$$Prob(\text{stable pattern}) \quad \approx \quad \left[1 - \sqrt{\frac{p}{2\pi N}}e^{-N/2p} \right]^N \tag{20.38}$$

$$\approx \quad 1 - N \sqrt{\frac{p}{2\pi N}} e^{-N/2p}. \tag{20.39}$$

The approximation in the second equation assumes that the probability of an error is small enough that second order and higher terms (equivalent to those cases where more than one error occurs in a pattern) are negligible.

In order for this second term to be small, we need to ensure that $\sqrt{(p/2\pi N)}e^{-N/2p}$ decreases faster than $1/N$ with increasing N. Choosing $p = N/2\ln N$ makes this term equal to $(1/N)\sqrt{1/4\pi \ln N}$, so the second term decreases as $1/\sqrt{\ln N}$. (Obviously, any choice for p which makes this second term decrease faster is also acceptable, but the choice made here would seem to be a minimum requirement, since if p is made any larger, the exponential term will not decrease fast enough.)

The condition for all stored patterns to be stable is then

$$p < \frac{N}{2\ln N}. \tag{20.40}$$

Notice that this condition depends on the patterns being random, both with respect to each other and internally. If the patterns are correlated, the number that can be stored may decrease significantly, due to the difficulty of separating two patterns that are almost identical.

20.6 Summary

Let us summarize the pros and cons of attractor neural networks interpreted as models of biological memory.

On the plus side, an ANN exhibits associative memory, in a form perceptrons and PDP nets do not manage.[2] This ability arises from the inherently dynamical structure of the ANN which allows it to continually refine an input pattern until a previously learned pattern is obtained. This property seems to mimic quite well the human ability to begin with a fragment of an idea or memory and reconstruct a complete memory through successive stages of recognition.

However, as a theory of learning, the ANN suffers from similar problems to those encountered in perceptrons and multilayer nets. We are offered a choice of specifying a set of synaptic weights which will guarantee that a net will learn a set of patterns, or using a perceptron-like learning rule to memorize the various images. The first method introduces many artificial assumptions, such as symmetric weights, the strengthening of a connection

---

[2]Perceptron-like nets can learn to classify patterns they have not seen before in the same category as patterns to which they are similar, but this isn't the same thing as a truly associative memory, which requires a dynamical process to reconstruct a full memory from a fragment.

between two neurons, neither of which fires, and so on. The second method, although more biologically plausible, requires far too many learning sessions to be a truly biological model—a criticism that applies here just as it did in the perceptron and PDP models treated earlier.

21

Unsupervised learning

21.1 Introduction

The neural networks we have considered so far have all required an external teacher to tell them the correct response for each input. The networks learn by adjusting their synaptic weights to make their outputs correspond more closely to that desired by the teacher.

Many biological neural networks learn things this way. This is, after all, how most schools and universities operate—the teacher trains a class of students by requiring them to produce certain responses when given certain inputs. If the students produce the correct responses (on exams, for example), the neural pathways that produced these responses are strengthened, while if an incorrect answer is given, the student fails the exam and is required to continue training his neural network, either by studying for a second exam or by retaking the course.

It is possible to train many other animals to produce the correct responses in much the same way. Animals that provide some parental care of their offspring use the teacher–student training method on their own. However, there are a great many things which animals and people must learn for themselves, without the aid of a teacher. Probably much of the early training of an infant's brain proceeds without a teacher. Interpreting a complex visual scene is something that all animals with eyes learn to do at an early age. It is something that people do almost at the subconscious level, since we use visual skills to avoid bumping into objects when we move about. So natural does this ability appear to us that we do not appreciate the enormous amount of computing power that we are using to do it. Recent attempts to develop robots using artificial neural networks that can successfully navigate through a space with only a few stationary objects have demonstrated that the task is not a trivial one. Yet, natural networks seem able to learn how to do these things without the aid of a teacher.

In this chapter, we will examine a few relatively simple models in which a neural network can be trained to recognize patterns, or groups of patterns, without the aid of a teacher. The only control the experimenter has over such a network is, firstly, specifying the geometry of the network (how many neurons there are and how they are connected together) and, secondly, specifying in a general way how individual neurons should respond to their inputs. The net is trained, in the usual way, by presenting patterns to the net and allowing it to modify its weights by some rule. The net is not required to produce any particular set of output patterns. Rather, we sit back and watch what the net will make of the patterns it is being fed as input.

We usually find that the net will learn to classify the input patterns into several groups based on some criteria that may or may not be obvious to the observer. For example, networks of this sort have been trained to distinguish between an empty street and a street that is crowded with people. Attempts at training such nets sometimes lead to unexpected results. One military application of such a net attempted to train the network to distinguish between pictures of a field containing tanks and the same field without tanks. After a lengthy training session in which pictures of the field in both conditions were presented to the network, it classified the pictures into two groups, but these groups seemed to have no relation to whether there were tanks present in the pictures or not. Eventually it was discovered that all the pictures in one classification had been taken on sunny days, and all those in the other classification had been taken on overcast days, or in the early morning or late evening when lighting was poor. The network had classified the images according to their brightness, completely ignoring the tanks.

The moral of this story is that if you want your network to classify its input in a particular way, you must choose the input in a way that highlights the distinctions you wish to emphasize.

21.2   Competitive learning

One of the simplest models which illustrates unsupervised learning is that by Rumelhart and Zipser (1986) of the PDP group. The network is a multilayer one similar to that used in the back-propagation system in Chapter 19.

The first layer of the network is an array of N_1 single input neurons. A pattern is presented to the net by stimulating some subset of these neurons. If the net is to analyse a series of pictures of a street with varying numbers of people on it, each picture could be digitized so that it becomes an array of black or white pixels, similar to a photograph in a newspaper. A black pixel would correspond to a stimulated input neuron, and white pixel to a quiescent one. Other kinds of data must be transformed so that they can be represented as such an array.

Every input neuron has an excitatory connection to every neuron in the second layer of the net. The second (and higher, if any) layer is where the processing of the input patterns begins. In the most general case, the second layer will contain N_2 neurons divided into g_2 groups, where the subscript 2 indicates the second layer. Inside each of these groups, there will be $n_{2,i}$ neurons, where $i = 1, \ldots, g_2$. Not all the groups need have the same number of neurons. Within each group, all neurons are connected to each other with *inhibitory* synapses. These inhibitory connections ensure that only the neuron with the largest input in a given group will be active, since it will inhibit the other members in the group more than the other members will inhibit it. Neurons from different groups in the same layer are not connected. The weights of the inhibitory connections within a group are fixed, so that they remain constant during the training process. The weights of the excitatory connections from the input layer to layer 2 (and from layer 2 to any higher layers) are variable. The notation for the weights presents something of a problem since each weight must connect a neuron from a particular group in the previous layer to a particular neuron in a particular group in the next layer. Thus to fully specify a weight we would need six subscripts: the neuron number, group number, and layer number for each of the two neurons that the weight connects. Although this notation would need to be used in a full description of the model, we will use a simplified notation here for the purposes of illustrating how the model works. We will define w_{ij} to be the weight connecting neuron i in one layer and neuron j in the next. The weights are normalized so that the sum of the weights for all signals coming into a single neuron in layer j is one:

$$\sum w_{ij} = 1 \qquad (21.1)$$

where the sum is taken over all neurons i that have a connection with neuron j in the next layer.

Before we describe how the weights are modified, we will examine what happens in such a network when an input pattern is presented.

Such a system gives rise to a 'winner takes all' situation within each group in layer 2. To see what this means, consider a specific layout (Fig. 21.1). Suppose that the input layer contains 5 neurons and the second layer consists of only one group containing two neurons. Let the weights be as given in the table:

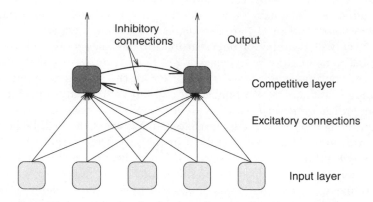

Figure 21.1   A simple competitive learning network.

Weights w_{ij}

i	j 1	2
1	0.2	0.5
2	0.0	0.1
3	0.6	0.1
4	0.1	0.2
5	0.1	0.1

Now suppose an input pattern where neurons $i = 1$, 3, and 5 are 'on' and neurons 2 and 4 are 'off' is presented to the net. In that case the signal received by neuron $j = 1$ in the second layer is $0.2 + 0.6 + 0.1 = 0.9$ and that received by neuron $j = 2$ is $0.5 + 0.1 + 0.1 = 0.7$. Thus neuron 1 receives the largest input and 'wins' the competition by inhibiting neuron 2. Neuron 1 will fire and neuron 2 will not.

Now if the input pattern is $i = 1$, 2, and 4, then neuron 1 receives a total of 0.3 and neuron 2 receives 0.8, so neuron 2 will win.

This simple network, as it stands, can already classify the input patterns into two groups: those that make neuron 1 fire and those that make neuron 2 fire. However, the classification would not be particularly meaningful, since the weights are more or less random, so the classification would be more or less random as well.

In what sort of a situation would we expect the net to produce a more meaningful classification if it were allowed to modify its weights? If all possible inputs were presented to the net with equal frequency, then there is no structure to the input data so we wouldn't expect the net to produce a meaningful distinction between different patterns. But suppose that certain patterns occur much more often than others. If we allow the weights to change in such a way that whenever an input pattern causes a neuron in the second layer to fire, the weights between the active input neurons and the active second layer neuron are strengthened, then sensitivity to that particular input pattern is increased. The next time that pattern, or one very similar to it, is presented to the net, the same neuron will respond even more vigorously. This is just the Hebbian learning rule again.

Now, if these common patterns fall naturally into two or more distinct groups (such as a set of pictures of empty and crowded streets), then each group may cause a different neuron in the second layer to fire, so that, with training, the net will be able to distinguish between input from each of these major groups.

The training rule proposed by Rumelhart and Zipser is as follows. Each time an input pattern is presented and a neuron in the second layer fires as a result of winning the competition over input from the first layer, the weights for the winning neuron are rearranged so that the weights on the active lines are increased and those on the inactive lines are decreased. Weights for lines leading from the input layer to inactive neurons in the second layer remain unchanged. Thus a particular neuron learns only if it wins the competition.

In order to maintain the normalization condition that the total weight on lines leading into each neuron be unity, an increase in weight on an active line must mean a decrease in weight on an inactive line. The prescription is, change each weight by an amount Δw_{ij}, where:

$$\Delta w_{ij} = \begin{cases} -\gamma w_{ij} & \text{if incoming line is inactive} \\ \gamma(1/a_k - w_{ij}) & \text{if incoming line is active.} \end{cases} \qquad (21.2)$$

Here γ is a scaling constant which specifies the learning rate. If $\gamma = 0$, no learning occurs, while if $\gamma = 1$, all inactive lines are effectively destroyed. In practice, a value of γ of around 0.1 is used. If γ is too large, the training process can become unstable, and if γ is too small, learning can take a very long time.

The quantity a_k is the number of active input lines in pattern k. Thus the algorithm requires each inactive line to transfer a fraction of its weight to an active line.

We can rewrite this rule in a more compact form if we define c_{ik} as follows:

$$c_{ik} = \begin{cases} 1 & \text{if input neuron } i \text{ is active in pattern } k \\ 0 & \text{if input neuron } i \text{ is not active in pattern } k \end{cases} \qquad (21.3)$$

Using this notation, the rule becomes:

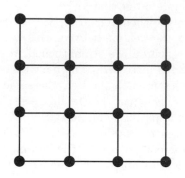

Figure 21.2   The input layer for the computer experiment. Black dots are neurons. An input pattern consists of two nearest neighbour neurons firing.

$$\Delta w_{ij} = \gamma \left(\frac{c_{ik}}{a_k} - w_{ij} \right) \tag{21.4}$$

Thus the first term is non-zero only if neuron i is active when pattern k is presented.

21.2.1   Computer experiments

In order to see how the competitive learning model behaves, let us examine a simple computer experiment described by Rumelhart and Zipser. The input layer consists of 16 neurons arranged in a four-by-four square (Fig. 21.2). There is a single higher level, consisting of only two neurons in a single inhibitory group. Thus the system should classify whatever patterns are presented in the input layer into two categories.

Each input pattern will consist of exactly two neurons firing. The neurons must be nearest neighbours either vertically or horizontally (not diagonally). There are thus 24 possible patterns (3 nearest-neighbour pairs in each row and column of the square). The weights are initially chosen randomly, subject to the condition that they are all positive, and that the total weight into each of the two second-layer neurons is unity. Then patterns are presented randomly to the input layer and the learning rule given above is applied. In practice, several thousand training steps are needed for the net to converge on a moderately stable set of weights.

After training, the weights are examined to see if any pattern can be found. What invariably happens is that the patterns are indeed divided into two groups. The square is usually divided in half vertically, horizontally, or diagonally, so that an input pattern lying in one half of the square will always cause the same neuron in the second layer to fire (Fig. 21.3). By

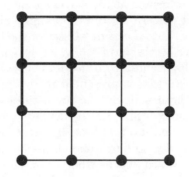

Figure 21.3 A possible classification of paired input patterns by a competitive learning network. Pairs of neurons connected by heavy lines cause one of the two neurons in the second layer to fire, pairs connected by thin lines cause the other neuron to fire.

examining the weights produced in a computer simulation, we find that weights from those neurons in that half of the square to the neuron that does *not* fire are essentially zero, while those to the neuron that *does* fire are non-zero, with various values.

It is reasonably straightforward to extend the computer model to cope with more complex input patterns, and larger numbers of input or higher level neurons. Rumelhart and Zipser describe some of these extensions, but the end result is similar to what we observed in the simple model above: the patterns are classified into compact groups. Let us examine the model in a bit more detail to see if we can discover why this is so.

21.2.2 Analysis of the pair model

Although an analytic investigation of the dynamics of the competitive learning model would be very difficult, we can get some idea of how the model behaves by looking at the conditions for equilibrium. Equilibrium will occur when training has proceeded long enough that none of the weights changes even if further patterns are presented to the input layer and the learning rule is still applied. In order for an equilibrium to be reached, however, we have to assume that the patterns are presented in some uniform way, in the sense that each pattern will occur at a constant average rate. For example, if we have 24 patterns, as in the pair system above, pattern 1 may appear 2 per cent of the time, pattern 2, 5 per cent of the time, and so on. If this were not so, then we could never guarantee that the weights would converge, since once they had settled into more or less constant values, we could suddenly change the sorts of patterns being presented to the net which would cause the weights to change in response.

If the patterns are presented at fixed average rates, we can define p_k to be the probability that pattern k will be presented on any single training cycle. Pattern k will activate a certain subset of the input layer which we will describe, as above, by the term c_{ik} which is 1 if pattern k activates neuron i in the input layer and zero if it does not.

Now, for each pattern that is presented to the input layer, one of the neurons in the second layer will win the competition over signals arriving from the input layer and will fire. Let us define v_{jk} to be the probability that neuron j in the second layer will fire if pattern k is presented to the input layer. There is really nothing random about this process, since we have a well-defined rule which tells us whether or not a given neuron in the second layer will fire: neuron j will fire only if it receives more input from the first layer than any other neuron. Thus, v_{jk} will take on the value 1 if neuron j receives the largest input for pattern k and zero otherwise.

A weight w_{ij} will be modified when pattern k is presented only if neuron j wins the competition. Since pattern k appears a fraction p_k of the time, the probability that weight w_{ij} will be modified due to the appearance of pattern k on any single training cycle is a product: (probability that neuron j fires given that pattern k is presented)×(probability that pattern k is presented) $= v_{jk}p_k$. The *average* change in the weight w_{ij} per pattern, defined to be $\langle \Delta w_{ij} \rangle$, will be, therefore

$$\langle \Delta w_{ij} \rangle = \sum_k \Delta w_{ij} v_{jk} p_k. \tag{21.5}$$

Using the rule (21.4), this becomes

$$\langle \Delta w_{ij} \rangle = \gamma \sum_k \left(\frac{c_{ik}}{a_k} - w_{ij} \right) v_{jk} p_k. \tag{21.6}$$

At equilibrium, we require the average change in the weights to be zero for all weights. This does not necessarily mean that the weights will *never* change if we continue to present patterns and apply the learning rule, only that, if the pattern frequencies stay the same and we apply a large number of patterns, no net change in the weights will ever occur, because any slight change of a weight due to, say, a run of one particular pattern will be countered by statistical fluctuations in the opposite direction at some later set of patterns. The equilibrium condition leads therefore to the condition:

$$\gamma \sum_k \left(\frac{c_{ik}}{a_k} - w_{ij} \right) v_{jk} p_k = 0 \tag{21.7}$$

or

$$\sum_k \frac{c_{ik}}{a_k} v_{jk} p_k = w_{ij} \sum_k v_{jk} p_k \tag{21.8}$$

from which we can get an expression for the weights at equilibrium:

$$w_{ij} = \frac{\sum_k c_{ik} v_{jk} p_k / a_k}{\sum_k v_{jk} p_k}. \tag{21.9}$$

Consider now the meaning of the terms. The denominator is the probability that neuron j will fire for any pattern, since it is the sum of the individual probabilities that neuron j will fire and that pattern k will be presented.

Let us consider the case where a_k is a constant, say a_0. This corresponds to the special case where all input patterns contain the same number of active neurons, such as the paired neuron patterns in the example of the square given earlier. In this case, we can write the equilibrium weights as:

$$a_0 w_{ij} = \frac{\sum_k c_{ik} v_{jk} p_k}{\sum_k v_{jk} p_k}. \tag{21.10}$$

Now consider the term $\sum_k c_{ik} v_{jk} p_k$. This term is just the denominator of eqn (21.10) with all terms where input neuron i does not fire removed. In other words, it is the probability that pattern k is presented, that this pattern causes neuron i in the input layer to fire, and that this pattern will cause neuron j in the second layer to fire. If all input patterns have the same number of active neurons, then a_k will be a constant, so that the numerator is just proportional to this probability. If the patterns have variable numbers of active neurons, the numerator in eqn (21.9) becomes a weighted sum, with a larger contribution from patterns with smaller numbers of active neurons.

The right-hand side of eqn (21.10) is the ratio of (probability that input neuron i is active AND second layer neuron j fires) to (probability that second layer neuron j fires). By the rules of conditional probability, this is just the conditional probability that input neuron i is active given that the second layer neuron j fires. Thus, in those models where all the patterns have the same number of active neurons (such as the pair model above) the equilibrium weights are proportional to these conditional probabilities. This is really just the Hebbian learning rule again: the strength of connection between two neurons (here i in the input layer and j in the second layer) is proportional to the probability that firing one will cause the other to fire.

We can now derive an expression for the response of any second layer neuron at equilibrium. If a pattern l is presented, then neuron j in the second layer will receive an input given by α_{jl}, where

$$\alpha_{jl} = \sum_i c_{il} w_{ij} = \sum_i c_{il} \left[\sum_k p_k c_{ik} v_{jk} / a_k \right] \div \left[\sum_k p_k v_{jk} \right] \tag{21.11}$$

where we have substituted the equilibrium expression (21.9) for w_{ij} in the last step. We can condense the notation a bit if we define the *overlap* r_{kl} between patterns k and l:

$$r_{kl} = \frac{1}{a_l} \sum_i c_{il} c_{ik}. \qquad (21.12)$$

If patterns k and l have no active neurons in common, $r_{kl} = 0$, while if the patterns are the same, or if one pattern is a subset of the other, then $r_{kl} = 1$. Intermediate overlaps give values of r_{kl} between 0 and 1. Substituting the definition 21.12 into 21.11 we obtain

$$\alpha_{jl} = \frac{\sum_k p_k r_{kl} v_{jk}}{\sum_k p_k v_{jk}}. \qquad (21.13)$$

At equilibrium, if the presented pattern l has a large overlap with one or more of the patterns which cause neuron j to fire, then these patterns will contribute a large input to neuron j (provided that these patterns with which pattern l has an overlap occur fairly often, so that p_k is not too small). If the pattern l has overlaps with patterns that do not cause j to fire, these overlaps make no contribution to the input to j, since v_{jk} is zero for such patterns.

Writing the input α_{jl} due to a pattern l in terms of overlaps with other known patterns reveals the ability of the network to classify patterns that it has not seen before. If a pattern l is sufficiently similar to (that is, has a large enough overlap with) one or more patterns that have been used in training the net, then the net should classify this new pattern in the same category as the training patterns. It is just this property that is being exploited when such nets are used to classify images such as empty or crowded streets, male and female faces, and so on.

As an example of how this analysis applies to a specific problem, we consider again the four-by-four square model. As mentioned above, there are 24 different pairs that can be presented to the net during training. Suppose we present all 24 patterns to the net randomly, and with equal frequency. Then $p_k = 1/24$ for all k. The pairs of neurons joined by heavy lines form 12 patterns which we will define to be pattern numbers 1 through 12, and the pairs of neurons joined by thin lines will form patterns 13 through 24. The precise numbering of the patterns is not important here. We will refer to a pattern by giving the numbers of the neurons it contains, so that pattern 1–2 is the pattern containing the pair of neurons numbered 1 and 2.

We saw above that computer simulations of this system usually result in the square being divided in half, so let us propose that a solution as shown in Fig. 21.4 is an equilibrium. Suppose patterns 1 through 12 cause

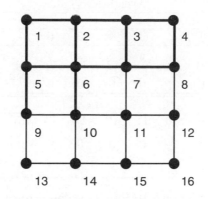

Figure 21.4   Input network used in text example.

neuron $j = 1$ in the second layer to fire (recall there are two neurons in layer two). Then

$$
v_{jk} = \begin{cases}
1 & \text{if } j = 1 \text{ and } k = 1, \dots, 12 \\
0 & \text{if } j = 1 \text{ and } k = 13, \dots, 24 \\
0 & \text{if } j = 2 \text{ and } k = 1, \dots, 12 \\
1 & \text{if } j = 2 \text{ and } k = 13, \dots, 24.
\end{cases} \tag{21.14}
$$

Since all the patterns contain two neurons, $a_k = 2$ for all k. Using this fact together with the constancy of p_k, the equilibrium weights are

$$
w_{ij} = \frac{\sum_k c_{ik} v_{jk}}{2 \sum_k v_{jk}}. \tag{21.15}
$$

Using the properties 21.14, we observe that $\sum_k v_{jk} = 12$ for both values of j, since each of the two neurons in the second layer has precisely 12 patterns that will cause it to fire. Therefore, the weights are given by:

$$
w_{ij} = \frac{1}{24} \sum_k c_{ik} v_{jk} \tag{21.16}
$$

We can now work out the weights to the two second layer neurons by inspecting the network shown in Fig. 21.4. To find $w_{1,1}$, we see that neuron 1 in the input layer forms part of two patterns (1–2 and 1–5), both of which cause neuron $j = 1$ in the second layer to fire, so that the term $c_{1k} v_{1k}$ will be 1 for two patterns and zero for the rest. Thus $w_{1,1} = 2/24$. By similar reasoning we can construct the following table for the weights.

Weights w_{ij}

j	i							
	1	2	3	4	5	6	7	8
1	$\frac{2}{24}$	$\frac{3}{24}$	$\frac{3}{24}$	$\frac{2}{24}$	$\frac{3}{24}$	$\frac{4}{24}$	$\frac{3}{24}$	$\frac{2}{24}$
2	0	0	0	0	0	0	$\frac{1}{24}$	$\frac{1}{24}$

j	i							
	9	10	11	12	13	14	15	16
1	$\frac{1}{24}$	$\frac{1}{24}$	0	0	0	0	0	0
2	$\frac{2}{24}$	$\frac{3}{24}$	$\frac{4}{24}$	$\frac{3}{24}$	$\frac{2}{24}$	$\frac{3}{24}$	$\frac{3}{24}$	$\frac{2}{24}$

Is this a correct solution? To test it, we need to calculate the input to each of the two neurons in the second layer α_{jl} for every pattern and check to see that the correct neuron will fire in each case. This is easy enough to do using the first equation in expression (21.11). For example, if pattern 6–10 is presented, neurons $i = 6$ and $i = 10$ in the input layer are firing, so the input to neuron $j = 1$ is $w_{6,1} + w_{10,1} = \frac{5}{24}$ and the input to neuron $j = 2$ is $w_{6,2} + w_{10,2} = \frac{3}{24}$. Clearly, neuron $j = 1$ receives the higher input, so it will fire, as required. We can continue in the same fashion and find everything checks out, so this is indeed a solution.

As we already know from the computer simulation, this is not the only solution to the equilibrium equations. We can rotate the pattern through any multiple of 90 degrees to generate new solutions, or we can partition the square diagonally. There are also solutions where the numbers of patterns in the two categories are not equal. For example, if we assigned pattern 5–9 to neuron $j = 2$ in the above example, the result is still a solution. In fact, the case where *all* input neurons are linked only to one of the two second-layer neurons is a solution as well, though not a particularly useful one for the purpose of classification.

However, even if we restrict our attention to one particular classification of patterns to second-layer neurons, there is more than one set of weights that will result in this division of patterns. The situation is similar to that encountered in the perceptron learning theorem in Chapter 18, where a range of weight values exists that will guarantee the correct division of patterns. If we take the weights calculated in the table above and perturbed them all slightly by, say, adding or subtracting 0.0001 to individual values in such a way as to preserve the overall normalization condition, the same firing pattern would result in the second layer. This result is apparent from examining the weights generated by the computer simulation, since only rarely does a weight come out to be an integral multiple of 1/24.

One property of major concern to users of such nets is the stability of such classifications. Rumelhart and Zipser analyse the stability of one of their experimental nets, but we will only consider the problem qualitatively here. The range of weight values giving rise to a particular partition of the patterns can be regarded as an attractor in the multidimensional space over which the weights are defined. As with any system of attractors, the stability of a point or a region in space is determined by how 'deep' the attractor well is, how close the wells are, and so on. Since the rules for determining the weights involve non-linear operations, it is possible that oscillations or even chaos could occur. Varying the geometry of the network could help or hinder the process of classifying patterns by separating the centres of attraction or removing instabilities that give rise to oscillations or chaos. Research into such networks is still in its early stages, so that these problems have not yet been fully investigated.

21.3 Summary

The competitive learning algorithm provides a model of unsupervised learning, in which a network is able to discover several features in a set of input patterns and classify patterns that it has not seen during training using the same classification scheme. Although, with the simple example in this chapter, such a network is only able to classify an image into one of two categories, it is a simple matter to increase the number of categories by increasing the number of neurons in the second layer, or increasing the number of clusters in this layer. In general, if we have g_2 groups in the second layer, and the ith group contains $n_{2,i}$ neurons, then, since only one neuron in each group can respond, there are a total of $n_{2,1} \times n_{2,2} \times \ldots \times n_{2,g_s}$ possible responses. In the simpler case where all groups contain n neurons, there are n^{g_s} possible responses.

The model does mimic one, as yet unexplained, biological phenomenon. In the embryo, the emerging neural network is more or less completely connected. As the animal matures, many of these connections atrophy and disappear, leaving the selectively connected neural system found in the adult animal. We have seen that, in a competitive learning model, we may begin with a random selection of synaptic weights and, as the system learns, many of these weights will become essentially zero. We do not know, of course, whether those connections in the embryonic nervous system that die off do so because of competitive learning, but it is an intriguing possibility.

The feature of this model that is perhaps the most irritating, from both the biological modeller's and the computer scientist's points of view, is the difficulty of predicting just what aspects of the patterns will be used for classification. The example at the beginning of this chapter of the military application that went awry is an all too common occurrence with competitive learning networks. To compound the problem, changing the network architecture or using different initial values for the synaptic weights can result in quite different classifications of the same set of input patterns. To be useful in a biological context, some form of natural selection is required. If the structure of the network is an inherited trait, we could imagine selection for those networks that gave the animal some form of competitive advantage. For example, a network that could learn to classify objects into the four categories *predators*, *food*, *mates*, and *everything else* would have great survival value, while another animal of the same species that had inherited a network which allowed to classify objects into *rocks*, *logs*, *clouds*, and *everything else* would have a low probability of survival as it would be prone to many embarrassing and probably fatal errors.

Finally, the competitive learning algorithm suffers from the same malady as all other nets we have studied so far: excessive learning time. Training a net even on a simple problem requires several thousand presentations of each pattern, just as the back propagation net and the perceptron required large amounts of training.

22

Evolutionary learning

22.1 Introduction

The models of learning that we have studied so far have all relied on the modification of synaptic weights, as suggested originally by Donald Hebb in 1949. The majority of these approaches treat the neuron as a point object whose only property is its threshold response to its input.

Real neurons are, of course, much more complicated than this, so we might expect that one way to improve a model of learning would be to incorporate more of what is known about the biology of nerve cells into the model. There are several large-scale models of neurons that attempt to do this for basic neuron function (without learning), but there are substantially fewer models that construct learning models based on biological neurons.

One novel approach to the problem is that of *evolutionary learning*, due to Michael Conrad and his group, including Roberto Kampfner and Kevin Kirby (see Kampfner and Conrad (1983), Conrad *et al.* (1989), and Kirby and Conrad (1991)). Their model enlarges the traditional point neuron so that it contains some internal structure. This idea is based on the experimental results alluded to in Chapter 15, where the the events following the arrival of an action potential at a synapse are described. Before describing the learning algorithm associated with these more detailed neurons, we shall investigate these events in a little more detail.

22.2 The enzymatic neuron

Recall from Chapter 15 that the arrival of an action potential at the presynaptic membrane (the membrane from which the impulse originates) causes packets of transmitter molecules to be released into the synaptic cleft. The molecules diffuse across the cleft and bind to sites on the postsynaptic membrane, where they initiate a series of events that may eventually lead to the postsynaptic neuron firing.

When a transmitter binds to a site on the post-synaptic membrane, it activates a molecule of adenylate cyclase (usually by changing its shape), which is a protein that catalyses the synthesis of cyclic adenosine monophosphate (or cAMP for short). cAMP molecules, in turn, activate another class of proteins called *kinases*, and the kinases change the shape of yet other proteins that are bound to certain sites in the membrane. These latter proteins control the permeability of the membrane to various ions, so that they can influence the membrane potential. Thus the arrival of transmitter molecules sets in motion a complex sequence of events that ultimately changes the membrane potential of various parts of the neuron.

The individual events in this process involve a combination of chemical reactions and diffusion, so that a fully realistic model should contain a detailed description of the rates of the various reactions and diffusion between various parts of the cell. In addition, there are several types of each molecule which have differing effects on each stage of the process. The most obvious difference is that between depolarization of the membrane, with the resultant contribution to an action potential, and hyperpolarization with its resultant inhibition.

Neurons are constantly receiving input from many sources. Each of these inputs sets in motion a chain of events similar to that described above, so that the membrane potential is a complex function of both space and time. If this combination of inputs gives rise, at some point in space and time, to a potential that exceeds the threshold of the neuron, it will generate an action potential. All the network models we have considered up to now ignore all these biochemical and physical details by simply summing up the inputs received (without regard to where on the neuron they are received) and testing if the sum is greater than the threshold.

The first model we shall consider attempts to incorporate some of the internal workings of the neuron, although it is still an idealized version of a real nerve cell.

The neuron is modelled as a cell with a number of discrete locations on its surface. Each of these locations is a possible binding site for a protein which can alter the membrane permeability. These proteins are called *excitases* because, in Kampfner and Conrad's model, only interactions that can excite the neuron are considered. In this model, these excitases will not necessarily be present at *all* locations, but only at those locations that give the neuron its desired responses to the set of input patterns that it is required to learn.

Each neuron may receive input from any other neuron in the net, as well as input from external sources. These inputs are not directed at any specific point on the neuron body—rather, each input can have an influence on all locations on the neuron. This corresponds to the experimental fact that a synapse at one location on the neuron's surface gives rise to events that can propagate throughout the cell and affect areas of the neural membrane far from the synapse.

The magnitude of the effect of any given input on a particular part of the neuron depends on the chemical and diffusive pathways that link the input to other locations on the membrane. In the simplest version of the model, this pathway is represented by a weight w_{ij} which gives the strength of the influence that input i has on location j. Unlike most other neural network models, this weight is considered to be fixed—the variability in the network (and hence its ability to learn) comes from the locations of the excitases, not from the nature of the chemical and diffusive pathways connecting various parts of the neuron. Despite the fact that synaptic weights have been observed to change in experiments on real neurons, this assumption is not as unrealistic as it may appear. This point will become clearer when we consider the learning algorithm below.

Suppose that there are l external inputs to a network containing n neurons. Then each neuron can receive input from up to $l + n$ sources (we are assuming that a neuron can send a signal to itself). If each neuron has p discrete locations on its surface, we need a two-dimensional array of synaptic weights of size $(l + n) \times p$ for each neuron.

In some cases, however, certain inputs will not be connected to a given neuron. Thus we need another array C_{ij} which tells us if input j is connected to neuron i. This array will be two-dimensional of size $n \times (l + n)$. A value of $C_{ij} = 1$ indicates a connection exists and of $C_{ij} = 0$ that no connection exists.

In a simple model, it is easiest to update the state of the network at discrete times. At each time, the states of all the neurons and input lines are checked to see which are active and which are not. Then, for each location on each neuron, the weighted sum S_{ij} of all the inputs to location j on neuron i is calculated by means of the formula

$$S_{ij} = \sum_{k=1}^{l+n} I_k C_{ik} w_{kj} \tag{22.1}$$

where I_k is the state of input k: $I_k = 1$ if the input is active and $I_k = 0$ if not.

Thus S_{ij} is the total input received by one location on one neuron due to all the inputs impinging on that neuron and propagating through the chemical and diffusive pathways to that location. All of the dynamics of the the reaction and diffusion are approximated by this single equation. The more detailed model that we shall consider below delves more deeply into these pathways and constructs explicit expressions for them, but for now we shall content ourselves with this simple version of affairs.

A signal S_{ij} at a location on the neuron will have no effect unless there is an excitase molecule embedded in the membrane at that point. In reality, if such a molecule is present, the effect of the signal is to produce a depolarization of the membrane in the general area of the molecule. If enough such local depolarizations are produced in a short enough time, they may accumulate and produce an action potential. To simplify things, we assume that each location on the membrane has its own threshold value, and that if the signal S_{ij} at the site exceeds the threshold, the neuron will fire.

22.3   The evolutionary learning algorithm

Now that we have constructed a simple model of an enzymatic neural network, how can we make it learn? In more conventional models, a set of input patterns to be learned is repeatedly presented to the network, the output from the net is compared to the desired output, and the synaptic weights are altered according to some rule (such as the perceptron learning theorem or the delta rule). However, as we mentioned above, the synaptic weights in the enzymatic neuron are assumed to be constant—they do not change with activity of the neuron. What can we alter to reflect that learning has occurred?

Kampfner and Conrad's evolutionary learning algorithm was inspired, as its name implies, by the theory of evolution by natural selection. The algorithm is based on the idea that there may be many identical networks in the brain, each of which can be used to perform the same task. There is certainly evidence that each part of the brain is not restricted to controlling only one part of the body: experiments on monkeys have shown that the section of the motor cortex (the part of the brain controlling muscular movement) which controls, say, one of the fingers will gradually shift to control neighbouring areas of the hand if the nerve to that finger is severed. However, there is no real direct evidence that a large set of identical networks exists for learning one particular task, as the evolutionary learning algorithm assumes. This section of the model must be taken as hypothetical.

The general idea is as follows. Suppose we have a collection of networks, identical in every way except in the distribution of excitase molecules. That is, each network contains the same number of neurons, the neurons have the same numbers of discrete locations, the same numbers of external inputs, and the same internal connection geometry. The weights connecting the inputs to the individual locations on the neurons are the same in all the networks. The only initial difference in the networks is that the excitase molecules have been sprinkled over the sites in the neurons at random. Because an excitase must be present at some site where the input signal exceeds the threshold in order for a neuron to fire, the variation in excitase locations will give rise to differing responses of the individual networks for a given set of input patterns. The situation at this stage is analogous to several members of a biological population invading new territory, where the various organisms have a random assortment of genotypes. Each genotype will have its own reaction to the environment in which it finds itself.

If we are to model these networks along the lines of evolution by natural (or even unnatural) selection, we must define the fitness of each network. In a typical learning situation, we have a set of desired outputs, one for each input pattern we present to the network. We can therefore present the set of input patterns to the network and compare the output it produces with the desired responses. A network whose responses are close to those desired will have a high fitness, while those with responses that are more distant from the desired set will have a lower fitness.

In a computer experiment, we must specify the set of desired responses artificially, but it is not too hard to imagine an organism in a natural environment where the 'desired' set of responses is determined by the condition that what the animal does in response to what it senses must produce some benefit for it—location of food or evasion of a predator, for example.

If the same input is presented to all the networks at the same time (remember the brain is a massively parallel computer), we will have some networks that produce better responses, and hence have a higher fitness, than others. We must now find a way to implement the next stage in evolution: selection.

In standard evolutionary theory, the principle of natural selection says, simply, that those organisms that have a higher fitness will produce more or healthier offspring than those with lower fitness. In the neural network context, we do not envision the production of any 'new' networks, in the sense of more neurons being formed. Rather, the properties of those networks with a higher fitness are propagated to the other, less fit, networks in the set. Again, the actual mechanisms in the brain whereby this might be accomplished are mainly hypothetical, since the process involves actually transporting some of these excitase molecules from fitter networks to others. It is known that neurons do exchange material by means of glial cells (the main type of cell in the brain other than neurons—glial cells are not involved in any nervous activity), but the sort of mechanism being postulated here has not been observed experimentally.

Suppose we have initialized a set of networks and have presented the complete set of training patterns once to each network in the set. Then, for each network, we can calculate a fitness (methods for doing this will be described below) based on that network's overall performance. We expect that some networks will do better than others, and that one, or possibly a few, networks will have the highest fitness. Since the only difference between any two networks is in the distribution of excitase molecules among the sites of the neurons, the fitness of a network must be due entirely to its configuration of excitases.

In line with the evolutionary principle of natural selection, those networks of less than optimal fitness will not survive. This is done, not by actually eliminating the neurons in a substandard network, but by eliminating the excitases in the network, thus converting each neuron into a blank slate. Then, some of the excitases from the fittest networks are moved to these freshly wiped networks. In this way, the abilities of the fittest networks are propagated to other networks in the set.

If this copying process were the only mechanism for changing the configuration of the networks, the overall fitness of any one network could never improve beyond that of the most-fit network existing after the initialization stage, although eventually all networks would come to equal this network in fitness. Just as in genetic evolution, some source of variation is needed. In a gene, variation is caused by mutation of the DNA. In evolutionary learning, variation is introduced by randomly inserting or deleting excitases into each network after the copying phase is complete. These variations may, of course, produce either beneficial or detrimental effects, but it is hoped that some of the fittest networks will have their fitness increased by one of these random insertions or deletions. If this does happen, the overall fitness of system is increased and this improvement will propagate to other networks in the set in the next round of learning.

At this point we should pause and review the biological relevance of this model. We have seen in Chapter 16 that there is experimental evidence for Hebb's idea that synaptic weights are altered in a learning situation, yet the evolutionary learning algorithm appears to deny this. But let us examine the concept of a synaptic weight in a little more depth. Most neural network models assume that the neuron is a point object with varying numbers of input lines and a single output line. A synaptic weight in such models is defined as a scaling factor which measures the effect of an input signal on the neuron on which it impinges. No details are given of just how this effect occurs. In the evolutionary learning model, the effect of an input on a neuron is determined by the (constant) weights connecting the input line to each of the sites on the neuron *and* by the distribution of excitases at these sites. Since the location of excitase molecules is varied as a result of learning, the effects of the various input lines on the neurons are being modified.

The evolutionary learning model thus offers a theory with some biological detail of what actually happens when a synaptic weight is modified as a result of learning. There are not yet enough details known experimentally about weight modification, so we cannot say that this is an accurate biological representation.

The other hypotheses in the evolutionary learning model are more problematical. Experimental evidence for sets of identical networks that can exchange membrane proteins in the precise manner required by the algorithm is very thin. On this level, therefore, the model should be interpreted as speculation.

22.4   Details of the model

We will now examine the details of the algorithm as originally specified by Kampfner and Conrad in 1983.

The algorithm, in outline, follows the steps described in the last section:

1. Initialize the network set.

2. Learning loop begins here. Present patterns to be learned to each network and evaluate the fitnesses.

3. Selection: determine the fittest network(s).

4. Deletion: delete excitases from those networks with suboptimal fitness.

5. Copying: copy some excitases from fittest to other networks.

6. Variation: Randomly insert or delete some excitases in each network. Repeat from step 2.

22.4.1   Initialization

To initialize the networks, we first need to decide how many neurons each network is to have, and how these neurons are to be connected. (Remember that all networks are to be identical except for excitase composition.) This can be done by initializing the connection array C_{ij}. We may also decide on the number of input lines and the neurons to which each line is to be connected.

If the networks have more than a single layer of neurons, it is only the final layer that will be examined for output. We must decide which neurons in the net are to have their outputs compared with the desired output set.

At this stage, the connection weights should also be generated. We will need two sets of weights: one to connect external input lines to the various neurons, and one to connect intranet signals, from one neuron to another. These weights could be specified in some systematic way, but it is easier to just generate them randomly.

The threshold level for each neuron must be specified here.

Kampfner and Conrad found that four main parameters could be used to specify the performance of one of these models. These are:

1. The number of networks in the set.

2. The maximum number of fittest networks allowed after each learning session. A limit is necessary on the number of most-fit networks, since these networks are not subject to the delete, copy and vary parts of the algorithm. If a significant fraction of the networks have the highest fitness, then very little variation will occur and the learning rate will be extremely slow or possibly even zero. If too few most-fit networks are maintained, their properties could be lost.

3. The probability of deletion of an excitase from a suboptimal network.

4. The probability of addition of an excitase from a suboptimal network.

These parameters should be specified in the initialization step.

The set of input patterns and the required responses for each must also be specified here.

22.4.2   Training and evaluation

In each learning cycle, the set of patterns needs to presented to each network only once in order that the performance of each network can be measured. At this stage, the measure of fitness must be defined.

Various methods for doing this have been proposed, but the simplest is probably a bit-by-bit comparison of the observed output of each neuron with the corresponding bit in the required output pattern. The *Hamming distance* between the two patterns can be used as a measure of fitness. The Hamming distance between two bit patterns is simply the number of corresponding bits that disagree, so that the Hamming distance between the patterns 011001 and 001101 is 2, since two bits (the second and fourth) disagree. If a network produced correct responses for all input patterns, its Hamming distance from the required pattern set would be zero, and it would have the highest possible fitness. In general, the larger the Hamming distance, the lower the fitness.

The procedure for evaluating a network is then to present each of the input patterns, calculate the Hamming distance of the output from the required output for each pattern, and sum the distances over the entire input set to obtain the fitness of the network. When all networks have been trained, a scan is made to determine the most-fit network(s). If more of these are found than are allowed according to the maximum number of most-fit networks, any extra most-fit networks can be labelled as such, since they are treated specially in later steps in the algorithm. At this stage, then, the networks have been divided into three groups: (i) most-fit networks; (ii) networks with the maximum fitness but surplus to the maximum number of allowed most-fit networks; and (iii) networks with less than the maximum fitness.

Other fitness functions may be considered here. The Hamming distance fitness treats all outputs equally. It may be desirable to emphasize certain output lines by assigning more fitness to a network where these lines give correct responses than to networks where the same number of lines, but in different locations, give correct responses. This is analogous to an examination where more marks are given for correct answers to some questions than others, perhaps because the examiner feels that certain questions are more important, or more difficult, than others.

Another possibility is that of defining fitness to be a non-linear function of Hamming distance. This would make no difference if we are only interested in which networks are the fittest, but if the acutal degree of fitness were used in the other sections of the algorithm, this non-linearity would play a role. This non-linearity has a practical application. Suppose you are an animal in the process of training your networks to recognize predators. If you are presented with the image of a lion and you mistake it for a tiger, this will probably not make much of a difference: in either case the correct response is to run away. However, if you mistake the lion for a large rock, the consequences could be fatal. Clearly the fitness of a network that produces potentially fatal errors should be much worse than that of a network that makes only minor mistakes.

22.4.3 Deletion

The procedure followed by Kampfner and Conrad is to delete *all excitases* from those networks whose fitness was suboptimal, and half the excitases from each site for those networks whose fitness was maximum, but were in excess of the maximum allowed number of most-fit networks.

As mentioned earlier, the deletion of excitases is an attempt to model the action of selection on the network system. The option of erasing all networks that are not of the highest fitness seems a bit drastic, though it no doubt leads to the fastest evolution rate. To model natural selection a bit more closely, the fitness of a network could be used as a measure of the probability of a network's excitases being deleted.[1] If fitness is measured by the Hamming distance between observed and required outputs, the probability of deletion might be defined as directly proportional to this distance, for example. Such a modification to the algorithm is relatively easy to make, and, although it would slow down the convergence of the model, it would be more realistic.

---

[1] This may remind you of the death function used in the spin glass model of the origin of life in Chapter 4.

22.4.4   Copying

After deletion of the excitases in the unfit networks, one excitase is inserted into each of these networks at each site where it appears in one of the fittest networks. Again, a more realistic model might introduce some probabilistic element into this reproductive stage. For example, each network may either donate or receive excitases from another network with a probability that depends on its fitness. The higher the fitness, the more likely a network is to be a donor rather than a recipient, thus maintaining the analogy with a naturally evolving system where a higher fitness means a greater probability of producing healthy offspring.

22.4.5   Variation

The analog to mutation may be performed by testing each site in each neuron to see if an excitase is added (with probability P_a) or deleted (with probability P_d). In the original model, the fittest networks are exempt from variation, which although it will speed up the evolution, is not particularly realistic. All networks should be subject to mutations, just as all organisms in nature are, even the fittest. It is possible that even the fittest networks could be improved by means of mutation.

22.5   Reaction–diffusion neurons

The basic model as described above is discussed in detail in Kampfner and Conrad's 1983 paper, which includes several network architectures of increasing complexity. The evolutionary learning algorithm is used to construct a simple robot which moves in the xy plane. The robot must learn to navigate so that it can locate the origin, even when it is being bumped occasionally.

For simple networks (such as a single neuron) that must recognize restricted pattern sets, the model behaves well, often requiring only 10 or 20 training cycles before it gives correct responses to all inputs. This learning rate compares very favourably with other models such as the perceptron and the delta rule, which can often require hundreds or even thousands of pattern presentations before they learn the correct responses. Recall that any model claiming biological realism must find a way for a network to learn using relatively few training sessions, since the speed of the brain is limited by the speed of the nerve impulse and synaptic transmission. Any model requiring hundreds or thousands of trials is just not feasible.

Despite the many aspects of the evolutionary learning algorithm that have, as yet, no experimental foundation, the model is a promising step towards a biologically realistic neural network.

One enhancement to the basic enzymatic neuron model presented above has been made by Kirby and Conrad (1984,1991). Up to now we have assumed that each input to the neuron is somehow connected to each excitase site on the membrane and that any input to the neuron was instantly propagated to all sites. The strength of the connection has been modelled by a single number: the weight w_{ij}. This weight incorporates a great many biochemical and electrical phenomena into a single number, with no explicit mention of just what is happening between the synapse and the excitase. Experimental evidence has shown that the chemical pathway from input to output is very complex, so it would be good to incorporate some of this detail into the model.

We now abandon the weight matrix w_{ij} and the concept of instant propagation of the effects of an input. Rather, we assume that each external input line is connected to one specific site on the neuron and that the arrival of an input signal affects only that site initially. As time elapses, the effects of the input diffuse outwards from the synapse, merge with the diffusing effects of other inputs, and possibly sum at some distant site to cause an action potential.

Recall that the chemical series of events that follows an input is: neurotransmitter binds to membrane protein which activates cAMP which diffuses through the neuron, locates a kinase protein which changes the form of another membrane protein which finally alters the permeability of the membrane, thus changing the membrane potential and, if the change is enough, producing an action potential. The action potential activates another chemical process within the neuron. The influx of ions activates an enzyme which destroys cAMP molecules, thus shutting down the system which produced the action potential in the first place. This feedback mechanism prevents the cell from continuously firing when a single input is received. We shall now examine how this chain of events is modelled.

We let $u_k(t)$ be the concentration of cAMP in site k at time t. We define $x_k(t)$ to be a binary function (it is either 1 or 0) which indicates if site k is receiving an input at time t. Whenever an input is received, the cAMP concentration in that compartment will jump, since the neurotransmitter which arrives as a result of the input will activate the membrane protein that synthesizes cAMP. In reality, of course, this synthesis will take a finite time, but it occurs very quickly compared with the other events we are considering. We can therefore assume that the change in cAMP concentration is a discontinuity in $u_k(t)$. That is, if an input to site k is received in time interval $[t, t + dt]$, then

$$u_k(t + dt) = u_k(t) + I \qquad (22.2)$$

where I is a constant indicating the amount of cAMP that is synthesized as a result of a single input pulse.

More generally, we can write the effect of an input on $u_k(t)$ as:

$$u_k(t + dt) = u_k(t) + I x_k(t) \qquad (22.3)$$

since $x(t)$ is 1 if input is received in the time interval $[t, t + dt]$ and 0 if not.

The removal of cAMP when the neuron fires can be handled in a similar fashion. We can define another binary function $F_k(t)$ which is 1 if the neuron fires in $[t, t + dt]$ and 0 if not. Then we can write the effect of firing on the cAMP concentration as:

$$u_k(t + dt) = [(h - 1)F_k(t) + 1]u_k(t) \qquad (22.4)$$

so that $u_k(t + dt) = hu_k(t)$ if the neuron fires $(F_k(t) = 1)$ and $u_k(t + dt) = u_k(t)$ if no firing occurs $(F_k(t) = 0)$. Here h is a constant $(0 \le h \le 1)$ which defines the fraction of cAMP remaining in the compartment after the neuron fires. Note that all compartments experience the loss of cAMP on firing, regardless of which excitase caused the action potential.

We can combine the effects of input and firing into a single equation:

$$u_k(t + dt) = [(h - 1)F_k(t) + 1]u_k(t) + I x_k(t). \qquad (22.5)$$

If the neuron receives no input and does not fire, $F_k(t) = x_k(t) = 0$ and $u_k(t + dt) = u_k(t)$.

During those times when no input or firing is occurring, cAMP is diffusing throughout the neuron. In a system continuous in space and time, diffusion is described by the diffusion equation:

$$\frac{\partial u(x, t)}{\partial t} = \nabla \cdot (D(x, t)\nabla u(x, t)) \qquad (22.6)$$

where $D(x, t)$ is the diffusion coefficient, which describes how readily diffusion occurs at each point in space and time.

We are dealing with a spatially discrete system, however, so we cannot use spatial derivatives. In general, eqn (22.6) cannot be solved analytically anyway, so it is necessary to approximate the solution by replacing continuous space and time by discrete intervals. For a quantity such as $u_k(t)$ which is defined in continuous time over a discrete set of spatial locations, we can approximate eqn (22.6) by

$$\frac{du_k}{dt} = \sum_j d_{jk}(u_j - u_k) \qquad (22.7)$$

where d_{jk} is the diffusion coefficient between sites j and k. That is, the rate of flow of the substance (du_k/dt) between two sites is proportional to the concentration difference $(u_j - u_k)$ between the sites. Since diffusion can only take place between neighbouring sites, $d_{jk} = 0$ if sites j and k do not share a boundary.

As an aside to those who may be familiar with the second difference approximation to the diffusion equation, we note that eqn (22.7) is an equivalent approximation. For example, if we are dealing with a one-dimensional system, the equation becomes

$$\frac{du_k}{dt} = \sum_j d_{jk}(u_j - u_k) \tag{22.8}$$

$$= d_{k-1,k}(u_{k-1} - u_k) + d_{k+1,k}(u_{k+1} - u_k) \tag{22.9}$$

$$= d_{k-1,k}u_{k-1} - (d_{k-1,k} + d_{k+1,k})u_k + d_{k+1,k}u_{k+1}. \tag{22.10}$$

If the diffusion coefficient is independent of position, this reduces to the more familiar form $du_k/dt = D[u_{k-1} - 2u_k + u_{k+1}]$.

Finally, even in the absence of input and firing, cAMP has background synthesis and degradation rates. The rate of synthesis A_k depends on the amount of activated membrane protein, which can vary from site to site, but is constant for any given site. The rate of degradation depends on the amounts of cAMP and degrading enzyme present. In a simple chemical kinetic model called the *Michaelis–Menten* model, it is assumed that there is a maximum rate at which degradation can occur because of the limited number of enzyme molecules present. The degradation is represented by a term of the form $u_k P/(u_k + K)$ where P and K are constants. We see that the maximum degradation rate occurs when $u_k \to \infty$, resulting in a rate of P. The constant K is called the saturation constant, and is the concentration of cAMP at which degradation proceeds at half the maximum rate.

Combining the synthesis and degradation terms with the diffusion terms gives a reaction–diffusion equation for cAMP in the absence of input or firing:

$$\frac{du_k}{dt} = \sum_j d_{jk}(u_j - u_k) + A_k - \frac{u_k P}{u_k + K}. \tag{22.11}$$

This is a system of non-linear (due to the last term) ODEs which can be solved numerically by standard computer packages. However, it must be remembered that the values of the u_ks will change discontinuously whenever an input is received or an action potential is generated. During the course of the numerical solution, the values of the firing functions $F_k(t)$ and the input functions $x_k(t)$ must be checked at each step and, if any of these have a value of 1, eqn (22.5) must be applied to alter the corresponding values of the u_ks.

With this reaction–diffusion mechanism in place, the model proceeds in a similar way to the first enzymatic neuron model described in the first part of this chapter. Since the concentration u_k of cAMP has a direct effect on the permeability of the membrane through its action on the kinases, the concentration of cAMP can be taken as a measure of the total input received by a site. When this level rises above the threshold for that site, the neuron will fire, just as in the previous model. Firing resets the cAMP concentrations as described above.

The evolutionary learning algorithm can be applied without change to a network of reaction–diffusion neurons, since the same mechanisms are postulated for transport and modification of the excitase compositions of the various neurons. A more complete description of the reaction-diffusion neuron and its application to evolutionary learning can be found in the papers by Kirby and Conrad (1984) and Kirby *et al.* (1991).

22.6   Summary

Despite several assumptions which, as yet, have little or no experimental foundation, the evolutionary learning model manages to overcome some of the problems with the other models we have considered in previous chapters. It incorporates some of the data on the internal structure of a neuron and the chemical events that occur when an action potential arrives at a synapse. It allows a network to learn a set of patterns with considerably fewer training cycles than the perceptron based networks, thus overcoming a major problem with these models. However, until more evidence is obtained to support its assumptions of the mechanisms of evolutionary learning, the main thesis of the model must be regarded as speculation.

A

Differential equations

This appendix will summarize a few techniques frequently used in analysing the fixed points of or solving ordinary differential equations.

A.1 Local stability analysis of fixed points

Given a system of differential equations such as

$$\dot{\xi}_i = \Lambda_i(\xi, \mathbf{k})$$

we may determine all the equilibrium points or fixed points by solving the set of purely algebraic equations arising from the conditions $\dot{\xi}_i = 0$ for $i = 1, \ldots, n$. This requires finding all sets of ξ_i for which $\Lambda_i(\xi, \mathbf{k}) = 0$. This in itself may be a formidable problem if the Λ_i are non-linear functions. If no exact solution can be found, numerical methods may have to be employed.

Assuming that we can find a fixed point, we would like to determine something about its dynamical nature. That is, if we found a natural system at or near such a point, would it tend to stay close to the equilibrium, or would it drift away from it? In a natural system, there will always be fluctuations in population numbers, so we cannot assume that if a system is placed precisely on one of the fixed points, it will automatically stay there for all time. Although no account is taken of these fluctuations in the dynamical equations, we can get some idea of their effects on systems that are close to an equilibrium point by means of *perturbation theory* or *local stability analysis*.

If the functions Λ_i that govern the dynamics of the system are assumed to be continuous functions, then even if they are non-linear, we may use a first-order Taylor series approximation to them near a fixed point. (From here on, we shall assume that, whenever reference is made to the function Λ_i, the dependence on ξ_i or x_i and k_i is understood.) In doing so, we shall replace the original system of non-linear differential equations by a system of linear equations for which there is an exact solution. We expect this solution to give, in most cases, an indication of the behaviour of the non-linear solution near the fixed point.

We define $\bar{\xi}_i$ to be the set of values at a fixed point, so that $\Lambda_i(\bar{\xi}_i) = 0$. Then for values of ξ_i near $\bar{\xi}_i$, the following expansion applies:

$$\dot{\xi}_i = \Lambda_i(\bar{\xi}) + \sum_j \left.\frac{\partial \Lambda_i}{\partial \xi_j}\right|_{\xi=\bar{\xi}_i} (\xi_j - \bar{\xi}_j) + \mathcal{O}((\xi - \bar{\xi}_i)^2) \qquad (A.1)$$

where the symbol $\mathcal{O}((\xi - \bar{\xi}_i)^2)$ indicates terms of the order of $(\xi - \bar{\xi}_i)^2$, that is, terms of higher order than linear. If the point ξ_i is close enough to $\bar{\xi}_i$, we expect these terms to be very small in comparison with the linear term, meaning that we can neglect them.

Now we define $z_i \equiv \xi_i - \bar{\xi}_i$ for $i = 1, \ldots, n$. Then, since the coordinates of the fixed point are constants, $\dot{z}_i = \dot{\xi}_i$. We also define the matrix B with elements

$$B_{ij} = \left.\frac{\partial \Lambda_i}{\partial \xi_j}\right|_{\xi=\bar{\xi}_i} = \left.\frac{\partial \Lambda_i}{\partial z_j}\right|_{\mathbf{z}=0}.$$

Then, since by the definition of a fixed point $\Lambda_i(\bar{\xi}) = 0$, eqn (A.1) becomes

$$\dot{z}_i = \sum_j B_{ij} z_j + \mathcal{O}(z^2).$$

If we ignore terms of higher than first order, we can write this as a matrix equation

$$\dot{\mathbf{z}} = B\mathbf{z}. \qquad (A.2)$$

This is a linear system of differential equations, which can be solved by the same technique we used in the process of deriving the solution to the quasi-species equations in Chapter 2. We shall briefly review the procedure.

Assume that B can be diagonalized, so that we can write

$$B = U\Omega U^{-1}$$

where Ω is a diagonal matrix whose diagonal elements $\Omega_{ii} \equiv \omega_i$ are the eigenvalues of B (which can, in general, be complex numbers), and the ith column of U is the eigenvector of B corresponding to the eigenvalue ω_i. We can then write equation (A.2) in the form

$$U^{-1}\dot{\mathbf{z}} = \Omega(U^{-1}\mathbf{z}).$$

Introducing $\zeta \equiv U^{-1}\mathbf{z}$ we obtain a system of uncoupled differential equations

$$\dot{\zeta}_i = \omega_i \zeta_i.$$

Each of these equations has a solution of the form

$$\zeta_i = A_i e^{\omega_i t}$$

where A_i is a constant determined by the initial conditions. The solution for z_i is then found from the relation

$$z_i = \sum_j U_{ij} \zeta_j$$

so that z_i is a linear combination of exponential terms.

The behaviour of the individual terms z_i as functions of time is thus determined by the eigenvalues of the matrix B. There are three main cases to consider.

1. $\mathcal{Re}\ \omega_i < 0$ (where $\mathcal{Re}$ means 'real part of'). In this case, the corresponding ζ_i will decay exponentially to zero.

2. $\mathcal{Re}\ \omega_i > 0$. The magnitude of the corresponding ζ_i will grow exponentially.

3. $\mathcal{Re}\ \omega_i = 0$. In this case, if $\mathcal{Im}\ \omega_i \neq 0$ ($\mathcal{Im}$ means 'imaginary part of'), ζ_i will oscillate with constant amplitude. (Recall the relation between a complex exponential and the trigonometric functions: $e^{ix} = \cos x + i \sin x$.)

We see, therefore, that if *all* the eigenvalues satisfy $\mathcal{Re}\ \omega_i < 0$, then all the ζ_i will decay to zero, and thus so will all the z_i. In this case, a small disturbance from a fixed point will be damped out over time and the system will return to the point. Such a fixed point is called an *asymptotically stable point*, or sometimes just a *sink*.

If *any* of the eigenvalues satisfies $\mathcal{Re}\ \omega_i > 0$, the corresponding ζ_i will grow exponentially. Any z_j that contains a term in that value of ζ_i will therefore also grow. In such a case, any small disturbance from the fixed point will be magnified, if the disturbance has a component in the direction of any z_j which contains one of these exponentially growing terms. Such a fixed point is therefore unstable.

It is possible (indeed, quite common) for a single fixed point to have a mixture of these two properties. If some of the eigenvalues have negative real parts, and others have positive real parts, then it is possible for some of the z_j to contain only negative exponential terms, while others have at least one term containing a positive exponential. Then, if a disturbance should occur in such a way that only a z_j with negative exponential terms should be upset, the system will return to the equilibrium. Of course, if any of z_j with positive exponentials should be disturbed, the disturbance will grow and the system will continue to drift away from equilibrium. A point with such a double property is called a saddle point. For our purposes, saddle points are much the same as totally unstable points, since with random fluctuations occurring it is virtually impossible for a perturbation to be so selective that it will excite only those values of z_j that contain only negative exponentials.

The third case referred to above, that for which $\mathcal{R}e\ \omega_i = 0$, unfortunately gives us very little information about the behaviour of the associated fixed point. The oscillatory behaviour of the linear system around such a fixed point is often not mirrored in the corresponding non-linear system. In fact, it is at just such points that many of the wilder properties of non-linear systems first manifest themselves. Although interesting mathematically, these properties are beyond our scope at the present time. In most practical systems, these properties must be explored by numerical solution of the equations.

Occasionally, one is unfortunate enough to come across a matrix B that cannot be diagonalized. A standard method of solution exists for such cases, but as it is a rather specialized case we simply refer the reader to a textbook on linear algebra such as Noble and Daniel (1988) for the details.

A.2   Numerical solution of ordinary differential equations

Very few differential equations that arise in real life can be solved analytically. Although analysis of the fixed points by techniques covered in the last section is sometimes sufficient, we often would like a full solution. We must use some form of numerical solution to obtain this. This section will explain the idea behind numerical solution of an ordinary differential equation by deriving the simplest such method (Euler's method). Finally, a more accurate technique will be given.

The sort of equation we wish to solve is a general first-order differential equation:

$$y' = f(x, y) \tag{A.3}$$

where $y' \equiv dy/dx$, and $f(x, y)$ is a general function of two variables.

Euler's method is based on a first-degree Taylor polynomial for $y(x)$:

$$y(x) \approx y(x_0) + y'(x_0)(x - x_0) = y(x_0) + f(x_0, y(x_0))(x - x_0). \tag{A.4}$$

The idea is to start with the initial conditions (x_0, y_0), where $y_0 \equiv y(x_0)$, and build up a solution by successive application of eqn (A.4). In particular, we build up the solution by finding values of y at equally spaced values of x. Let $h \equiv x - x_0$. Then Euler's method for numerically solving the equation A.3 is

$$y_{n+1} = y_n + hf(x_n, y_n) \tag{A.5}$$

given initial conditions $y = y_0$ at $x = x_0$.

As a simple example, we may solve the equation

$$y' = xy \tag{A.6}$$

with initial condition $y(0) = 1$. The value of h must be chosen, so we will try $h = 0.1$.

Constructing a table, we may estimate $y(0.5)$:

n	x_n	y_n	$f(x_n, y_n)$
0	0	1	0
1	0.1	1	0.1
2	0.2	1.01	0.202
3	0.3	1.0302	0.30906
4	0.4	1.061106	0.4244424
5	0.5	1.10355024	

This particular differential equation can be solved exactly to give

$$y(x) = e^{x^2/2} \tag{A.7}$$

which has the value $y(0.5) = 1.133148\ldots$, so the solution is not particularly accurate in this case.

The accuracy of any numerical method can be improved (up to a point) by reducing the step size h. However, since any such method must be calculated with finite accuracy (on a calculator or computer), if h is made too small, round-off error can ruin the result just as surely as too large a step size. A useful technique for deciding when you have an accurate answer is to begin with a value of h that is fairly large and then repeat the calculation, each time halving the value of h. When two successive runs give the same answer, you can be fairly certain that the process has converged and you have a good approximation to the solution.

Numerical analysis, however, is always fraught with difficulties, especially if the differential equation is what is known as *stiff*. A stiff equation has a solution with regions that change very rapidly, so that even a small value of h may not be small enough to catch all the twists and turns in the solution curve. For most equations, Euler's method with successive halving of the step size will give a reasonable answer.

One final method worth mentioning here is the *Runge–Kutta* method, since this method is frequently used in commercially available computer packages. The method requires several stages of calculation, as follows.

$$y_{n+1} = y_n + \frac{h}{6}(k_1 + 2k_2 + 2k_3 + k_4) \tag{A.8}$$

where

$$k_1 = f(x_n, y_n) \tag{A.9}$$
$$k_2 = f(x_n + h/2, y_n + hk_1/2) \tag{A.10}$$
$$k_3 = f(x_n + h/2, y_n + hk_2/2) \tag{A.11}$$
$$k_4 = f(x_n + h, y_n + hk_3) \tag{A.12}$$

This method is more accurate than Euler's method, and so should converge faster, although it is a bit more work to program (and harder to remember!).

B

A statistics primer

This appendix is designed as a quick introduction to the concepts from probability and statistics that are used in this book. It will provide all the factual information needed in this respect but, in the limited space of this appendix, the experience attained from a full course in the subject cannot, of course, be acquired. There are a great many introductory statistics texts available (see, for example, Clarke and Cooke (1983) or Walpole and Myers (1989)). The reader who still feels uncertain about the subject after reading this appendix should consult one of these texts.

B.1 Probabilities and random events

Most of us probably feel that we have a good idea of what a *random* event is. We would list examples such as tossing a coin, rolling dice, or an unplanned meeting with an old friend in the street. We feel that the occurrence of these events cannot be predicted, although we usually do not take the analysis any deeper than that. It is possible to become deeply philosophical about just how random such events as coin tossing or dice throwing really are, since, in principle, if you know the initial conditions of a coin toss and the laws of physics well enough, you should be able to predict the outcome. Or should you? Quantum theory predicts that certain events (usually on the subatomic scale) have an inherently uncertain nature, so maybe the outcome of a coin toss is, to a certain extent, truly unknowable.

If all this talk about tossing coins seems a bit irrelevant to the main theme of this book, theoretical biology, think again. In most of the models in this book, random numbers are used to simulate events in a complex biological system. We are assuming that certain events in an organism are unpredictable, and the only way we can decide what happens is to determine the probabilities of all the possible outcomes of the event and make our choices bases on these probabilities. It is important to decide just what we mean when we say that these events are 'unpredictable' or 'random'.

In one sense, we might actually mean that each event is unpredictable in the quantum mechanical sense that physical theory really cannot predict what will happen. In some cases, since we are dealing with events on the molecular scale, this is true. However, more often we use the concept of probability as a convenient fiction in dealing with large numbers of similar events. Whenever the outcome of an event, such as the toss of a coin, can have more than one value, with the proportions of times each value is assumed tending to a constant the more often the event is performed, it is often convenient to assume that the event really is random and to use these proportions as probabilities that each outcome will occur. In doing so, we are ignoring all the finer workings that could have a bearing on the outcome. For example, suppose we observe that in several hundred tosses of a coin, 60 per cent of the time tails came up and 40 per cent of the time heads came up. By simply saying that the probability of a head is 40 per cent and that of a tail is 60 per cent, we are ignoring any reasons as to why this might be so. This is not to say that we can never investigate the nature of the coin tossing experiment further if we state that a head and a tail have fixed probabilities—in fact, an observation of the probabilities of an event often leads to further investigation into the reasons for the distribution of outcomes. However, if all we want is a way of generating a realistic set of outcomes in a simulation without bothering about the details of the processes determining the outcome, the assignment of a set of probabilities to the outcomes is a convenient way to achieve this.

In order to construct a mathematical theory of probability, we have to be a bit more precise about the sorts of systems in which random events arise. We will always consider a definite experiment, such as the tossing of a coin, which has a certain possible set of outcomes, such as heads and tails. The set of all possible outcomes is called the *sample space* of the experiment. The set can be discrete, as in the case of a coin toss or a throw of dice, or it can be continuous if the experiment depends on a continuous variable. The latter case could occur is we wished to predict the probability of the temperature at noon tomorrow, or the winning time of a horse in a race. For the moment, however, we will restrict ourselves to discrete sample spaces.

Having defined our sample space, we can now define the probability of each event in the space. If we repeated the same experiment a great many (ideally, infinitely many) times, we would find that each member of the set occurred a certain fraction of the time. We define the probability p of event E, written $p(E)$ or sometimes $prob(E)$, to be just this fraction. Defining a probability in this way imposes certain restrictions on its value. In particular, we must always have

$$0 \le p(E) \le 1 \tag{B.1}$$

Now we must examine how carefully we have specified our sample space. Suppose our experiment consists of tossing a coin twice and the sample space associated with the outcome is defined to be (i) a head occurs at least once; (ii) a tail occurs at least once; (iii) neither a head nor a tail occurs in either toss. You may think that these three possibilities satisfy the definition of a sample space since they do seem to cover all possible outcomes of the experiment. If you do this experiment many times with a fair coin (one which is equally likely to come up heads as tails), you will find that the probability of (i) and (ii) are both about 0.75 and, if you discount the possibility of the coin landing on its edge or rolling off the table, out the door and disappearing down a drain, the probability of (iii) is zero.

The problem with this sample space is that it does not separate the possible outcomes into *mutually exclusive* subsets. We can tell this from the probabilities alone. If we *had* classified all possible outcomes into mutually exclusive subsets, then any one outcome of the experiment must be in one, and only one, of the subsets. Since the sample space must include all possible outcomes, the sum of the probabilities of each element of a sample space where the subsets consist of mutually exclusive events must be 1:

$$\sum p(E) = 1 \qquad (B.2)$$

where the sum is over all events E.

This condition is obviously not true for the sample space given above for the double coin-tossing experiment, since the sum of the probabilities is 1.5. The problem is that outcomes (i) and (ii) are not mutually exclusive: the outcome head–tail belongs to both (i) and (ii) for example, and is therefore counted twice when the probabilities are being added up. From now on, we will restrict our sample spaces to consist only of mutually exclusive subsets, unless otherwise stated.

Sample spaces, despite this restriction, are not necessarily unique. Two possible correct sample spaces for the double coin-toss are:

$$S_1 = \{HH, HT, TH, TT\} \qquad (B.3)$$

where H indicates a head and T indicates a tail, and

$$S_2 = \{2 \text{ heads, exactly 1 head, no heads}\}. \qquad (B.4)$$

The first sample space consists of four subsets, each of which contains a single outcome, while the second space contains three subsets, one of which (exactly 1 head) contains two outcomes (HT and TH). Both of these spaces are acceptable, since they both partition the set of all possible outcomes into mutually exclusive (or disjoint, to use set terminology) subsets.

In general, then, we have the additional condition on a set of probabilities:

$$\sum_{E\in \text{ sample space}} p(E) = 1 \qquad \text{(B.5)}$$

where the sum is taken over all events E in the sample space.

A generalization of this result can be applied to probabilities of combinations of mutually exclusive events. If A and B are mutually exclusive, then the probability that the outcome of an experiment is either A or B is the *sum* of $p(A)$ and $p(B)$:

$$p(A \text{ or } B) = p(A) + p(B) \qquad \text{(B.6)}$$

For example, the probability that two coin tosses yields either two heads or two tails is

$$p(HH \text{ or } TT) = p(HH) + p(TT) \qquad \text{(B.7)}$$

However, this addition rule is *not* true if the events are not mutually exclusive. For example,

$$p(\text{at least 1 head or at least 1 tail}) \neq p(\text{at least 1 head}) + p(\text{at least 1 tail}).$$
$$\text{(B.8)}$$

In fact, the probability of at least one head or at least 1 tail is 1.0, since any outcome must include one head or one tail, but as we saw above, adding the individual probabilities gives 1.5, which is too large to be a probability.

B.2   Independence and conditional probability

Two events are said to be *independent* when the outcome of one event has no effect on, and is not affected by, the other. The independence (or otherwise) of two events must be established with care, and is a matter that is outside the realm of probability theory, since it depends on the experimental setup and the definitions of the events. For example, it is usually considered safe to assume that two coin tosses are independent, but the probability that tomorrow's weather will be wet or cold has a strong dependence on the nature of today's weather. Arguments could be mounted against both these positions: tossing the first coin creates air currents which could affect the result of the second toss if it is done soon enough after the first, or the tosser's hand could be a bit more fatigued after the first toss, causing a different amount of force to be applied to the second coin. Both of these effects are expected to be negligible, so that independence is a reasonable assumption. In the case of the weather, although it is true that sharp swings in the weather do occur, it is far more common for one day to be followed by another with very similar weather.

This tendency is so strong, especially in certain areas (such as deserts) that independence of daily weather is demonstrably false.

The moral of these examples is that you must carefully examine the nature of the experimental quantities to determine if independence applies. It is tempting to assume independence, since it usually makes calculations much easier.

The probability that two independent events C and D both occur is the product of the probabilities of each event. To see this, consider the coin-tossing experiment yet again. The probability that two heads in a row are seen can be evaluated as follows. The probability that the first toss gives a head is 0.5 on a fair coin. The probability that the second toss is a head is also 0.5, independently of what happened on the first toss. Now since the two tosses are independent, we would expect only half the second batch of heads to have occurred in experiments where the first toss yielded a head, so the overall probability is $0.5 \times 0.5 = 0.25$.

In general we have, for independent events C and D:

$$p(\text{both } C \text{ and } D) = p(C)p(D). \tag{B.9}$$

Thus the probability of two independent events both occurring is always *less than or equal to* the probability that either of them occurs alone.

These results can be generalized to the case of non-independent events by the use of *conditional probability*. To illustrate this, we shall return to the example of weather forecasting. To simplify things, suppose we consider only two types of weather: hot and cold. We take a series of measurements of daily weather over a period of several years and record the following data:

- $p(hot) = 0.4$; $p(cold) = 0.6$. (40 per cent of the days were classified as 'hot' and 60 per cent as 'cold'.)

- If a day is hot, the next day will be hot with probability 3/4 and cold with probability 1/4.

- If a day is cold, the next day will be hot with probability 1/6 and cold with probability 5/6.

Now suppose we wish to find the probability that two consecutive days will be cold. The probability that the first day is cold is simply $p(cold) = 0.6$, since this day is chosen at random. Now that we know the first day is cold, however, we can use this information to calculate the probability that the second day is also cold. We know this from the data to be 5/6. Since 5/6 of cold days are followed by cold days, and 0.6 of first days in pairs will be cold, the overall probability of a pair of cold days is the product, or $0.6 \times 5/6 = 0.5$.

This argument is rather cumbersome, so let us introduce the standard notation used in such cases. We define a *conditional probability* $p(A|B)$ to be the probability that event A occurs *given* that event B has already occurred. The vertical bar in the notation $p(A|B)$ is read as 'given'. Using this notation, we can rewrite the data above as follows, using the definitions $p_h = p(hot)$ and $p_c = p(cold)$.

- $p_c = 0.6$, $p_h = 0.4$.

- $p(h|h) = 3/4$; $p(c|h) = 1/4$.

- $p(c|c) = 5/6$; $p(h|c) = 1/6$.

Then the probability of a pair of cold days, which we shall write $p(cc)$, is given by

$$p(cc) = p(c|c)p_c \tag{B.10}$$

In general, for two events A and B, which need not be independent, the probability that both A and B occur is

$$p(A \text{ and } B) = p(A|B)p(B) \tag{B.11}$$

or

$$p(A \text{ and } B) = p(B|A)p(A). \tag{B.12}$$

Which of these two forms to use depends on what data you have. In the above example, if A is the event 'second day in a pair is cold' and B is the event 'first day in a pair is cold', eqn (B.11) would be used, since we do not know $p(A)$, the probability that the second day in a pair is cold.

A couple of useful properties of conditional probabilities can be seen using a little thought.

First, if events A and B are, in fact, independent, then $p(A|B) = p(A)$, since the probability of A occurring does not depend on whether or not B has occurred. In this case, eqns (B.11) and (B.12) both reduce to the product rule for combining probabilities of independent events.

Second, we must have

$$\sum_B p(A|B)p(B) = p(A) \tag{B.13}$$

where the sum is over all events in the sample space. This follows, because, in any pair of events A and B, event A, if it occurs at all, must be paired with *some* other event from the sample space so, if you sum over all possible events B, you must just get the probability that A occurs.

Similarly,

$$\sum_A p(A|B)p(B) = p(B). \tag{B.14}$$

This follows by a similar argument, or by combining eqns (B.11) and (B.12) to obtain

$$p(A|B)p(B) = p(B|A)p(A). \tag{B.15}$$

B.3 Distribution functions and density functions

Once we have decided on a sample space for describing the outcome of an experiment, we must assign a probability to each member of the space in such a way that, for a discrete sample space, the sum of the probabilities is 1.0. Although we have used the notation $p(E)$ to mean 'the probability of event E', we can also interpret this same notation as a mathematical function, called the *distribution function*. If the events E can be specified numerically, we may be able to derive a mathematical formula for $p(E)$ but in many cases the elements of the sample space must just be listed descriptively (as in 'head' and 'tail' or 'hot' and 'cold'), so the only way to define the function is to list its elements as we have done in examples above.

So far, we have assumed that all our sample spaces were finite sets of possibilities. We now consider how to handle continuous sample spaces. Let us return to weather prediction for an example to guide us. Instead of merely predicting whether a day will be hot or cold, we would like to predict the actual temperature T, in degrees centigrade, at noon.

The first problem is to specify the sample space. Since T is a continuous variable, we cannot list all its values, since there are an infinite number of them. We must specify an interval instead. In principle, temperatures can range anywhere from absolute zero up to infinity, but a range of $[-100, 100]$ should handle all situations, at least in any settled area on planet Earth. Having decided on the sample space, the next problem is a bit trickier: how do we assign probabilities to each temperature in this interval? We cannot assign a definite probability to every real number in an interval, because the sum of all the probabilities in a sample space must be 1.0. If we assign a non-zero probability to each of an infinite set of temperatures, the sum will be infinite, which is certainly larger than 1.0.

The solution to this problem lies in using a bit of common sense. Any measurement has a limited accuracy. It is not possible to tell whether a temperature is exactly 12.0 degrees or, say, 12.01 degrees, or any value in between, if the accuracy of your thermometer is only 0.1 degree. In practice, we say that the temperature is 12.0 ± 0.1 degrees and leave it at that.[1] All we really need, then, is a theory that gives us the probability that

---

[1]If you are worried that the temperature must actually have some precise value even if we can't measure it, you may take solace from the fact that quantum theory predicts that you can't measure any continuous quantity exactly anyway. This is a fundamental property of physics.

T lies within some *interval*, such as [12.0, 12.1], rather than the probability that T has some *precise* value.

To this end, we define a function $f(T)$, called the *probability density function*, or pdf for short. It must be emphasized that $f(T)$ is *not* the probability that the temperature has the precise value T. (Often $f(T)$ will assume values greater than 1.0.) Rather, as its name implies, it gives the density of probability around the value T. The 'units' of $f(T)$ (to stretch the meaning of the word 'units') would be 'probability per unit degree'. To find the probability of a temperature lying in a certain interval of infinitesimal size dT starting at T, that is, $[T, T + dT]$, we multiply the density by the interval length:

$$Prob(T \in [T, T + dT]) = f(T)dT. \tag{B.16}$$

To find the probability that T lies within a finite interval, say $[T_1, T_2]$, we must sum up the probabilities that T lies in all the infinitesimal intervals making up this finite interval. This we do using integration:

$$Prob(T \in [T_1, T_2]) = \int_{T_1}^{T_2} f(T)dT. \tag{B.17}$$

Let us consider probability density functions in general. We consider a function $f(x)$ defined over a domain $x \in X$, where X is the sample space. X need not be a continuous interval—it could be the union of several separate continuous intervals, for example.

We cannot chose just any form for a pdf. Since it must produce a probability when integrated over any subinterval of the sample space, it must be non-negative over its entire domain:

$$f(x) \geq 0 \qquad x \in X. \tag{B.18}$$

Since x must lie somewhere within X, we must have the condition

$$\int_X f(x)dx = 1 \tag{B.19}$$

where the integral is taken over the entire sample space X.

The probability that $a < x < b$ is

$$p(a < x < b) = \int_a^b f(x)dx \tag{B.20}$$

Note that it is irrelevant whether we include the endpoints of the interval, that is, whether we ask for $p(a < x < b)$ or $p(a \leq x \leq b)$. The difference between these two quantities consists of two intervals of zero width, which means there is no difference in probability.

As an example, suppose we define the following pdf for our temperature prediction experiment:

$$f(T) = \begin{cases} 0 & -100 \leq T \leq -30 \\ \frac{1}{40}\left(1 - \frac{T^2}{900}\right) & -30 < T < 30 \\ 0 & 30 \leq T \leq 100 \end{cases} . \tag{B.21}$$

The pdf predicts that the temperature will never be less than -30 or greater than 30. The temperature is most likely to be near zero. The factor of $1/40$ is included so that $\int_{-100}^{100} f(T)dT = 1$.

Another commonly used function is the *cumulative distribution function* (cdf for short) usually denoted $F(y)$, which gives the probability that the random variable in question is less than the value y. That is, if a random variable x has pdf $f(x)$, then

$$p(x < y) = F(y). \tag{B.22}$$

This is just the probability that $x \in (-\infty, y)$, so we have

$$F(y) = \int_{-\infty}^{y} f(x)dx. \tag{B.23}$$

If the domain of $f(x)$ does not extend to $-\infty$, the lower limit on the integral should be replaced with the lower limit of the domain.

For example, the probability that the temperature is less than 10 degrees is, using eqn (B.21),

$$p(T < 10) = F(10) = \int_{-100}^{10} f(x)dx = \int_{-30}^{10} \frac{1}{40}\left(1 - \frac{x^2}{900}\right)dx = 0.741 \tag{B.24}$$

to 3 decimal places.

A couple of useful properties of the cdf are obvious from its definition:

$$F(-\infty) = 0; \qquad F(\infty) = 1 \tag{B.25}$$

These conditions state that it is impossible for any quantity to have a value less than $-\infty$ or greater than ∞.

Since $F(y)$ is the integral of a non-negative function $f(x)$, it can never decrease: it either remains constant or increases over any interval.

B.4 Mean and variance

Although all the information about a random system, apart from actual experimental measurements, is contained in its distribution function, it is often convenient to characterize the distribution using a few simple parameters. Two of these are the *mean* and *variance*.

If an event E occurs with probability $p(E)$ then, in N trials, it will occur, on average, $Np(E)$ times. Note that this is not necessarily an integer, which illustrates that a mean does not necessarily give a value that can occur as the result of a single experiment.

The mean of a discrete distribution is just the arithmetic average. Suppose a discrete random variable n has a distribution function $p(n)$. Then the mean of n is defined as

$$\bar{n} \equiv \sum_m m p(m) \tag{B.26}$$

where the sum is taken over the sample space of n.

The mean of any function of a random variable can be found the same way. Given a function $g(n)$ of a discrete random variable n, then the mean of g is

$$\overline{g(n)} = \sum_m g(m) p(m). \tag{B.27}$$

For a continuous random variable x, the mean is calculated using an integral instead of a sum:

$$\bar{x} = \int_{-\infty}^{\infty} x f(x) dx \tag{B.28}$$

and for a function $g(x)$ of the random variable:

$$\overline{g(x)} = \int_{-\infty}^{\infty} g(x) f(x) dx. \tag{B.29}$$

The mean gives us an idea of the average behaviour we should expect if we repeated an experiment many times, but it gives us no idea of the scatter in the results. A good qualitative idea of the spread to be expected in experimental results can be found from a plot of the pdf. If $f(x)$ is spread out over a wide range of values, we would expect a lot of scatter in the data, while if it is peaked about the mean, we would expect very little scatter. We need some way to measure this scatter more quantitatively. For this we can use the variance.

The variance, denoted σ^2, is defined as the mean of the square of the difference between the random variable x and its mean $\bar{x}$:

$$\sigma^2 \equiv \sum_m (m - \bar{m})^2 p(m) \tag{B.30}$$

for a discrete distribution, and

$$\sigma^2 \equiv \int_{-\infty}^{\infty} (x - \bar{x})^2 f(x) dx \qquad (B.31)$$

for a continuous distribution.

Expanding either of these definitions and using the definition of the mean of a function, we obtain the more common expression for the variance:

$$\sigma^2 = \overline{x^2} - \bar{x}^2. \qquad (B.32)$$

The variance is the difference between the mean of the square and the square of the mean.

A few properties of the variance easily seen from its definition follow. Since the variance is the sum or integral of a non-negative quantity (a square), it can never be negative. The variance is only zero if all experiments always give the same the same result, that is, there is no uncertainty as to the outcome. In general, the larger the scatter in the data, the larger the variance.

B.5 Binomial and Poisson distributions

We will now examine a few commonly occurring distribution functions.

The binomial and Poisson distributions are both discrete distribution functions.

The binomial distribution may already be familiar to the reader from a study of permutations and combinations, as the binomial coefficient

$$\binom{N}{m} \equiv \frac{N!}{m!(N-m)!} \qquad (B.33)$$

is the number of ways of choosing m objects from a total of N objects without regard for the order in which they are chosen. The binomial coefficient also figures prominently in the binomial distribution.

Suppose we return to our coin-tossing experiment again. This time we toss the coin a total of, say, 10 times and want the probability that there are precisely 2 heads in the 10 tosses. Let the probability of a head be p and that of a tail be $q = 1 - p$. One way we could get 2 heads is if the first 2 tosses give heads and all the rest tails. The probability of this happening is $p^2 q^8$. We could also have had the first toss give a head, the second a tail, the third a head, and all the rest tails. The probability of this is $pqpq^7 = p^2 q^8$ as before. We can see that it doesn't matter in which order the heads and tails appear, all that matters is that we have 2 heads and 8 tails. The probabilities of all of the various ways this can happen are the same. Since all the ways of getting 2 heads are mutually exclusive, we can obtain the total probability of finding 2 heads in 10 tosses by multiplying the probability of one such occurrence, namely $p^2 q^8$, by the number of ways this can be achieved. This is just the combinatoric problem of counting the number of ways of choosing 2 objects from a total of 10 without regard to order, which is the binomial coefficient $\begin{pmatrix} 10 \\ 2 \end{pmatrix}$. Hence the total probability is $\begin{pmatrix} 10 \\ 2 \end{pmatrix} p^2 q^8$.

The binomial distribution applies to any system in which each experiment can have two outcomes, one with probability p and the other with probability $q = 1 - p$. If N trials of the experiment are carried out, the probability that m of them will have the first result is:

$$Prob(m) = \begin{pmatrix} N \\ m \end{pmatrix} p^m (1 - p)^{N-m}. \tag{B.34}$$

It can be shown that the mean and variance of the binomial distribution are given by

$$\bar{m} = Np \tag{B.35}$$

and

$$\sigma^2 = Np(1 - p). \tag{B.36}$$

The *Poisson distribution* applies to systems where events occur a constant mean rate, either in time or space. A commonly used example of a so-called *Poisson process* is that of cars passing a fixed point on a lonely country road. If an average of, say, 5 cars pass the point every hour, but with the time intervals between successive cars being random, then we have a Poisson process. The randomness of the time intervals is essential, for there are many systems in which events happen at a constant rate with regular intervals between them, such as the ticking of a clock.

The theory of the Poisson distribution is considerably more complicated than that of the binomial distribution, so we will simply quote the results here. If a Poisson process occurs with a mean rate of λ events per unit time then the probability[2] that n events occur in time t is

$$Prob(n, t) = \frac{e^{-\lambda t}(\lambda t)^n}{n!}. \tag{B.37}$$

In the car example above, $\lambda = 5$ cars per hour, so the probability of 9 cars in 2 hours is then

$$Prob(9, 2) = \frac{e^{-10}10^9}{9!} = 0.125 \tag{B.38}$$

to 3 decimal places.

---

[2]'Time' may be substituted by 'length' or any other appropriate unit.

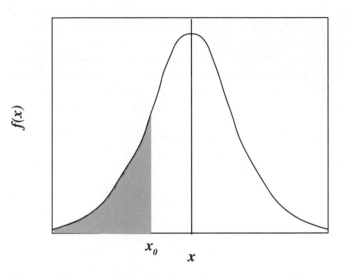

Figure B.1   The normal distribution. The maximum of the curve occurs at $x = \mu$. The probability of a random value of x being less than x_0 is the shaded area.

The Poisson distribution has the curious property that its mean is equal to its variance. The mean number of events in a time t may be shown to be:

$$\bar{n}(t) = \lambda t = \sigma^2(t). \tag{B.39}$$

B.6   The normal distribution

By far the most common continuous distribution function is the normal, or Gaussian, distribution. Its density function is given by

$$f(x) = \frac{1}{\sqrt{2\pi}\sigma} e^{-(x-\mu)^2/2\sigma^2} \tag{B.40}$$

where μ is the mean ($\mu = \bar{x}$) and σ^2 is the variance of the distribution.

A graph of $f(x)$ (Fig. B.1) shows that it is a symmetric bell-shaped curve with a maximum at $x = \mu$ and a width that depends on the variance σ^2. The total area under the curve is, of course, 1.0, although advanced integration techniques are needed to prove this, since $f(x)$ has no integral in terms of simple functions.

Because the pdf of the normal distribution is not an easily integrable function, tables of its values often need to be used in calculating probabilities, although some pocket calculators now have the normal distribution built in. The tables are usually given in terms of the special distribution with a zero mean ($\mu = 0$) and unit variance ($\sigma^2 = 1$). It is fairly straight-forward to transform these values into probabilities for arbitrary means and variances, however.

Let us illustrate the technique by calculating probability that the normal variable x, with mean μ and variance σ^2, lies in the interval $[a, b]$. This is given by the integral

$$Prob(a < x < b) = \int_a^b \frac{1}{\sqrt{2\pi}\sigma} e^{-(x-\mu)^2/2\sigma^2}\,dx. \qquad (B.41)$$

Now, make the substitution

$$z \equiv \frac{x - \mu}{\sigma}. \qquad (B.42)$$

This transforms the integral to

$$Prob(a < x < b) = \frac{1}{\sqrt{2\pi}} \int_\alpha^\beta e^{-z^2/2}\,dz. \qquad (B.43)$$

The new limits on the integral are

$$\alpha = (a - \mu)/\sigma; \qquad \beta = (b - \mu)/\sigma. \qquad (B.44)$$

Now the new integral is a probability that a random variable z drawn from a normal distribution with mean zero and variance 1.0 lies in the interval $[(a - \mu)/\sigma, (b - \mu)/\sigma]$.

The zero-mean, unit-variance tables of the normal distribution are usually given in terms of the cumulative distribution function $F(y)$, which is the probability that $z < y$. If we want the probability that z actually lies in an interval $[\alpha, \beta]$, we need only observe that

$$Prob(\alpha < z < \beta) = Prob(z < \beta) - Prob(z < \alpha). \qquad (B.45)$$

A complete numerical example will help to tie all this together. Given a normal variable x with mean $\mu = 2.0$ and variance $\sigma^2 = 5.3$, find the probability that $x \in [1.2, 1.8]$.

First, we must convert this to a problem dealing with a zero-mean unit-variance normal distribution. To do this, we use the substitution

$$z = \frac{x - \mu}{\sigma} = \frac{x - 2.0}{2.302}. \qquad (B.46)$$

The new problem is then to find $P(-0.347 < z < -0.0869)$. In terms of a tabulated cdf, this will be $P(z < -0.0869) - P(z < -0.347)$. Looking these quantities up in a table we find $P(z < -0.0869) = 0.4653$ and $P(z < -0.347) = 0.3643$. Our final answer is then

$$P(x \in [1.2, 1.8]) = 0.1010. \tag{B.47}$$

The importance of the normal distribution stems from a result in statistical theory called the *central limit theorem*. To see the significance of this theorem, suppose we conduct an experiment on a system with an unknown distribution function. Let $\bar{X}$ be the mean of n measurements, that is, the mean result obtained after running the experiment n times. The central limit theorem states that, if n is large enough, $\bar{X}$ will approach a normal distribution arbitrarily closely. Further, the mean and variance of the normal distribution are related to the mean and variance of the distribution from which each experimental result was originally obtained, as follows. The means are the same and, if the original distribution has variance σ^2, the normal distribution will have variance σ^2/n.

The central limit theorem thus implies that the distribution obtained in measurement of any experimental quantity will be approximately normal, provided enough measurements are taken. In practice, surprisingly few measurements are needed—often only 6 or 7 will do.

C

Computer simulation

C.1 Introduction

This appendix is intended as an introduction to the basics of writing computer simulations to model the sorts of systems described in this book. It is assumed that you are familiar with some reasonably high-level computer language such as Pascal or C, so no attempt is made to teach the syntax of any language. The first parts of this appendix will be kept free of references to any specific language. The intention of the first section is to introduce some essential knowledge about data structures (the way computers store information) which are needed if you are to write intelligent simulations.

The final section of this appendix will describe in detail the implementation of one of the models discussed earlier in the book to give an example of how a complete computer simulation may be written. Computer programming is to a large extent a personal endeavour, in the sense that different programmers have different ways of writing functions to perform the same tasks, but there are certain aspects of programming style which are (or should be) common to all programs. Some of these principles will be discussed as we go along.

In order to describe the writing of a simulation in detail, a specific language must be used. The language used here is C. This is partly due to the author's personal taste, since other languages such as Pascal or Fortran could have been used equally well. C is becoming increasingly common in all areas of computing, taking over from Cobol in financial applications, Fortran in science, and so on. Its increasing popularity is partly due to its power (it allows more control over the memory being managed by your program than many other languages) and partly because it is the language designed to mesh with the UNIX[1] operating system, which is making equally large strides in the computing community. The power of C comes at a cost, however: it is not the easiest language to learn, especially if you have never done any programming before. If you are a novice programmer, or have only programmed in interpreted languages

---

[1] UNIX is a trademark of Bell Labs.

such as BASIC, you may be better off learning Pascal before graduating to C. All the simulations in this book could be written in Pascal, at the expense of a bit more typing.

This appendix begins with a description of how numbers are stored in the binary code common to all computers. Following this, we examine several data structures frequently used in computer modelling: arrays, structures (called records in Pascal), and pointers and linked lists. Following this is a section on aspects of good programming style. Finally we look at a detailed example of writing a computer simulation.

C.2   Data representation in a computer

In digital computers information is stored and transmitted using a binary code. This code consists of a sequence of symbols which are of the off/on type, that is, each symbol is one of two types: off or on. A code is written on paper in binary notation, with the two states represented as '0' and '1'.

C.2.1   Binary, octal, and hexadecimal representation of integers

Although all data are stored in a binary code we will start by examining the representation used for integers.

Let's review ordinary decimal notation. Consider a decimal (base 10) number like 170. The digits 1, 7 and 0 are arranged with the least significant digit (the one that represents the smallest quantity) on the right, in the *units* place, then the tens place, hundreds place, and so on. The notation 170 means that we are talking about a quantity of magnitude $1 \times 10^2 + 7 \times 10^1 + 0 \times 10^0$. Note that the base (10) of the notation is raised to successively higher powers as we move from right to left.

In binary or base 2, the digits are also arranged with the least significant on the right and most significant on the left. The rightmost binary digit or *bit* as it is called is the units place, just as for decimal numbers. However, since we are using base 2 instead of 10, successive places to the left are the twos, fours, eights, sixteens, and so on, that is, successive powers of 2. In base 10, we use 10 symbols (0 through 9) to represent numbers. In base 2, we only need 2 symbols (0 and 1). So for example, the number 101_2 in binary is $1 \times 2^2 + 0 \times 2^1 + 1 \times 2^0 = 5_{10}$ where the subscript 10 on the 5 indicates that it is a base 10 number.

It is customary, when writing binary numbers, to write out the digits in groups of 4, even if the numbers require fewer than 4 digits. Thus, the first 8 binary integers are 0000, 0001, 0010, 0011, 0100, 0101, 0110, 0111, 1000. A sequence of 8 bits is called a *byte*. A group of 4 bits is sometimes called a *nybble*.

To write a decimal number in binary notation, it is best to follow a definite and precise set of steps. Any precisely defined method for doing something is called an *algorithm*. The algorithm for representing a decimal number in binary is as follows.

1. Set N equal to the decimal number.

2. Divide N by 2. Set R equal to the remainder and set N equal to the integer part of the division (replacing the old value of N).

3. Write down R to the left of any previous remainders.

4. If $N > 0$ repeat from step 2. Otherwise stop.

To illustrate, we convert 42 to binary. Following the algorithm we have

- $N = 42$.

- $N/2 = 21$ so $R = 0$ and we set $N = 21$.

- Write down R: 0.

- $N > 0$ so continue.

- $N/2 = 10$ with remainder $R = 1$. Set $N = 10$.

- Write down R to left of previous value: 10.

- $N > 0$ so continue.

- $N/2 = 5$. $R = 0$, new $N = 5$.

- Write down R: 010.

- $N > 0$ continue.

- $N/2 = 2$, $R = 1$, $N = 2$.

- Write down R: 1010.

- Continue.

- another couple of cycles eventually gives $42_{10} = 101010_2$.

In standard notation, this number would be written as two groups of 4 digits: 0010 1010.

To convert from binary to decimal it is easiest to start with the least significant bit (lsb) and work towards the most significant bit (msb). For example to convert the binary number 0110 1001, we would do the following. $0110\ 1001 = 1 \times 2^0 + 0 \times 2^1 + 0 \times 2^2 + 1 \times 2^3 + 0 \times 2^4 + 1 \times 2^5 + 1 \times 2^6 = 1 + 8 + 32 + 64 = 105_{10}$.

Obviously, writing and reading long strings of bits can be tedious and confusing. For this reason, two other ways of writing numbers are commonly used: octal and hexadecimal. Octal numbers are base 8 and hexadecimal (or hex for short) are base 16. Because both bases are powers of 2 ($8 = 2^3$, $16 = 2^4$), conversion to and from binary is easy, as we shall see. However, first we must deal with the symbols used in these two bases. Octal requires 8 symbols (0 through 7) so this is no problem. Hex, however, requires 16 symbols. For the numbers 0 through 9 we may use the decimal symbols, but new symbols need to be defined for the numbers 10 through 15. In practice, the uppercase letters A through F are used. Thus to count from 1 to 15 in hex, we write 1, 2, 3, 4, 5, 6, 7, 8, 9, A, B, C, D, E, F.

The places in octal are powers of 8, so we have the units (8^0) place, the eights, sixty-fours, 512s, etc. Similarly, in hex we have powers of 16: 1s, 16s, 256s, etc. Conversion from decimal to octal or hex proceeds the same way as to binary, except you replace the division by 2 in the algorithm with division by 8 or 16. For example, to convert 42 to octal, we have

- $N = 42$.

- $N/8 = 5$ with $R = 2$. Set $N = 5$.

- write 2.

- continue.

- $N/8 = 0$, remainder $R = 5$. Set $N = 0$.

- write 52.

- $N = 0$ so stop.

so that $42_{10} = 52_8$.
To convert 42_{10} to hex:

- $N = 42$.

- $N/16 = 2$, $R = 10$, set $N = 2$.

- write (in hex notation) A.

- continue.

- $N/16 = 0$ with $R = 2$ and set $N = 0$.

- write 2A.

- stop.

and $42_{10} = 2A_{16}$.

Converting from octal or hex to decimal, we use the same method as for binary. For example, $371_8 = 1 \times 8^0 + 7 \times 8^1 + 3 \times 8^2 = 1 + 56 + 192 = 249_{10}$. And $A4F_{16} = 15 \times 16^0 + 4 \times 16^1 + 10 \times 16^2 = 2639_{10}$.

The conversion between octal and binary is easy, either way. Since the base of octal is 2^3, each group of 3 bits, starting from the lsb on the right, corresponds to one octal digit. Thus to convert from binary to octal, partition the binary number into groups of 3 bits, starting from the right.

Example. Convert 1101 0101 to octal. We write the partition as 011|010|101 where we've padded out the leftmost group with an extra zero. Now we simply convert each group of three bits to a single octal digit: 325_8.

To convert from octal to binary, simply write out the binary form of each octal digit in order, using 3 bits for each digit.

Example. Convert 471_8 to binary. Using $4_8 = 100_2$, $7_8 = 111_2$ and $1_8 = 001_2$ we have $471_8 = 100111001_2$. Rewriting in the usual 4-digit grouping we have 0001 0011 1001.

To convert from binary to hex, we observe that the base of hex is 2^4, so we can take the bits in the binary number in groups of 4. To convert 0001 0011 1001 to hex we simply write the hex digit for each group of 4, in order: $0001\ 0011\ 1001 = 139_{16}$. Finally to convert hex to binary, just write out the binary equivalent of each hex digit, using 4 bits per digit. Convert A4F to binary: 1010 0100 1111.

To convert between octal and hex, it is easiest to go via binary. For example, to convert A4F to octal, write it in binary first: 1010 0100 1111, then convert to octal: $101|001|001|111 = 5117_8$. Similarly to convert from octal to hex, use binary. Converting 347_8 to hex, we write $347_8 = 011100111_2 = 11100111 = E7_{16}$.

C.2.2   Integer overflow

Simple arithmetic such as addition and multiplication can be done in binary using rules similar to those familiar to you in decimal. However, the computer modeller should be aware of some of the things that can produce errors while doing arithmetic.

In most standard languages, numeric variables have a certain amount of space allocated to them. Standard integer variables in C usually have 32 bits allocated to them. If these integers are *unsigned* (that is, they are all positive or zero), an integer variable can hold any integer between 0 and $2^{32} - 1 = 4\,294\,967\,295$. However, standard integer variables in most languages allow both positive and negative integers in the same amount of space. Because of the way negative integers are represented (a format called *two's complement*), the range of integers than can be stored in n bits is $[-2^{n-1}, 2^{n-1} - 1]$. For a 32-bit integer variable, the values are $[-2147483648,\ 2147483647]$. If a program includes a calculation that causes an integer variable to exceed either of these limits, *integer overflow* will result. The effects of overflow vary, depending on the language and the operating system. Some machines will print an error message and kill the program. Others will perform the calculation to obtain an incorrect result and simply proceed with the process. If the latter case occurs, your program may give you wildly incorrect answers (negative population sizes, for example) for no apparent reason. Such bugs can be extremely difficult to detect, because the internal logic of the program is correct.

The problem arises because the two's complement method of representing negative integers assumes that any integer in which the most significant bit is set to 1 is to be interpreted as a negative number. Thus it is possible to do an addition of two integers i and j, both of which are less than $2^{n-1} - 1$, but whose sum $i + j$ is greater than $2^{n-1} - 1$ and obtain a number whose most significant bit is set to 1. If unsigned integers were being used, the answer would be correct, but with two's complement, the result is interpreted as a negative quantity. You can easily test to see if your compiler produces errors of this sort by writing a simple program which adds together two numbers that will give an answer larger than the maximum permissible integer. If the answer is negative, you are suffering from integer overflow.

When writing programs in which you expect integers to get large, it is worth putting in some checks to ensure that integer overflow never occurs. If it does not seem reasonable to rewrite the program in a way that avoids large integers, you may have to write your own routines to add and multiply such integers together to avoid overflow, but usually this can be avoided.

C.3   Floating point numbers

We now consider how real numbers—those with fractional parts—are represented on a computer. In decimal, we can always write any real number in the form $m \times 10^e$ where m is the *mantissa*, and is usually taken to be some number in the interval $[0.1, 1)$, and e is the *exponent*, which is an integer (positive or negative or zero). For example, $12\,345 = 0.12345 \times 10^5$, $0.0000982 = 0.982 \times 10^{-4}$, and so on.

Computers use the same sort of notation for storing real numbers, except they are stored in base 2 instead of base 10. In base 2, a number can always be written in the form $m \times 2^e$, where m is in the interval $[0.5, 1)$ and e is an integral exponent. To express a number in this form we divide or multiply it by 2 until we obtain a number in the interval $[0.5, 1)$, recording the number of divisions or multiplications required. For example, to express $12\,345$ in this form, we divide by 2 14 times so that $12\,345 = 0.7534790039... \times 2^{14}$. A fractional number is multiplied by 2 in the same way. To convert 0.0000982, we multiply by 2 13 times so that $0.0000982 = 0.8044544 \times 2^{-13}$.

C.3.1 Converting fractions from decimal to binary

To see how a computer stores binary real numbers, we must first see how a fraction is written in binary. Again, the motivation comes from decimal notation. The digits in a decimal fraction, such as 0.1328, can be determined by successively multiplying the fraction by 10 and recording the integral parts. For example, $0.1328 \times 10 = 1.328$. The integral part is 1, so the first digit in the decimal representation is 1. Now we take the remaining fractional part, 0.328, and repeat the procedure. $0.328 \times 10 = 3.28$, so the next digit is 3 and so on. This is all blindingly obvious because the fraction was originally written in base 10, so we aren't really learning anything new.

However, we can use the same technique to convert a decimal fraction to binary (or octal or hex or any other base). To read off the binary form of the fraction 0.1328, we multiply by 2 instead of 10. Thus we get $0.1328 \times 2 = 0.2656$ with integral part 0 so the first digit in the binary fraction is 0. Now take $2 \times 0.2656 = 0.5312$ so another 0. Continuing we get $2 \times 0.5312 = 1.0624$ so the next digit is a 1. Now we take fractional part and multiply by 2 again: $2 \times .0624 = 0.1248$ so we get another 0. Thus to 4 binary places, we have $0.1328_{10} = 0.0010_2$. Continuing for a few more places, we get 0.001000011111111100... Just as with decimal fractions, any binary representation of a rational number will either terminate or give a repeating pattern of numbers after a while.

To convert to a hex or octal fraction, just use 16 or 8 as the mutliplier in place of 2.

To convert back from binary (or hex or octal) to decimal, suppose we write a general binary fraction as $0.b_1 b_2 b_3 b_4 \ldots$ where each b_i is either 0 or 1. Then the value of the fraction is given by $b_1 \times 2^{-1} + b_2 \times 2^{-2} + b_3 \times 2^{-3} + \ldots$. So to convert 0.01101 to decimal, we write $0 \times 2^{-1} + 1 \times 2^{-2} + 1 \times 2^{-3} + 0 \times 2^{-4} + 1 \times 2^{-5} = 0.25 + 0.125 + 0.03125 = 0.40625$.

Example: convert 0.A4F from hex to decimal. Here we have $10 \times 16^{-1} + 4 \times 16^{-2} + 15 \times 16^{-3} = 0.644287\ldots$

C.3.2 Storage of floating point numbers

Floating point numbers are stored in three pieces: the sign, the exponent and the mantissa. Unlike integers, two's complement notation is not used for representing floating point; rather, a separate bit is used to indicate the sign. The sign bit is 0 if the number is positive or zero and 1 if the number is negative.

Floating point numbers usually come in at least two precisions: single and double. A single precision number is allotted 32 bits, a double 64. The layout is as follows for single precision:

```
31    |    30 ... 23    |    22 ... 0
Sign        Exponent         Mantissa
```

The exponent, being an integer, is written in two's complement. Thus, since eight bits are given to the exponent, the largest exponent that can be represented is $2^7 - 1 = 127$ and the smallest is $-2^7 = -128$. Thus the largest number representable is about $2^{127} \approx 10^{38}$ and the smallest is about $2^{-128} \approx 10^{-39}$.

Example Express 1897.634 in floating point. First we must convert the number to the form $m \times 2^e$. Upon dividing by 2 11 times we get $0.9265791015 \times 2^{11}$. The exponent is therefore 11 and will be written as 0000 1011.

To determine the mantissa, we multiply the fractional part successively by 2, recording the integral part at each step. We get 0.11101101 to eight binary places. Finally, since the number is positive, the sign bit is 0. The representation is 0|00001011|11101101....

In double precision the extra 32 bits are all allocated to the mantissa, so that the exponent is still 8 bits. Thus the range of numbers that can be represented in double precision is the same as that in single precision. Only the accuracy of the numbers is increased. The accuracy of single precision is $\pm 2^{-23}$ or around $\pm 10^{-7}$ in the mantissa. Since numbers are usually input into the computer in decimal and converted to binary floating point internally, you can only expect the binary representation to correspond to the number you input to within this error tolerance. Double precision is accurate to $\pm 2^{-55}$ or about 10^{-17}. Thus double precision is actually more than twice as accurate as single precision. These initial conversion errors can be greatly magnified in subsequent calculations.

Some computer languages support even higher precision in which even more bits are allocated to the mantissa. Some precisions give more bits to the exponent so that larger and smaller numbers can be represented.

C.3.3 Floating point arithmetic

To see how round-off errors arise in floating point arithmetic we will consider the addition problem $5.981 \times 10^{-3} + 0.152$. The exact answer is 0.157981. The first number is equivalent to 0.765568×2^{-7}. Using an 8-bit mantissa and the procedure above for converting this to a binary number, we obtain a mantissa of 1100 0011. Similarly, $0.152 = 0.608 \times 2^{-2}$, giving a mantissa of 1001 1011. Now in order to add the mantissas, the exponents of the two terms must be the same. Since the mantissa must always be less than one, we must convert the number with the smaller exponent so that its exponent equals the larger exponent. In this case the smaller exponent is -7 and the larger is -2. We can change the exponent of -7 to -2 if we divide the mantissa by the difference, that is, by 2^5. This is equivalent to shifting the mantissa 5 bits to the right, filling in the left with zeroes. Thus mantissa of the first number becomes 0000 0110. We can now add the two mantissas directly: 0000 0110 + 1001 1011 = 1010 0001. This mantissa converts back to $2^{-1} + 2^{-3} + 2^{-8} = 0.62890625$ in decimal. Mutliplying by the exponent of 2^{-2} gives the final answer of 0.157226562. We see that we have retained only 3 decimal places of accuracy, which is what we expect, since an 8-bit mantissa is only accurate to within $\pm 2^{-8} \approx 0.004$.

The implications of round-off error for modelling should be fairly obvious: don't attempt to add or subtract two floating point numbers that are very different in size. In an extreme case, if one number is much much smaller than the other, an addition may make no difference to the larger number. This problem can lead to infinite loops. For example, if you are following the behaviour of a population between two times, say $t_1 = 2 \times 10^{10}$ and $t_2 = 2.001 \times 10^{10}$, you may wish to achieve greater accuracy in the simulation by using smaller time steps. Using a time step of $\Delta T = 10$ will never change the time variable if you are using a single precision floating point variable to record the time, since $\Delta T < 10^{-7} \times 2 \times 10^{10}$, so adding the time increment to the time variable will not change the time at all.

In other cases, the round-off error may accumulate over the course of many calculations with the result that the final answer is meaningless. Again, such errors may be very difficult to detect, since the algorithm has been correctly coded and it is only the values of the variables that are causing the problem. You should try to plan things so that you do not need to add variables of greatly different sizes. If this is unavoidable, you may need to use higher precision in your variables.

C.4   Text data: ASCII

While numbers are always represented in base 2 for the purposes of calculation in a computer, any data that are stored as text uses a different code. For example, the source code to a program or a file that contains lists of numbers or other alphanumeric data is stored as sequences of characters, not as base 2 numbers. The main code used for storing character data is ASCII.

ASCII stands for American Standard Code for Information Interchange. It contains a binary code for all the characters generated by the keyboard, and a few others that are not generated by all keyboards.

The standard ASCII set consists of 128 binary codes, from 000 0000 to 111 1111. The msb of the byte is not written because it is sometimes reserved for a *parity* bit (an error check) and on some micro computers another 128 special symbols (graphic characters or mathematical symbols) are defined using this eighth bit. Since its use varies from one system to another, we will explicitly write only the first 7 bits.

Table of ASCII codes

Note: The prefix 'C-' means 'hold down control key';

e.g. 'C-G' means control-G.

Dec	Char	Binary	Hex	Comments
0	NUL	000 0000	00	C-@ (Null byte)
1	SOH	000 0001	01	C-A (Start of heading)
2	STX	000 0010	02	C-B (Start of text)
3	ETX	000 0011	03	C-C (End of text)
4	EOT	000 0100	04	C-D (End of transmission)
5	ENQ	000 0101	05	C-E (Enquiry)
6	ACK	000 0110	06	C-F (Acknowledge)
7	BEL	000 0111	07	C-G (Ring terminal bell)
8	BS	000 1000	08	C-H (Backspace)
9	HT	000 1001	09	C-I (Horizontal tab)
10	LF	000 1010	0A	C-J (Line feed)
11	VT	000 1011	0B	C-K (Vertical tab)
12	FF	000 1100	0C	C-L (Form feed)
13	CR	000 1101	0D	C-M (Carriage return)
14	SO	000 1110	0E	C-N (Shift out)
15	SI	000 1111	0F	C-O (Shift in)
16	DLE	001 0000	10	C-P (Data link escape)
17	DC1	001 0001	11	C-Q (Device control 1)
18	DC2	001 0010	12	C-R (Device control 2)
19	DC3	001 0011	13	C-S (Device control 3)
20	DC4	001 0100	14	C-T (Device control 4)
21	NAK	001 0101	15	C-U (Negative acknowledge)
22	SYN	001 0110	16	C-V (Synchronous idle)
23	ETB	001 0111	17	C-W (End of transmission block)
24	CAN	001 1000	18	C-X (Cancel)
25	EM	001 1001	19	C-Y (End of medium)
26	SUB	001 1010	1A	C-Z (Substitute)
27	ESC	001 1011	1B	C-[(Escape)
28	FS	001 1100	1C	C-\ (File separator)
29	GS	001 1101	1D	C-] (Group separator)
30	RS	001 1110	1E	C-^ (Record separator)
31	US	001 1111	1F	C-_ (Unit separator)

Dec	Char	Binary	Hex	Dec	Char	Binary	Hex
32	(space)	010 0000	20	73	I	100 1001	49
33	!	010 0001	21	74	J	100 1010	4A
34	"	010 0010	22	75	K	100 1011	4B
35	#	010 0011	23	76	L	100 1100	4C
36	$	010 0100	24	77	M	100 1101	4D
37	%	010 0101	25	78	N	100 1110	4E
38	&	010 0110	26	79	O	100 1111	4F
39	'	010 0111	27	80	P	101 0000	50
40	(	010 1000	28	81	Q	101 0001	51
41	)	010 1001	29	82	R	101 0010	52
42	*	010 1010	2A	83	S	101 0011	53
43	+	010 1011	2B	84	T	101 0100	54
44	,	010 1100	2C	85	U	101 0101	55
45	-	010 1101	2D	86	V	101 0110	56
46	.	010 1110	2E	87	W	101 0111	57
47	/	010 1111	2F	88	X	101 1000	58
48	0	011 0000	30	89	Y	101 1001	59
49	1	011 0001	31	90	Z	101 1010	5A
50	2	011 0010	32	91	[	101 1011	5B
51	3	011 0011	33	92	\	101 1100	5C
52	4	011 0100	34	93	]	101 1101	5D
53	5	011 0101	35	94	^	101 1110	5E
54	6	011 0110	36	95	_	101 1111	5F
55	7	011 0111	37	96	'	110 0000	60
56	8	011 1000	38	97	a	110 0001	61
57	9	011 1001	39	98	b	110 0010	62
58	:	011 1010	3A	99	c	110 0011	63
59	;	011 1011	3B	100	d	110 0100	64
60	<	011 1100	3C	101	e	110 0101	65
61	=	011 1101	3D	102	f	110 0110	66
62	>	011 1110	3E	103	g	110 0111	67
63	?	011 1111	3F	104	h	110 1000	68
64	@	100 0000	40	105	i	110 1001	69
65	A	100 0001	41	106	j	110 1010	6A
66	B	100 0010	42	107	k	110 1011	6B
67	C	100 0011	43	108	l	110 1100	6C
68	D	100 0100	44	109	m	110 1101	6D
69	E	100 0101	45	110	n	110 1110	6E
70	F	100 0110	46	111	o	110 1111	6F
71	G	100 0111	47	112	p	111 0000	70
72	II	100 1000	48	113	q	111 0001	71

Dec	Char	Binary	Hex	Dec	Char	Binary	Hex
114	r	111 0010	72	121	y	111 1001	79
115	s	111 0011	73	122	z	111 1010	7A
116	t	111 0100	74	123	{	111 1011	7B
117	u	111 0101	75	124	|	111 1100	7C
118	v	111 0110	76	125	}	111 1101	7D
119	w	111 0111	77	126	~	111 1110	7E
120	x	111 1000	78	127	DEL	111 1111	7F

The first 32 ASCII codes (000 0000 to 001 1111 or 0 to 31 in decimal) are reserved for special codes, most of which are invisible if printed on a terminal screen. They are also interpreted differently by some programs (such as text editors). For example, 13 is a carriage return, which positions the cursor at the beginning of a line, 10 is a line feed, which moves the cursor down one line and so on. On many keyboards many of these codes can be produced by holding down the control key and pressing one of the alphabet keys A to Z. You should be careful in trying this, though, since some codes have special meanings to certain terminals and can cause them to do strange things!

ASCII 32 to 47 are punctuation codes and other special symbols like $, %, and so on. ASCII 48 to 57 are codes for the digits 0 to 9. Note that the binary code for the numbers is 011 0000 through 011 1001, that is, the lower nybble is a base 2 number equal to the digit character it represents. ASCII 58 to 64 are a few more punctuation symbols. ASCII 65 to 90 code for the upper-case letters A through Z in order. The binary codes for the letters are 100 0001 through 101 1010. The 5 least significant bits cover the decimal numbers 1 through 26. ASCII 91 through 96 are more punctuation symbols. ASCII 97 through 122 are the lower-case letters. Again, the 5 least significant bits are base 2 1 through 26. Finally, ASCII 123 through 126 are punctuation and ASCII 127 is the code for the DELETE key.

C.5 Arrays

Computer models frequently make use of data structures in which several variables are grouped together under a single name. In order to write efficient programs, both from the point of view of memory and time usage, it is important to understand how these composite structures are stored and accessed.

The first data structure we shall examine is the *array*. Arrays are available in most computer languages, and are usually declared as a single variable name to which a certain number of elements are allocated as in `vector[50]`, which refers to an array named *vector* holding 50 elements of some specific data type, such as integers. Arrays of more than one dimension are frequently allowed. For example, a matrix may be represented by a two-dimensional array `matrix[30][20]` which could store the elements of a 30 × 20 array.

The individual array elements are accessed in a program by simply specifying the index of element required. For example, the statement

`x = matrix[27][19]`

would (in some languages) assign the contents of element [27][19] from the two-dimensional array matrix to the variable x.

C.5.1   Implementation of arrays

There are two fundamental operations that can be performed on an array: *reading* one of its elements or *writing* into one of its elements. Arrays allow direct or random access to their elements, meaning that it takes the same computing time to read or write any of the elements. This is in contrast to linked data structures (such as a linked list using pointers) where access to the list always starts at the beginning and proceeds item by item until the desired location is reached. In a linked list, the time taken to access an item depends on how far down the list it is. In addition, the elements of a linked list cannot be referred to by an index; you must write your own procedure to find a given location.

Although arrays have the advantages of a faster access time and easier notation for referring to a given element, they have the disadvantage that their sizes must be fixed at compilation time. If you plan to use an array to store a list, you must know in advance how large the list can get and declare the array size to handle the largest list. This can be wasteful of memory if most of the lists are smaller than the maximum size. It can also cause the program to crash if a list longer than the maximum allowed for is encountered.

To see how the advantages and disadvantages of arrays arise, we need to consider how they are stored in the computer's memory. When you declare a single variable such as an integer, you are giving instructions to the compiler that it should reserve space in memory for this variable. The compiler then interacts with the operating system (the program that manages the entire computer system) to find where in memory there is some free space for this variable to be stored. Each word[2] in the computer's RAM (random access memory) has an *address*, which is just an integer saying which location in memory the word occupies.

For individual variables like single integers and reals, each of which occupy a single word (usually 32 bits), only single free words need be found. These words are usually in consecutive addresses in memory, though they

---

[2]As variables vary in length, we shall use the term *word* to denote the space occupied by any variable. Not all words are same length.

need not be. The compiler records the address assigned to each variable by the operating system so that the program can find its way around once it is run. However, if you request space for an array of say N elements, the compiler must find N free consecutive addresses for this array. The first element in the array, say vector[1] above, is stored at the first address reserved, called the *base address* for the array. Let us call the base address b. Successive elements are stored at sequential locations from b. Thus vector[2] is stored at location $b + 1$, vector[3] at $b + 2$ and so on until vector[50] is stored at location $b + 49$.[3]

When you refer to a particular array element in your program, its location in memory is calculated by the program from the base address b and the index i. For example, if you refer to vector[10], the the index is 10 and the program finds the address of vector[10] by adding 9 to b. It is for this reason that access to all locations requires the same time, since a single addition is required to determine the address of any element.

Because there must be a direct correspondence between the index and the address, array indexes must be ordinal types. You cannot use, for example, real numbers as indexes since there is no such correspondence between reals and addresses.

Not all variable types occupy the same amount of space. For example, characters are single bytes. Some languages provide higher precision variables (such as double floating point variables in C or double precision variables in Fortran) which occupy twice as much space. Arrays can be defined for all of these types. The address calculation must take the different size of the variable types into account. In general, suppose we wish to store an array each of whose elements occupy s bytes. Then to find the byte address a of the element with index i we would use the formula

$$a = b + s * (i - 1). \tag{C.1}$$

For example, we may wish to store an array heavy[20] of 20 double precision reals each of which occupies 64 bits, or 8 bytes. Then $s = 8$, so that the 12th element begins at location $a = b + 88$, where the base address b would be determined by the operating system when the program is compiled.

C.5.2 Address translation formulas

The storage of one-dimensional arrays is simple because only a single offset need be calculated to locate each element. Higher-dimensional arrays

---

[3]The relation between the offset and the array index will be most familiar to C programmers, since the first element of an array in C is always assigned index number 0. Thus the vector array would be *declared* as vector[50], but *accessed* by referring to elements vector[0] through vector[49].

need to be stored in some specific order: although a two-dimensional array such as `matrix[30][20]` looks plain enough on paper, the computer must store everything in a one-dimensional form in its memory, since memory is accessed by means of a single address. We therefore must have a way of mapping the two-dimensional array into one-dimension for storage.

There are various conventions for doing this, depending on the language you are using. In some languages, such as Pascal and C, you can choose, via the way you define the array, which storage method you want.

Let us look at two-dimensional arrays first. Suppose you wish to store the numbers in a 3×5 matrix in an array *matrix[3][5]*. The elements in the first row of the matrix will be `matrix[1][1]`, `matrix[1][2]`, ... `matrix[1][5]`. The second row is `matrix[2][1]`, `matrix[2][2]`, and so on. One way to store the array is to store it by rows (sometimes referred to as *row major* order). Then the elements would be stored in the order [1][1]; [1][2]; [1][3]; [1][4]; [1][5]; [2][1]; [2][2]; ... [3][4]; [3][5]. In some languages this is the default storage order; in others they are stored in columns.

To work out the actual address of a particular element in a matrix of size r rows by c columns, just use the same procedure as for one-dimensional arrays. Suppose for simplicity that the matrix stores integers of size 1 word. The matrix will start at a base address b, determined by the compiler, which will vary from one compilation to the next. If the matrix is stored row-wise, then element `[i][j]` will be the jth word in the ith block of c words. If $i = 1$, so the element is in the first row, then the address will be $b + j - 1$. If $i > 1$, then we must first skip over the first $i - 1$ rows. Since each complete row has c columns, it will take up c words. Thus in general, element $[i, j]$ will be at address $b + c(i - 1) + j - 1$. This formula is an example of an *address translation formula* or *array mapping function*, that is, a function which tells you the memory location for a particular array element.

In most applications, we don't care what the actual base address b is, since that is a byte address which refers to the computer's internal memory. What is more common is a requirement to know the relative position of element `[i][j]` in the one-dimensional storage array. In this case, we may take $b = 1$, since it now refers to the first element of the one-dimensional array, no matter where it may be stored in memory. The array mappping function above then may be written more conveniently as

$$a = c(i - 1) + j \qquad \qquad \text{(C.2)}$$

where a is the location of element `[i][j]` in the one-dimensional array.

Sometimes it is convenient to use a lower dimension to represent data than the form of the data immediately suggests. For example, in a lower triangular square matrix (of size $n \times n$), all entries above the diagonal are zero. Declaring such a matrix as `lowtri[n][n]` wastes nearly half of the n^2 words reserved in memory, since we know they are always zero. If n is large, this can be a considerable waste of space. Such a matrix can be stored as a one-dimensional array if you write your own address calculation function. If you store only the non-zero entries by row, then you will be storing entries [1][1]; [2][1]; [2][2]; [3][1]; [3][2]; [3][3]; ... To get element [i][j], where $i \geq j$, you must skip over $i-1$ rows ranging in size from 1 element in row 1 to $i-1$ elements in row $i-1$. Thus the number of elements to be skipped over is $\sum_{r=1}^{i-1} r = \frac{1}{2}i(i-1)$. Having reached the correct row, the required element will be a further j elements along, so we have the array mapping function for storing a lower triangular matrix by rows as a one-dimensional array:

$$a = \frac{1}{2}i(i-1) + j \qquad (C.3)$$

C.6 Structures and records

Frequently we wish to represent an object with several attributes as a single entity in a program. For example, in constructing a program to simulate the spin glass model of the origin of life discussed in Chapter 4, we need to represent an RNA molecule as a sequence of bases. Each of these bases has an identity (one of two types) and may or may not be connected to up to three other bases: one on either side in the same strand, and a complementary base on another strand. The entire RNA molecule is composed of a sequence of these bases so such a sequence is one property of the molecule that we wish to record. However, each molecule will have a number of other properties, such as whether it is dead or alive, whether it is part of a complex, and so on.

We could write a program in which each of these properties was stored in an individual array, with the index of the array being a label for the molecule to which it refers. However, it is much clearer to represent all these properties of a molecule as separate parts of a single data structure. Several languages provide such a composite structure, although the feature is not as widespread as the array. There is no common term for such a structure in those languages that do support it. In C, it is known simply as a *structure*, while in Pascal it is called a *record*. We will use the term 'structure' here.

As an example, let us consider a structure that might be defined to represent an RNA molecule. First we need a structure to represent a single base within the molecule.[4] A suitable structure is[5]

---

[4]Structures may contain other structures, so the structure representing the RNA molecule may contain as one of its entries a structure representing a base.

[5]The syntax we use for a structure is not that found in any specific computer language. Readers should consult a book on their favourite language to find the syntax peculiar to that language.

```
base = structure {
  char identity
  pointer leftbase
  pointer rightbase
  pointer compbase
}
```

This definition states that a data type named **base** is a structure with four parts or *fields* as they are usually called. In this case the first field is a character variable (of type **char**), and the last three are pointer variables (they contain addresses of other locations in memory). Pointers are really just integers, although they have a different interpretation. The meanings of the four fields are: **identity** is the chemical identity of the base represented by the structure, **leftbase** and **rightbase** are pointers[6] to the bases to its left and right on the same strand, and **compbase** is the pointer to the base on the complementary strand to which it is bound. Any of the latter three fields could, of course, be empty, since any of the neighbours of a base could be absent. A special symbol would be reserved to indicate this.

A master structure representing the entire RNA molecule might be defined as

```
rnamol = structure {
  integer length
  sequence[20] base
  boolean dead
  boolean complex
}
```

This definition declares a new data type called **rnamol** which is a structure containing four fields. The first field is an integer in which the length of the strand (the number of bases) is stored. The second field is defined to be an array of 20 elements, each of which is a structure of type base. This field would be used for storing the sequence of the RNA molecule. The array size of 20 elements imposes an upper limit on the length of any molecule that can be handled in the program. The last two fields are declared as boolean variables, which means they can take on only two values: true and false. They are flags telling us whether or not the molecule is dead or alive, and whether or not it is part of a complex.

This example illustrates that a structure is able to combine several different data types under one heading. It also illustrates that it is possible to define arrays of structures (as in **sequence[20] base**) and that fields

---

[6]See the next section for a discussion of pointers.

of structures may be arrays. By combining arrays and structures, it is possible to organize the variables in a program in such a way that it is easy to locate the precise piece of information required. It is advisable to make as much use of these data constructs as possible.

Once a structure has been defined, we may define variables in terms of them. The declarations we have given in the examples above are not definitions of variables, that is, they do not actually reserve any space in RAM in which data can be stored. They merely define a new data type which can be used later in declarations of variables. These data types are similar in spirit to simpler data types such as integers, floating point numbers and characters: they determine how much space a variable of that type will need in memory, and how that space is divided up.

For example, we could define an array of 1000 RNA molecules using a statement like

```
rna[1000] rnamol
```

The compiler would need to reserve enough consecutive space in RAM for 1000 variables, each of type **rnamol**. To see how much space this is, let us assume that integers, pointers and boolean variables all require 4 bytes each and that a char variable requires a single byte. Then one **base** structure requires 13 bytes (3 pointers and a character). One **rnamol** structure requires an integer (4 bytes), 20 **base** structures (260 bytes), and two booleans (8 bytes) for a total of 272 bytes. The entire array of 1000 molecules therefore requires 272 000 bytes.

These calculations of storage space requirements are usually of little interest to the programmer, since they are all done by the compiler, and the storage locations are recorded so that the variables can be found during execution of the program. However, in biological simulations, it is quite common for the programmer to attempt to explore the model's behaviour for large population sizes. If each member of a population is represented as a structure, as with an RNA molecule in our example, it is important to know how much space the simulation will require, in order that you do not write a program that requires more memory than the computer has. If the machine you are using is *multitasking*, which means that it is capable of running more than one job at a time, the memory requirements of all running jobs must be satisfied. If you are running a text editor, a mail program, and a game in addition to your simulation, the amount of memory available for the simulation may be considerably less than the total RAM of the machine. Even on single-tasking machines, such as many personal computers, not all of the RAM is normally available for the current program.

It is important for the modeller to be aware of the capabilities of the computer system on which the simulation is to be run. If you plan to run a large simulation, you should estimate how much memory the program will expect. If this estimate comes anywhere near the total amount of memory available on your machine, there is a good chance the program will run out of memory at some point. For example, the computer on which I am typing this appendix contains 8 megabytes[7] of RAM. On such a machine, a simulation of the spin glass origin of life model in which the system was restricted to no more than 1000 molecules should run without any problems, since the 272 000 bytes used by the data declarations is only about 3 per cent of the total RAM available. However, increasing the population size to 10 000 could cause problems, since this would require one third of the total RAM. If many other programs are running on the same machine, the simulation may not have enough memory to run. Running a simulation with a population of 100 000 is impossible, since this would require about 27 megabytes.

C.7   Pointers and linked lists

Arrays and structures are efficient data structures to use in those situations where the numbers and types of objects in the simulation do not change much, either within a single run or over several runs. The major restriction of the array is that its size must be fixed when the program is written, as the space for the entire array is reserved by the compiler and cannot be changed during the execution of the program. This can be a problem if the program is to be used to run simulations of systems with different population sizes. If arrays are to be used in this case, either the program must be written to accomodate the largest possible population, or the source code must be changed and recompiled every time the array size is to be changed. The former case is a waste of memory if the program is to be run mainly for small or medium-sized populations and only occasionally for large populations. The latter possibility is not very practical, especially if the program is to be run by users other than the author.[8]

One solution is to abandon the array as the data structure used to implement lists and use *linked lists* instead. A linked list, implemented using pointers, is an example of a *dynamic data structure*, which means storage for the elements of the list is allocated during the execution of the program, and not by the compiler. This has the obvious advantage that you need not specify the size of the list in advance, so that the program can handle populations of varying sizes without any alteration or wasting space on array elements that are never used.

---

[7]A megabyte is not exactly one million bytes. Since most numbers referring to computer hardware are powers of 2, a megabyte is the power of 2 nearest to one million, which is $2^{20} = 1\,048\,576$ bytes.

[8]There are few things in life more difficult or frustrating than trying to alter someone else's computer program.

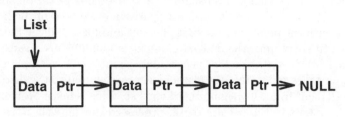

Figure C.1   A linked list. The pointer `List` points to the first element of the list. The last element of the list contains a `NULL` pointer.

The only space that needs to be reserved by the compiler to get a linked list started is a single variable in which a *pointer* to the location of the first list element may be stored. A pointer is simply an integer which is the address of a location in memory. Thus the number stored in this initial variable is used by the program to find the first element in the list. If the list is empty, as it will be when the program is started, the pointer will be set to a special value (usually called `nil` or `NULL`) which indicates an empty list.

To enter the first element in the list, we must first reserve some space for it. This is done by calling a special function or procedure (e.g. the `new` function in Pascal or `malloc()` in C) whose job is to find some free area of memory which is large enough to hold a single list entry. List entries may be single variables such as integers or characters, or they may structures or arrays. The function that reserves the space for the entry will have a way of determining the size of the entry so it knows how much space to find. Once the space is located, the address of this location will be placed in the initial pointer variable so the program can find the place where the data have been stored.

No matter what fields comprise each list entry, there must always be at least one field which points to the next entry in the list. When an entry is added to the list, this pointer field will be set to `NULL`, but when the next entry is added, its address will be inserted in the pointer field of the preceding element. In this way a linked list is built up, one entry at a time (see Fig. C.1).

There are several points worth stressing about linked lists:

- Since the address of each element is stored in the pointer field of the preceding element, successive elements do not need to be adjacent in memory. Linked lists can thus fit into odd vacant corners of a computer's RAM.

- Because the elements of a list may be scattered over various parts of the RAM, the only way to find any particular element of the list is to start with the pointer to the first element and follow all the links from entry to entry until the desired element is found. This means that a linked list is *not* a random access data structure like an array—the time it takes to locate a list element is proportional to the distance of the element from the beginning of the list. This is not a problem if all the elements in the list are to be processed during each iteration in the program, but if you must access some specific, scattered locations in the list frequently and others rarely or not at all, a list can be very inefficient.

- Storing data in a linked list always takes more space than storing the same data in an array of the same length, because each list entry must include the pointer to the next entry. Pointers usually take up 4 bytes of RAM, so this amount of space must be added to each location. This is usually a small price to pay for the added flexibility of dynamic data allocation, but if the list is expected to get very long, it is worth considering.

- Although a linked list removes the restriction of a maximum size on a population due to a fixed array declaration, caution must be used if the population is expected to get very large since the program may attempt to use more memory than the machine has available. Usually the special memory allocation function used to find space for new list elements will return some error flag if all the memory is exhausted, so your program should observe this flag and take appropriate action if memory runs out.

C.8 Programming style

Programming style is to a large extent a personal affair. After you have written several large programs, you develop your own favourite ways of writing certain types of code, defining variables and functions and so on. All of this is normal and acceptable, but it is still safe to say that every programmer's style should adhere to some fundamental principles of proper code construction. Although people have their own mannerisms in the use of their native language, all users of a language should adhere to the rules of grammar and proper language constructs in order that they may be understood by other users of the same language.

Although there are often several different ways of writing computer code to solve a particular problem, computer languages are less flexible than normal languages such as English. If an English word is misspelled, the sense of the sentence is often obvious from the context and no misunderstanding arises. Misspelled variable names or missing semicolons in a computer program, however, may result in the program being rejected by the compiler or, more seriously, a syntactically correct program which gives incorrect results. In order to avoid as many errors as possible while writing a program, as well as to make the code understandable to others (and yourself, six weeks later!) you should strive for a clear, logical approach to programming. This section gives some guidelines which will help you achieve this goal.

To begin, we will list some points which should be followed in any program of any size—even simple ten-line programs to calculate a table of square roots.

- Try to avoid unconditional branching (as exemplified in most languages by the `goto` statement). Use conditional statements such as `if...else`, `while`, and so on. Conditional statements always allow you see where you are in a program if something goes wrong as well as forcing you to plan your program more logically before you start writing the code. Unconditional branches lead to large, messy blocks of code in which the direction of program flow is very difficult to follow. The bit of extra thought required to use conditional statements for all branching is more than repaid by the ease in debugging the program later.

  There are some rare occasions where a `goto` statement may be used. The most common is as an error trap inside a deeply nested loop. If some error condition occurs inside, say, a triply nested `while` loop, a `goto` is a convenient way of breaking out of the entire loop structure and sending the program to a location where errors can be processed. If a `goto` is used, it is advisable to make it the last instruction in the program before it prints an error message and quits.

- Familiarize yourself with the difference between *local* and *global* variables, and use each in its proper place. Global variables are those which are defined outside of all functions and procedures, so that they are recognized everywhere within the program. Local variables are active only within the function in which they are declared. Global variables should only be used for objects which have global meaning, and are expected to be used in all or most of the functions in the program. In a simulation, typical global variables would be the arrays or linked lists which hold the characteristics of the population. Variables such as loop counters, temporary storage variables, and so on, that are used only locally within a particular function should be declared as local variables in the function.

Even though the syntax rules of some languages allow it, you should avoid using the same name for a global and a local variable, simply because it will confuse anyone trying to understand the code.

- Use 'obvious' names for your variables. If you are calculating the average of a set of ages, for example, where the ages are stored in an array, you should call the array elements something like `age[i]` and the variable in which the average is stored '**average**', rather than `x[i]` and `y`, say.

Use constants or external definitions to represent fixed numbers rather than just writing in the number itself. For example, if you encountered the statement

```
c = 6.283185 * r
```

you may not immediately recongnize what is happening, but if you use a constant and more obvious variable names:

```
#define PI = 3.141592
```

```
    . . . . . . . .
```

```
    circum = 2*PI*radius;
```

it is more obvious what's going on.

- Use comments intelligently. Every program and function should begin with a commented description saying what the program or function does. Each variable should have a comment on the line where it is declared to say what it is used for. Major program sections should have comments indicating what is happening at that point. Although comments are useful, avoid overusing them. For example, the line

```
i = i+1;   /* increment i by 1 */
```

does not need the comment. Such comments are more distracting than useful.

- Make your program 'user-friendly'. Always give clear prompts when the user is expected to input data. Try to anticipate the mistakes a user will make when entering data and provide helpful error handling code to cope with them. For example, if the user is supposed to input a number n which must lie between two values, say 0 and 100, a prompt of the form

```
Enter n (0 <= n <= 100):
```

is more useful than a prompt saying `Input number:` or, worse, no prompt at all. If the user types in a number outside the acceptable range, print a helpful error message and ask for the number again, rather than simply allowing the program to crash.

C.8.1 Structured programming

The most important aspect of good programming style has been left until last because it deserves a section on its own. All programs, especially larger ones, should be constructed by using the *top-down* or *structured* approach. The term 'top-down' means that you start with a simple, one-sentence description of the project as a whole and successively subdivide the project into logical blocks or steps until you arrive at a collection of simple tasks, each of which can be coded using a single function or procedure. A good guide to the level of subdivision required is that individual functions should each comfortably fit in their entirety on the screen—about 20 or 30 lines of code. In most cases, if the function is considerably longer than this, it contains more than a single task and should be subdivided further.

The main function in a program should contain a series of function calls, each of which initiates a block of code in the next layer below the top. Each of these functions will in turn call other functions until the level of the single tasks is reached. The structure of the program is similar to that of a tree: the main routine provides the trunk which gives rise to several branches, which in turn give rise to smaller branches and so on, until the leaves at the ends of the branches are encountered. Each leaf is a single task which can be programmed in a simple, short function.

On many computer systems, it is possible to write each function in a separate file and link all the files together with the compiler to produce the final executable code. This is a convenient way of constructing a major package since each file can be kept to a single screenfull in size, and if the files are properly named, it is easy to find a particular section of code if modifications need to be made. In addition, declarations of constants, data structures and global variables should be placed in a separate header file which is included in the other files at compilation time.

A utility, often called `make`, is available for the maintenance of large programs constructed along these lines. The `make` utility requires a file called a *makefile* containing a set of instructions which `make` will follow to build the complete package. Once this makefile is written, the programmer need only type a single command (`make`) to compile and link the entire program. `make` has the advantage that it will only compile those files that have been changed since the last compilation, providing a considerable

saving in compilation time if only one or two out of a dozen or so files have
been changed.

Many commercial compilers of languages such as Pascal, C, and Fortran
now include a `make` utility, which is well worth using. As well, there are
several public domain (that is, free) compilers available for some of the most
common languages on many computer systems. Public domain software
may be obtained through several companies who will charge you only for
the cost of the floppy disk and a small handling charge, or if you have access
to an international computer network, such software may be obtained free
of charge at various sites around the world. Consult a favourite computer
magazine (or your systems administrator, if you have access to a computer
network) for details.

C.9   Example: Supervised learning in a neural network

As an example of the construction of a complete simulation package, we
will present, in full, the code which can be used to run simulations of the
supervised neural network discussed in Chapter 19. Obviously, we cannot
present a complete description of a simulation without writing some real
computer code, so at this stage we must introduce a specific computer
language. The program presented in this section is written in C. Readers
unfamiliar with C, but familiar with a language such as Pascal, should still
be able to follow most of what appears here. It is, of course, also assumed
that the reader has studied Chapter 19, so that the model is familiar.

We will use a top-down approach to writing the program, and store
each function in a separate file, as described above.

To begin, we need a single statement of what the program is to achieve.
We would like a program that allows us to set up a feed-forward neural
network which can be trained using the generalized delta rule and used to
classify input patterns.

Before we write any of the functions, we must decide how we are to
represent the data to be used in the programs. We would like to make the
network as general as possible, which means we would like the freedom to
specify the number of layers of neurons, and the number of neurons in each
layer. Since some of the models using the generalized delta rule involve
connections beyond the nearest neighbour layer, we need the freedom to
construct connections over any number of layers.

All this freedom means that we cannot be certain how many layers
or how many cells we will need in any given run of the program. As
discussed above, in programs where the amount of data storage is unknown
in advance, dynamic data structures are a more useful data representation.
However, a true linked list is not a convenient way of representing a neural
network, since, as we can see from the equations describing the generalized

delta rule, we need to access individual cells in various layers at different times in the algorithm. A sequential data structure in which we had to trace a path from the beginning of the list every time we wanted to access a particular element would be very inefficient.

Fortunately, C allows us to declare arrays dynamically. In C, the name of an array such as `vector` in the array declared as `int vector[50]` is actually a pointer to the first element of the array. The number in square brackets in an array reference is an offset from the first location, so that `vector[5]` refers to the memory location 5 words along from the location to which the name `vector` points (which is actually the sixth element in the array). Thus if we reserve a block of memory sufficiently large to hold 50 integers and define a pointer called `vector` which points to the beginning of this block, we have dynamically allocated an array of 50 integers. It is this technique we will use to define our neural network, since it gives us the freedom to define networks of any size and to access elements within them in a random fashion.

To construct the data structures, we must consider what information needs to be stored. Let us consider an individual neuron. From an examination of the equations used in the model, we see that each cell receives input from previous layers and produces a single output value which is carried to following layers through connections with varying weights. Also, in training the net using the delta rule, we will need to calculate the value of $\delta_{i,j}$. We therefore build a structure containing the output, $\delta_{i,j}$ and the weights to other layers:

```
typedef struct {
  float output;      /* output value for cell */
  float delta; /* for back propagation */
  float **weight;    /* weights from cell to other layers */
} celltype;
```

The field `**weight` is actually a pointer to a set of weights rather than an array of weights, since we do not know in advance how many weights we will need.

Now to construct the layers, we will store the number of cells in the layer and a pointer to a linked list of the cells present in that layer:

```
typedef struct {
  int number;    /* number of cells in layer */
  celltype **cell;   /* pointers to cells */
} layertype;
```

Finally, we will define a pointer to a list of pointers to all the layers:

```
layertype **layer;
```

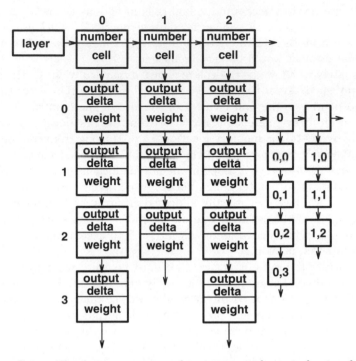

Figure C.2   The data structure used to represent the neural network. All the **weight** fields point to lists of weights; only one such list is shown for clarity.

This is a rather complex set of data declarations, and is easier to understand if we draw a diagram of the structure (Fig. C.2).

There are a number of other global variables and declarations, all of which are placed in a header file, *gendelta.h*, which we list here in its entirety. The other variables will be discussed as they are used.

```
/* Declarations for generalized delta rule */

#define MAXRAND 2147483648.0 /* maximum random number from rand() */

#define TEST 0 /* flags for testing or training net */
#define TRAIN 1

#define SINGLE 0 /* weights for single level or whole net */
#define FULL 1

#define RANDOM 0 /* Weight initialization */
```

```
#define READFILE 1

typedef struct {
  float output;      /* output value for cell */
  float delta; /* for back propagation */
  float **weight;    /* weights from cell to other layers */
} celltype;

typedef struct {
  int number;    /* number of cells in layer */
  celltype **cell;    /* pointers to cells */
} layertype;

layertype **layer;

int numlayers;    /* Number of layers */

typedef struct listptr { /* Structures used for input patterns */
  struct listptr *NextElem;
  int Point;
} ListType;

typedef struct nodeptr {
  struct nodeptr *NextNode;
  ListType *Input;
  ListType *Output;
} NodeType;

NodeType *Train;   /* list of input/output
                      patterns to be learned */

struct {
  int *patt;
  int count;
} RandPatt;    /* Stores random pattern with a
                  count of active cells */

float *required; /* Output required for given input */
float scale; /* Scale factor eta in weight adjustments */
int singfull; /* Weights for next level or whole schmeer */
int testtrain; /* Train net or test it? */
int randfile; /* Random weights or read from file? */
```

   With the declarations out of the way, we may now turn to the main function. The program is to be used in two main ways: to *train* a net to recognize a set of patterns or to *test* a trained net to see how well it performs. In both cases, we need to define the architecture of the network and construct the cells and their connections. Thus this is a logical block of the program which belongs in a function of its own. Also, for both options, we need to initialize a set of patterns which will be used as input to the network. This defines another function.

   Once the net is constructed, we proceed to use it. If the net is to be trained, we will present a certain number numpat of patterns to the net, determine the required output for each pattern, generate the output of the network, apply the back propagation algorithm and alter the weights. If the net is only being tested, we must still generate the output for each input pattern, but we do not apply the back propagation algorithm or change the weights.

   After all patterns have been processed, we write the weights out to a file for future use.

   The complete main function is listed below:

```
/* Generalized delta rule */
#include"gendelta.h"
#include<stdio.h>

void
main()
{
  int seed,i,j,numpat;
  NodeType *Node;

  printf("Enter number of patterns: ");
  scanf("%d",&numpat);
  printf("Test net or train it? (0/1) ");
  scanf("%d",&testtrain);
  printf("Weights for next level only or whole net? (0/1) ");
  scanf("%d",&singfull);
  printf("Random weights or read from file? (0/1) ");
  scanf("%d",&randfile);

  time((long *)&seed); /* Initialize random number generator */
  srand(seed);

  startup(); /* Set up network */
  SetPatterns(&Train); /* Set up input patterns */
```

```
  Node = Train->NextNode;
  for(i=0; i<numpat; i++) {
    ReqdOutput(&Node);
    GenerateOutput();
    if (testtrain == TRAIN) { /* TRAIN mode: train net */
      CalculateDeltas();
      AdjustWeights();
    } else { /* TEST mode: print output values */
      for(j=0; j<layer[0]->number; j++)
printf("%f ",layer[0]->cell[j]->output);
      printf("\n");
    }
  }
  WriteWeights();
}
```

Several flags are requested from the user to start things off. These flags are declared in the header file **gendelta.h** and are used in other functions to choose between possible actions. Note that if 'obvious' names are used for functions, comments are unnecessary at many places.

The most complex function is that which initializes the network, since it must dynamically construct the arrays for storing characteristics of cells and weights. The function **startup** is as follows:

```
#include"gendelta.h"
#include<stdio.h>

void
startup()
{
  FILE *fp,*wts;
  int i,j,k,m,kstart;

  fp = fopen("startup.dat","r");
  if (randfile == READFILE) wts = fopen("weights.dat","r");
                      /* read in scale factor */
  fscanf(fp,"%f",&scale);
                      /* read in no of levels; cells per level */
  fscanf(fp,"%d",&numlayers);
  layer = (layertype **)malloc(numlayers * sizeof(int));
  for(i=0; i<numlayers; i++) {
    layer[i] = (layertype *)malloc(sizeof(layertype));
    fscanf(fp,"%d",&(layer[i]->number));
    layer[i]->cell =
```

```
        (celltype **)malloc(layer[i]->number * sizeof(int));
    for(j=0; j<layer[i]->number; j++) {
                                /* Need biases to all cells */
        if (i == numlayers-1 && j == 0) kstart = 0;
        else {
kstart = (singfull == SINGLE) ? i-1 : 0;
if (kstart < 0) kstart = 0;
        }
        layer[i]->cell[j] = (celltype *)malloc(sizeof(celltype));
        layer[i]->cell[j]->weight =
          (float **)malloc(i * sizeof(int));
        for(k=kstart; k<i; k++) {
layer[i]->cell[j]->weight[k] =
            (float *)malloc(layer[k]->number*sizeof(float));
if (randfile == RANDOM)
  for(m=0; m<layer[k]->number; m++)
    layer[i]->cell[j]->weight[k][m] =
              2*rand()/MAXRAND-1.0;
else
  for(m=0; m<layer[k]->number; m++)
    fscanf(wts,"%f",&(layer[i]->cell[j]->weight[k][m]));
        } /* for k */
      } /* for j */
    } /* for i */
    required = (float *)malloc(layer[0]->number * sizeof(float));
}
```

The parameters describing the structure of the net are read in from the file startup.dat, rather than from the keyboard. Most of the parameters will be the same from one run to the next, and the user will find it tedious to have to type in the same set of parameters every time the program is run.

The flag randfile is checked to see if the weights are to be read in from the file weights.dat or generated randomly.

The pointer layer is to be a pointer to an array of pointers, each of which points to one of the layers in the network. The number of layers is read into the variable numlayers and enough space to store numlayers pointers (remember that a pointer is just an integer, so we reserve space for integers) is reserved using the C library function malloc(), which reserves the specified number of bytes and returns a pointer to the first byte so reserved.

We now enter the first loop, in which the properties of each layer will be determined. The pointer to each layer (layer[i]) is initialized to point

to enough space to describe a layer (recall we defined the data structure
layertype in the header file). Each layer pointer points to a structure with
two fields: the number of cells in the layer and a pointer to a list of the cells
in that layer. We read in the number of cells from the startup file and then
use malloc() to reserve enough space for pointers to each of these cells.
We only reserve a pointer to each cell at this stage, rather than space for a
complete description of the cell, because we do not yet know the contents
of the other layers in the network, so we do not know how much space will
be needed for the weights connecting this cell to the rest of the net.

Once we have determined the number of cells in the layer and reserved
space for pointers to each cell, we can enter the second loop (with index
j), in which we will initialize the properties of the individual cells. This
section of the code resolves several options. First of all, the generalized
delta rule requires that all cells be given a threshold value (which can
change as the net is trained) in addition to all the other weights. This
threshold may be interpreted as a signal from one special cell, the *bias
cell*, which always fires a signal to every other cell in the network. This
cell is located in position 0 in the input layer.[9] The if statement which
starts off the second loop checks to see if it is the bias cell that is currently
being processed. If so, the parameter kstart is set to 0. This parameter
determines the connectivity of the network, since it states the most distant
layer to which cells in the current layer are to be connected. If kstart =
0 cells are to be connected to all layers from the one just above them all
the way to the output layer, so weights will have to be defined for all these
connections. The flag singfull determines whether we are constructing a
net where each layer is connected only to the next layer above it, or to all
layers above it. If we are constructing the bias cell, however, it must always
be connected to all other cells, so it is treated specially at this point.

The else statement considers the singfull flag for all non-bias cells,
and sets kstart appropriately. We need to know to how many layers each
cell will be connected at this stage because we must reserve space for the
weights from this cell a bit later on.

The statement after the else initializes the pointer layer[i]->cell[j]
to point to a structure of type celltype, which is defined in the header
file. Once space for the cell's description has been obtained, we must now
construct the weights from this cell to the other cells with which it connects.
First we reserve space for pointers to the lists of weights from cell j in layer
i to all other layers. This statement actually reserves a pointer for all
layers from the next layer to the output layer, even if the network is only a

---

[9]For convenience in other parts of the program, we have numbered the layers so
that the input layer is layer numlayers - 1 and the output layer is layer 0. This is the
opposite numbering convention to that used in the equations in Chapter 19, but it makes
the programming easier.

nearest neighbour network. This is for clarity of notation in the program: we plan to refer to a weight from cell j in layer i to cell m in layer k by the name `layer[i]->cell[j]->weight[k][m]` which we can only do if we have defined weight pointers from indexes 0 up to k, even if indexes 0 to $k-1$ are never used. This does waste some space if we are dealing with nearest-layer nets, but the alternative of having to write special code to change the notation in the two cases is not really worth thinking about.

With the space for the weight pointers obtained, we now reserve spaces for each weight required and initialize the weight values, either by generating a random number in the interval $[-1, 1]$ or by reading them in from the file `weights.dat`.

Finally, a pointer to an array in which the `required` output is stored is initialized. This completes the construction of the network.

The complexity of these data structures may make you wonder if it is really worth using dynamic instead of static arrays. If you plan to use only small networks, perhaps arrays would be easier. However, a program using dynamic arrays may be used for large or small networks without the user having to worry whether enough space has been declared to handle a network of a large size, or that a vast amount of memory is being needlessly reserved when only a small network is being used.

The next module in the main routine is `SetPatterns`. This function sets up the data structures and loads in the input patterns. In this program, the patterns are presented to the network in sequence, so there is no need to randomly access individual patterns in the list. In this case we may use a linked list to store the patterns, since we do not know in advance how many patterns we will be presenting to the network.

The data structures to be used to store the patterns are declared in the header file and are given here for convenience:

```
typedef struct listptr {
  struct listptr *NextElem;
  int Point;
} ListType;

typedef struct nodeptr {
  struct nodeptr *NextNode;
  ListType *Input;
  ListType *Output;
} NodeType;
```

`NodeType *Train;  /* list of input/output patterns to be learned`

The variable `Train` is a pointer to a structure of type `NodeType` which contains input and output patterns, both represented as linked lists of type

ListType. This way of representing patterns allows an arbitrary number of patterns, each of arbitrary length, to be stored.

The code for the routine SetPatterns follows:

```c
/* Creates a new list with a head node */
#include"gendelta.h"
#include<stddef.h>
#include<stdio.h>

void
MakeList(List)
  ListType **List;
{
  *List = (ListType *)malloc(sizeof(ListType));
  (*List)->NextElem = NULL;
}


/* Creates a new list with a head node */
void
MakeNode(Node)
  NodeType **Node;
{
  *Node = (NodeType *)malloc(sizeof(NodeType));
  (*Node)->NextNode = NULL;
  (*Node)->Input = NULL;
  (*Node)->Output = NULL;
}


/* Reads in patterns that network is supposed to recognize */

void
StorePattern(fp,List)
    FILE *fp;
    ListType *List;
{
  int pt;

  while ((fscanf(fp,"%d",&pt) != EOF) && (pt > 0)) {
    MakeList(&(List->NextElem));
    List = List->NextElem;
    List->Point = pt;
  }
}
```

```
void
SetPatterns(Train)
  NodeType **Train;
{
  NodeType *TempNode;
  ListType *TempIn, *TempOut;
  FILE *in, *out;
  int pt;
  void MakeList(),MakeNode();

  in = fopen("input.dat","r");
  out = fopen("output.dat","r");
  MakeNode(Train);
  TempNode = *Train;   /* overall head node: never used */
  while (fscanf(in,"%d",&pt) != EOF) {
    MakeNode(&(TempNode->NextNode)); /* New node */
    TempNode = TempNode->NextNode;
    MakeList(&(TempNode->Input)); /* Create new pattern lists */
    MakeList(&(TempNode->Output));
    TempIn = TempNode->Input;
    TempOut = TempNode->Output;

    TempIn->Point = pt;  /* Store number of items in lists */
    fscanf(out,"%d",&pt);
    TempOut->Point = pt;

    StorePattern(in,TempIn);
    StorePattern(out,TempOut);
  }
}
```

The module SetPatterns calls a number of subsidiary routines, which are included in the code fragment above. The input patterns are to be read from the file input.dat and the corresponding output patterns (the patterns which the net *should* produce upon being presented with the corresponding input pattern) are read from the file output.dat.

The routine MakeNode creates a new node in the list of patterns. It is used first to create the first node in the list, which is a *head node* pointed to by Train. A head node is an extra node before the first 'true' node in a list which is often created as a programming convenience. It avoids writing extra code to cope with the special case when the node being processed is the first node in the list.

The while loop creates new nodes for successive patterns and uses the routines MakeNode and MakeList to reserve the initial space in memory for the nodes and patterns, while the function StorePattern stores the actual patterns.

The remaining functions in the simulation merely implement the steps specified by the generalized delta rule, so we need not discuss them in depth. They are presented below for completeness.

The routine ReqdOutput clears the network's input layer and loads the current input pattern into it, then loads the required output pattern into the array required. If the net is being run in TEST mode, the output is printed.

```
/* Determines required output for given input */
#include"gendelta.h"
#include<stddef.h>
#define ON 0.9
#define OFF 0.1

void
ReqdOutput(Node)
  NodeType **Node;
{
  int i;
  ListType *TempIn, *TempOut;

  layer[numlayers-1]->cell[0]->output = 1.0;   /* Cell 0 is bias */
  if(testtrain == TEST) printf("Input: ");

/* Initialize required vector */
  for(i=0; i<layer[0]->number; i++)
    required[i] = OFF;
/* Clear input layer */
  for(i=1; i<layer[numlayers-1]->number; i++)
    layer[numlayers-1]->cell[i]->output = 0.0;
/* Load input pattern */
  TempIn = (*Node)->Input->NextElem;
  TempOut = (*Node)->Output->NextElem;
  while (TempIn != NULL) {
    layer[numlayers-1]->cell[TempIn->Point]->output = 1.0;
    TempIn = TempIn->NextElem;
  } /* while */
```

```
/* Load required output */
  while (TempOut != NULL) {
    required[TempOut->Point - 1] = ON;
    TempOut = TempOut->NextElem;
  }
  if (testtrain == TEST) {
    for(i=1; i<layer[numlayers-1]->number; i++)
      printf("%f ",layer[numlayers-1]->cell[i]->output);
    printf("\n");
  }
  *Node = (*Node)->NextNode;
  if((*Node) == NULL) *Node = Train->NextNode;
}
```

The routine `GenerateOutput` applies the signal propagation algorithm to carry the input signal through the net until it produces signals in the output layer.

```
/* Determines output for given input */
#include"gendelta.h"
#include<math.h>

void
GenerateOutput()
{
  int i,j,k,m,kend;

  for(i=numlayers-2; i>=0; i--) {
    kend = (singfull == SINGLE) ? i+1 : numlayers-1;
    for(j=0; j<layer[i]->number; j++) {
      layer[i]->cell[j]->output = (kend == numlayers-1) ? 0.0 :
layer[numlayers-1]->cell[0]->weight[i][j]; /* Make sure of bias *
      for(k=i+1; k<=kend; k++) {
for(m=0; m<layer[k]->number; m++) {
  layer[i]->cell[j]->output += layer[k]->cell[m]->weight[i][j] *
    layer[k]->cell[m]->output;
} /* for m */
      } /* for k */
      layer[i]->cell[j]->output =
1.0/(1.0 + (float)exp(-(layer[i]->cell[j]->output)));
    } /* for j */
  } /* for i */
}
```

If the net is being trained, the two routines `CalculateDeltas` and `AdjustWeights` are used to apply the back propagation algorithm. Both of these routines merely translate the equations into C, using the data structures defined in the header file.

First we calculate the δ_{ij} values:

```
/* Calculates deltas used in back propagation */
#include"gendelta.h"

void
CalculateDeltas()
{
  int i,j,k,m,kstart;

/* Delta for output layer */
  for(i=0; i<layer[0]->number; i++)
    layer[0]->cell[i]->delta =
      (required[i] - layer[0]->cell[i]->output) *
      layer[0]->cell[i]->output *
      (1.0 - layer[0]->cell[i]->output);
/* Now for lower layers */
  for(i=1; i<numlayers-1; i++) {
    kstart = (singfull == SINGLE) ? i-1 : 0;
    if (kstart < 0) kstart = 0;
    for(j=0; j<layer[i]->number; j++) {
      layer[i]->cell[j]->delta = 0.0;
      for(k=kstart; k<i; k++) {
for(m=0; m<layer[k]->number; m++) {
  layer[i]->cell[j]->delta += layer[k]->cell[m]->delta *
    layer[i]->cell[j]->weight[k][m];
} /* for m */
      } /* for k */
      layer[i]->cell[j]->delta *= layer[i]->cell[j]->output *
(1 - layer[i]->cell[j]->output);
    } /* for j */
  } /* for i */
}
```

Now we adjust the weights:

```
/* Applies delta rule to adjust weights */
#include"gendelta.h"

void
```

```
AdjustWeights()
{
  int i,j,k,m,kstart;

  for(i=1; i<numlayers; i++) {
    for(j=0; j<layer[i]->number; j++) {
                          /* Need biases to all cells */
      if (i == numlayers-1 && j == 0) kstart = 0;
      else {
kstart = (singfull -- SINGLE) ? i-1 : 0;
if (kstart < 0) kstart = 0;
      }
      for(k=kstart; k<i; k++) {
for(m=0; m<layer[k]->number; m++) {
  layer[i]->cell[j]->weight[k][m] +=
    scale * layer[k]->cell[m]->delta *
          layer[i]->cell[j]->output;
} /* for m */
      } /* for k */
    } /* for j */
  } /* for i */
}
```

Finally, we call the routine `WriteWeights` to store the weights generated after the training session:

```
/* Writes out weights */
#include"gendelta.h"
#include<stdio.h>

void
WriteWeights()
{
  FILE *wts,*human;
  int i,j,k,m,kstart;

  wts = fopen("weights.dat","w");
                /* Human readable listing of weights */
  human = fopen("humread.dat","w");
  for(i=0; i<numlayers; i++) {
    kstart = (singfull == SINGLE) ? i-1 : 0;
    if (kstart < 0) kstart = 0;
    for(j=0; j<layer[i]->number; j++) {
                /* Need biases to all cells */
```

```
      if (i == numlayers-1 && j == 0) kstart = 0;
      else {
kstart = (singfull == SINGLE) ? i-1 : 0;
if (kstart < 0) kstart = 0;
      }
      for(k=kstart; k<i; k++) {
fprintf(human,"From layer %d cell %d to layer %d\n",i,j,k);
for(m=0; m<layer[k]->number; m++) {
  fprintf(wts,"%f ",layer[i]->cell[j]->weight[k][m]);
  fprintf(human,"%f ",layer[i]->cell[j]->weight[k][m]);
}
fprintf(wts,"\n");
fprintf(human,"\n");
      } /* for k */
    } /* for j */
  } /* for i */
}
```

Bibliography

Abbott, L. F. (1988). A model of autocatalytic replication. *J. Molecular Evolution*, **27**, 114-120.

Amit, D. J. (1989). *Modeling brain function: The world of attractor neural networks*. Cambridge University Press, Cambridge.

Amitrano, C., Peliti, L., and Saber, M. (1989). Population dynamics in a spin-glass model of chemical evolution. *J. Molecular Evolution*, **29**, 513-525.

Anderson, P. W. (1983). Suggested model for prebiotic evolution: The use of chaos. *Proc. National Academy of Science (USA)*, **80**, 3386-3390.

Atlan, H. (1989). Automata network theories in immunology: their utility and their underdetermination. *Bull. Math. Biol.* **51**, 247-253.

Bell, G. I. (1970). Mathematical model of clonal selection and antibody production. *J. Theoretical Biology*, **29**, 191.

Bell, G. I. (1971a). Mathematical model of clonal selection and antibody production II. *J. Theoretical Biology*, **33**, 339-378.

Bell, G. I. (1971b). Mathematical model of clonal selection and antibody production III. The cellular basis of immunological paralysis. *J. Theoretical Biology*, **33**, 379-398.

Bernal, J. D. (1960). *Nature*, **186**, 694-695.

Bresch, C., Niesert, U., and Harnasch, D. (1980). Hypercycles, parasites and packages. *J. Theoretical Biology*, **85**, 399-405.

Burnet, F. M. (1959). *The clonal selection theory of acquired immunity*. Cambridge University Press, Cambridge.

Byrne, J. H. and Berry, W. O. (1989). *Neural models of plasticity: experimental and theoretical approaches*. Academic Press, San Diego.

Cairns-Smith, A. G. (1982). *Genetic takeover and the mineral origins of life*. Cambridge University Press, Cambridge.

Cairns-Smith, A. G. (1985). *Seven clues to the origin of life: a scientific detective story.* Cambridge University Press, Cambridge.

Clarke, G. M. and Cooke, D. (1983). *A basic course in statistics,* (2nd edn). Edward Arnold, London.

Clough, B. and Mungo, P. (1992). *Approaching zero: Data crime and the computer underworld.* Faber and Faber, London.

Conrad, M. and Strizich, M (1985). Evolve II: A computer model of an evolving ecosystem. *BioSystems,* **17**, 245-258.

Conrad, M., Kampfner, R. R., Kirby, K. G., Rizki, E. N., Schleis, G., Smalz, R., and Trenary, R. (1989). Towards an artificial brain. *BioSystems,* **23**, 175-218.

Coutinho, A. (1989). Beyond clonal selection and network. *Immunological Reviews,* **110**, 63-87.

Cox, D. R. and Miller, H. D. (1977). *The theory of stochastic processes.* Chapman and Hall, London.

Crick, F. (1984). Memory and molecular turnover. *Nature,* **312**, 101.

Darnell, J., Lodish, H., and Baltimore, D. (1986). *Molecular cell biology,* Scientific American Books, New York.

Dawkins, R. (1986). *The blind watchmaker.* Harlow Longman Scientific & Technical, London (Also available from Penguin Books (1988).)

Dawkins, R. (1976). *The selfish gene,* Oxford University Press, Oxford.

De Boer, R. J. and Hogeweg, P. (1989). Idiotypic networks incorporating T-B cell co-operation. The conditions for percolation. *J. Theoretical Biology,* **139**, 17-38.

De Boer, R. J. and Perelson, A. S. (1991). Size and connectivity as emergent properties of a developing immune network. *J. Theoretical Biology,* **149**, 381-424.

DeLisi, C. (1983). Mathematical modeling in immunology. *Ann. Rev. Biophys. Bioeng.* **12**, 117-138.

Dudai, Y. (1989). *The neurobiology of memory: concepts, findings, trends,* Oxford University Press, Oxford.

Eigen, M. (1971). Selforganization of matter and the evolution of biological macromolecules. *Naturwiss.,* **58**, 465-523.

Eigen, M. and Schuster, P. (1977). The hypercycle—a principle of natural self-organization. Part A: Emergence of the hypercycle. *Naturwiss.*, **64**, 541-565.

Eigen, M. and Schuster, P. (1977). The hypercycle—a principle of natural self-organization. Part B: The abstract hypercycle. *Naturwiss.*, **64**, 541-565.

Eigen, M. and Schuster, P. (1977). The hypercycle—a principle of natural self-organization. Part C: The realistic hypercycle. *Naturwiss.*, **64**, 541-565.

Eigen, M. and Schuster, P. (1979). *The hypercycle: a principle of natural self-organization.* Springer-Verlag, Berlin.

Fox, S. W. and Dose, K. (1977). *Molecular evolution and the origin of life.* Dekker, New York.

Gardner, E. (1988). The phase space of interactions in neural network models. *J. Physics; A: Mathematical and General,* **21A**, 257-270.

Gardner, M. (1970). Mathematical games: The fantastic combinations of John Conway's new solitaire game 'Life'. *Scientific American,* October 1970, 112-117.

Gardner, M. (1983). *Wheels, life and other mathematical amusements.* Freeman, New York.

Gillespie, D. T. (1976). Stochastic simulation of chemical processes. *J. Computational Physics,* **22**, 403.

Gillespie, D. T. (1977). Exact stochastic simulation of coupled chemical reactions. *J. Physical Chemistry* **81**, 2340-2361.

Golub, E. S. and Green, D. R. (1991). *Immunology: a synthesis,* (2nd edn). Sinauer, Sunderland, Mass.

Grossberg, S. (1988). *Neural networks and natural intelligence.* MIT Press, Cambridge, Mass.

Gunther, N. and Hoffmann, G. W. (1982). Qualitative dynamics of a network model of regulation of the immune system: a rationale for the IgM to IgG switch. *J. Theoretical Biology,* **94**, 815-855.

Harada, K. and Fox, S. W. (1964). Thermal syntheses of natural amino acids from a postulated primitive terrestrial atmosphere. *Nature,* **201**, 335-336.

Hebb, D. O. (1949). *The organization of behaviour: a neuropsychological theory.* Wiley, New York.

Hoffmann, G. W. (1974). On the origin of the genetic code and the stability of the translation apparatus. *J. Molecular Biology*, **86**, 349-362.

Hoffmann, G. W. (1975a). The stochastic theory of the origin of the genetic code. *Annual Review of Physical Chemistry*, **26**, 123-144.

Hoffmann, G. W. (1975b). A theory of regulation and self-nonself discrimination in an immune network. *Eur. J. Immunol.* **5**, 638-647.

Hopfield, J. J. (1982). Neural networks and physical systems with emergent selective computational abilities. *Proc. Natl. Acad. Sci. USA*, **79**, 2554.

Hull, D. E. (1960). Thermodynamics and kinetics of spontaneous generation. *Nature*, **186**, 693-694.

Ishida, K. (1986). Fluctuations and mutation in hypercyclic organization. *J. Theoretical Biology*, **118**, 3-13.

Jerne, N. K. (1974a). Towards a network theory of the immune system. *Ann. Immunol. (Inst. Pasteur)*, **125C**, 373-389.

Jerne, N. K. (1974b). Clonal selection in a lymphocyte network. In *Cellular selection and regulation in the immune response* (ed. G. M. Edelman), p. 39. Raven Press, New York.

Jones, B. L., Enns, R. H., and Rangnekar, S. S. (1976). On the theory of selection of coupled macromolecular systems. *Bull. Math. Biol.* **38**, 15-28.

Jones, B. L. and Leung, H. K. (1981). Stochastic analysis of a nonlinear model for selection of biological macromolecules. *Bull. Math. Biol.*, **43**, 665-680.

Kampfner, R. R. and Conrad, M. (1983). Computational modeling of evolutionary learning processes in the brain. *Bull. Math. Biol.*, **45**, 931-980.

Kandel, E. R. and Schwartz, J. H. (1985). *Principles of neural science*, (2nd edn). Elsevier, New York.

Karlin, S. and Taylor, H. M. (1980). *A first course in stochastic processes.* Academic Press, New York.

Kauffman, S. A. (1986). Autocatalytic sets of proteins. *J. Theoretical Biology*, **119** 1-24.

Kauffman, S. A. (1988). Origins of order in evolution: Self-organization and selection. In R. Livi, *et al.* (eds), *Chaos and complexity.* World Scientific, Singapore, pp. 349-387.

Kauffman, S. A., Weinberger, E. D., and Perelson, A. S. (1988). Maturation of the immune response via adaptive walks on affinity landscapes. *Theoretical immunology, Part one; SFI studies in the science of complexity.* In A. S. Perelson (ed.), Addison-Wesley. pp. 349-382.

Kauffman, S. A. (1989). Adaptation on rugged fitness landscapes. In Stein, D. (ed.) *Complex systems. SFI studies in the science of complexity.* Addison-Wesley, Reading, Mass., pp. 527-617.

Kauffman, S. A. and Levin, S. (1987). Towards a general theory of adaptive walks on rugged landscapes. *J. Theoretical Biology*, **128**, 11-45.

Kauffman, S. A. and Weinberger, E. D. (1989). The NK model of rugged fitness landscapes and its application to maturation of the immune response. *J. Theoretical Biology*, **141**, 211-245.

Kirby, K. G. and Conrad, M. (1984). The enzymatic neuron as a reaction-diffusion network of cyclic nucleotides. *Bull. Math. Biol.*, **46**, 765-783.

Kirby, K. G., Conrad, M., and Kampfner, R. R. (1991). Evolutionary learning in reaction-diffusion neurons, *Applied Mathematics and Computation*, **41**, 233-263.

Kirkwood, T. B. L. and Holliday, R. (1975). The stability of the translation apparatus. *J. Molecular Biology*, **97**, 257-265.

Kirkwood, T. B. L., Holliday, R., and Rosenberger, R. F. (1984). Stability of the cellular translation process. *International Review of Cytology*, **92**, 93-132.

Koch, C. and Segev, I. (eds) (1989). *Methods in neuronal modeling: from synapses to networks.* MIT Press, Cambridge, Mass.

Kohonen, T. (1977). *Associative memory—a system-theoretical approach.* Springer, New York.

Kohonen, T. (1984). *Self-organization and associative memory.* Springer-Verlag, Berlin. (Reprinted in 1988)

Kohonen, T. (1988). The "neural" phonetic typewriter. *Computer*, **21**, No. 3, 11-22.

Langton, C. G. (1986). Studying artificial life with cellular automata, *Physica D*, **22**, 120-149.

Langton, C. G. (ed.) (1989). *Artificial life* (Volume 6). In *Proceedings of the Santa Fe Institute studies in the sciences of complexity*. Addison-Wesley, Reading, Mass.

Langton, C. G., Taylor, C., Farmer, J. D., and Rasmussen, S. (eds) (1992). *Artificial life II* (Volume 10). In *Proceedings of the Santa Fe Institute studies in the sciences of complexity*. Addison-Wesley, Reading, Mass.

Levine, D. S. (1991). *Introduction to neural and cognitive modeling*. Lawrence Erlbaum Associates, Hillsdale, New Jersey.

Levy, S. (1992). *Artificial life: the quest for a new creation*. Jonathan Cape, London.

Little, W. A. (1974). The existence of persistent states in the brain, *Math. Biosci.*, **19**, 101.

McCulloch, W. S. and Pitts, W. (1943). A logical calculus of the ideas immanent in nervous activity. *Bulletin of Mathematical Biophysics*, **5**, 115-133. (Reprinted in 1990 in *Bulletin of Mathematical Biology*, **52**, 99-115.)

Miller, S. L. (1953). A production of amino acids under possible primitive Earth conditions. *Science*, **117**, 528-529.

Miller, S. L. (1986). Current status of the prebiotic synthesis of small molecules. *Chemica Scripta*, **26B**, 5-11.

Miller, S. L. and Urey, H. (1959). Organic compound synthesis on the primitive earth. *Science*, **130**, 245.

Minsky, M. and Papert, S. (1969; reprinted with epilog 1988). *Perceptrons*. MIT Press, Cambridge, Mass.

Murray, J.D. (1989). *Mathematical Biology*. Springer-Verlag, Berlin.

Neumann, A. U. and Weisbuch, G. (1992). Window automata analysis of population dynamics in the immune system. *Bull. Math. Biol.*, **54**, 21-44.

Noble, B. and Daniel, J. W. (1988). *Applied linear algebra,* (3rd edn). Prentice-Hall, Englewood Cliffs, New Jersey.

Oparin, A. I. (1938). *The origin of life.* Macmillan, New York.

Orgel, L. E. (1973). *The origins of life: molecules and natural selection.* Wiley, New York.

Pandey, R. B. (1991). Cellular automata approach to interacting cellular network models for the dynamics of cell population in an early HIV infection. *Physica A,* **179**, 442-470.

Perelson, A. S. (1988). Toward a realistic model of the immune system. In A. S. Perelson (ed.), *Theoretical Immunology, Part Two, SFI Studies in the Sciences of Complexity,* Addison-Wesley, Reading, Mass., pp. 377-401.

Perelson, A. S. (1989). Immune network theory. *Immunological Reviews,* **110**, 5-36.

Ray, T. S. (1992). An approach to the synthesis of life. In C. G. Langton, *et al.* (eds), *Artificial life II,* Addison-Wesley, Reading, Mass., pp. 371-408.

Robertson, D. L. and Joyce, G. F. (1991). The catalytic potential of RNA. In A. S. Perelson, and S. A. Kauffman (eds), *Molecular evolution on rugged landscapes: proteins RNA and the immune system* (Volume 9 in *Proceedings of the Santa Fe Institute studies in the sciences of complexity.* Addison-Wesley, Reading, Mass., pp. 265-278.

Roitt, I. M., Brostoff, J., and Male, D. *et al.* (1989). *Immunology,* (2nd edn). Gower Medical, London.

Rokhsar, D. S., Anderson, P. W., and Stein, D. L. (1986). Self-organization in prebiological systems: simulations of a model for the origin of genetic information. *J. Molecular Evolution,* **23**, 119-126.

Rosenblatt, F. (1962). *Principles of Neurodynamics.* Spartan Books, Washington, D.C.

Rumelhart, D. E. and McClelland, J. L. (1986). *Parallel Distributed Processing: Explorations in the Microstructure of Cognition* (2 vols.). MIT Press, Cambridge, Mass.

Rumelhart, D. E. and Zipser, D. (1986). Feature discovery by competitive learning. In Rumelhart and McClelland (1986). vol. 1, chapter 5.

Rumelhart, D. E., Hinton, G. E., and Williams, R. J. (1986). Learning internal representations by error propagation. In Rumelhart and McClelland (1986). vol. 1, chapter 8.

Shepherd, G. M. (ed.) (1990). *The synaptic organization of the brain,* (3rd edn). Oxford University Press, New York.

Stein, D. L. (1984). A model for the origin of biological information. *International Journal of Quantum Chemistry: Quantum Biology Symposium*, **11**, 73-86.

Stein, D. L. and Anderson, P. W. (1984). A model for the origin of biological catalysis. *Proc. National Academy of Science (USA)*, **81**, 1751-1753.

Stent, G. S. and Calendar, R. (1978). *Molecular Genetics: An Introductory Narrative*, (2nd edn). Freeman, San Francisco.

Stryer, L. (1988). *Biochemistry*, (3rd edn). W. H. Freeman, New York.

Walpole, R. E. and Myers, R. H. (1989). *Probability and Statistics for Engineers and Scientists*. Macmillan, New York.

Watson, J. D. (1981). *The double helix: A personal account of the discovery of the structure of DNA*. Weidenfeld and Nicolson, London.

Weinand, R. G. (1990). Somatic mutation, affinity maturation and the antibody repertoire: A computer model. *J. Theoretical Biology*, **143**, 343-382.

Weinand, R. G. and Conrad, M. (1988). Maturation of the immune response: A computational model. *J. Theoretical Biology*, **133**, 409-428.

Weisbuch, G., DeBoer, R. J., and Perelson, A. S. (1990). Localized memories in idiotypic networks. *J. Theoretical Biology*, **146**, 483-499.

Wicken, J. S. (1985). An organismic critique of molecular Darwinism. *J. Theoretical Biology*, **117**, 545-561.

Index